HEALTH CARE INFORMATION SYSTEMS

A Practical Approach for Health Care Management

Second Edition

KAREN A. WAGER
FRANCES WICKHAM LEE
JOHN P. GLASER

FOREWORD BY
LAWTON ROBERT BURNS

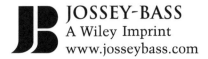

JOSSEY-BASS
A Wiley Imprint
www.josseybass.com

Published by Jossey-Bass
A Wiley Imprint
989 Market Street, San Francisco, CA 94103-1741—www.josseybass.com

The first edition of this book was previously published as *Managing Health Care Information Systems: A Practical Approach for Health Care Executives.*

Readers should be aware that Internet Web sites offered as citations and/or sources for further information may have changed or disappeared between the time this was written and when it is read.

Limit of Liability/Disclaimer of Warranty: While the publisher and author have used their best efforts in preparing this book, they make no representations or warranties with respect to the accuracy or completeness of the contents of this book and specifically disclaim any implied warranties of merchantability or fitness for a particular purpose. No warranty may be created or extended by sales representatives or written sales materials. The advice and strategies contained herein may not be suitable for your situation. You should consult with a professional where appropriate. Neither the publisher nor author shall be liable for any loss of profit or any other commercial damages, including but not limited to special, incidental, consequential, or other damages.

Jossey-Bass books and products are available through most bookstores. To contact Jossey-Bass directly call our Customer Care Department within the U.S. at 800-956-7739, outside the U.S. at 317-572-3986, or fax 317-572-4002.

Jossey-Bass also publishes its books in a variety of electronic formats. Some content that appears in print may not be available in electronic books.

Library of Congress Cataloging-in-Publication Data

Wager, Karen A., 1961-Health care information systems : a practical approach for health care management / Karen A. Wager, Frances Wickham Lee, John P. Glaser ; foreword by Lawton Robert Burns. – 2nd ed.

p. ; cm.

Rev. ed. of: Managing health care information systems / Karen A. Wager, Frances Wickham Lee, John P. Glaser. 1st ed. c2005. Includes bibliographical references and index.

ISBN 978-0-470-38780-1 (pbk.)

1. Medical informatics. 2. Health services administration. I. Lee, Frances Wickham, 1953- II. Glaser, John (John P.) III. Wager, Karen A., 1961- Managing health care information systems. IV. Title.

[DNLM: 1. Medical Informatics–organization & administration. W 26.5 W131h 2009]

R858.W34 2009

610.68–dc22

Printed in the United States of America
SECOND EDITION

PB Printing   10 9 8 7 6 5

CONTENTS

Key Terms   441
Learning Activities   441

16 HEALTH IT LEADERSHIP   **443**
Case 1: Board Support for a Capital Project   445
Case 2: The Decision to Develop an IT Strategic Plan   447
Case 3: Selection of a Patient Safety Strategy   448
Case 4: Strategic IS Planning for the Hospital ED   450
Case 5: Planning an EMR Implementation   452
Case 6: Considerations for Voice over IP Telephony   454
Case 7: Implementing a Capacity Management Information System   455
Case 8: Implementing a Telemedicine Solution   456
Case 9: Replacing a Practice Management System   457
Case 10: Conversion to an EMR Messaging System   459
Case 11: Concerns and Workarounds with a Clinical Documentation
System   460
Case 12: Strategies for Implementing CPOE   462
Case Study 13: Implementing a Syndromic Surveillance System   464
Case Study 14: The Admitting System Crashes   466
Case Study 15: Breaching the Security of an Internet Patient Portal   467
Case Study 16: Assessing the Value and Impact of CPOE   469

Appendixes

A   Overview of the Health Care IT Industry   471
B   Sample Project Charter   483

References   **493**

Index   **504**

TABLES, FIGURES, AND EXHIBITS

TABLES

FIGURES

EXHIBITS

To our students

FOREWORD

Information systems (IS) constitute the source of many of the problems in the health care industry. Health care is one of the most transaction-intensive industries (estimated at thirty billion transactions annually), given all the encounters between patients and providers, providers and other providers, providers and insurers, suppliers and providers, and so on. Yet compared to other industries, health care has historically underinvested in IS—and it shows. The transactions between parties in health care take place not so much electronically as through a mixture of telephone, paper, fax, and EDI media. The result is that much information is never captured, is captured incorrectly, is captured inefficiently, or is difficult to retrieve and use. Moreover, the industry relies heavily on legacy systems that cannot communicate with one another, not only between organizations but often within the same organization.

What is required to fix this messy situation? To paraphrase an old adage, the system may be the solution. The U.S. health care industry is in need of a massive infusion of capital to fund the adoption of new information technology (IT). Kaiser Permanente is well into the implementation of a paperless system that has already cost $5 billion, which provides a glimpse of the scale involved. Who will offer providers (where much of the IS help is needed) the financial assistance to underwrite these investments? Physicians are now getting help from their hospitals, thanks to a ruling by the Internal Revenue Service that allows hospitals to foot 85 percent of the costs of an EMR in doctor offices. Both hospitals and physicians will need support from their trading partners (for example, manufacturers who sell them products) and a big nudge from private sector insurers and (especially) the federal government in terms of how they pay for health care. Private payers are linking reimbursement to performance metrics via pay-for-performance (P4P) programs. The federal government is also linking reimbursement to e-prescribing and quality data reporting. Linking IT use to reimbursement is a further step in the right direction. In addition, provider organizations will need to provide incentives to their own physicians to employ IT—for example, by linking IT use to credentialing decisions. Finally, to convince all parties to adopt the necessary IT systems, we will need rigorous studies that document the cost and quality returns from these investments and the parties to which these returns accrue. This is not a small task; the value of IT investments still remains a messy discussion.

This book provides an incredibly thorough overview of information systems and their importance in the health care industry. It provides an overview of the health care IT industry; a history of health care IS in the United States; a review of the fundamental characteristics of information, the uses to which it is put, and the processes it supports; and a highly detailed discussion of the primary clinical and managerial applications of information (including electronic medical records), the value of information and IS to multiple stakeholders, and most important, the management of information and IS. This approach is particularly helpful when one considers that the vast majority of health system executives underwent their graduate training at a time when information systems were in their infancy and thus when no such text existed. The second edition now also includes a dozen mini-cases documenting the challenges of IT implementation. This is incredibly valuable, since the technology costs are usually outweighed by the process costs of installation and achieving adoption by end users. This volume is thus a great primer, offering a systematic presentation of a complex, important topic.

The reader will benefit from the collaborative effort that went into this volume. The first two authors are academics with considerable experience in teaching health care information management; the third is the chief information officer at one of the most prominent hospital (and integrated) systems in the United States. The combined talents of these two academics and one practitioner (all of whom have doctoral degrees) are reflected in the scope and depth presented here. This book is both systematic and practical, serving the needs of graduate students and current executives in the industry. What I have found particularly helpful is its ability to show how information and IS integrate with the other functions of the health care provider organization. The reader comes away from this book with a more profound understanding of how information serves as the lifeblood of the institution and as the real glue that can cement together professionals and departments within a health care organization and that can also tie the organization more closely to its upstream trading partners (manufacturers, wholesalers, and group purchasing organizations) and downstream trading partners (insurers and managed care organizations). At the end of the day, information and IS construct the real pathway to the utopia sought by providers during the past decade: integrated health care.

This book is required reading for all those who toil in the field of health care management—whether as managers, professionals, consultants, suppliers and customers, students, or scholars. The topic of IS in health care is simply too important, and until recently too often ignored, to be left to haphazard learning. I commend the authors for their great contribution to the field of health care management and information management.

March 2009

Lawton Robert Burns
The James Joo-Jin Kim Professor
The Wharton School

ACKNOWLEDGMENTS

We wish to thank Amanda Price, a student in the master's degree program in health administration at the Medical University of South Carolina (MUSC), for her assistance in preparing the final manuscript for this book. We also wish to thank the following MUSC students in the doctoral degree program in health administration, who contributed their information systems management stories and experiences to us so we could use them as case studies: Penney Burlingame, Barbara Chelton, Stuart Fine, David Freed, David Gehant, Patricia Givens, Victoria Harkins, Randall Jones, Catrin Jones-Nazar, Ronald Kintz, James Kirby, George Mikatarian, Lorie Shoemaker, and Gary Wilde.

THE AUTHORS

Karen A. Wager is associate professor and executive director for student affairs in the College of Health Professions at the Medical University of South Carolina (MUSC), where she teaches management and health information system courses to graduate students. She has over twenty-five years of professional and academic experience in the health information management field and has published numerous articles, case studies, and book chapters. Recognized for her excellence in interprofessional education and bringing practical research to the classroom, Wager received the 2008 MUSC outstanding teaching award in the educator-lecturer category. She is past president of the South Carolina chapter of the Healthcare Information and Management Systems Society (HIMSS) and past president of the South Carolina Health Information Management Association. In her current position Wager spends part of her time working with the clinical leadership team at the MUSC Medical Center to assess the impact of clinical information systems on quality, safety, and staff efficiency. She holds a DBA degree with an emphasis in information systems from the University of Sarasota.

Frances Wickham Lee is director of instructional operations for the Clinical Effectiveness and Patient Safety Center, a statewide organization dedicated to improving patient safety and clinical education through the use of health care simulation, and associate professor in the College of Health Professions at the Medical University of South Carolina (MUSC) in Charleston. Prior to joining the MUSC faculty in 1991, she served on the faculty at Western Carolina University. Her academic career spans thirty years, and she has taught courses related to health information management and information technology to both undergraduate and graduate students. She has published a variety of articles and has been a contributing author for several health information management books. She received her undergraduate degree from the University of Tennessee Center for the Health Sciences, her MBA degree from Western Carolina University, and her DBA degree from the University of Sarasota.

John P. Glaser is vice president and chief information officer at Partners Health-Care, Inc. Previously, he was vice president, information systems, at Brigham and Women's Hospital, and before that he managed the health care information systems consulting practice at Arthur D. Little. He was the founding chairman of the College of Healthcare Information Management Executives (CHIME), is a past president of the Healthcare Information and Management Systems Society (HIMSS) and of the eHealth Initiative, and has been a member of the board of the American Medical Informatics Association (AMIA). He is a senior adviser to the Deloitte Center for Health Solutions and a fellow of HIMSS, CHIME, and AMIA. CHIME has established a scholarship in his name. He has been awarded the John Gall award for health care CIO of the year and has been elected to *CIO* magazine's CIO Hall of Fame. Partners HealthCare has received several industry awards for its effective and innovative use of information technology. Glaser has published over one hundred fifty articles and three books on the strategic application of information technology in health care. He holds a PhD degree in health care information systems from the University of Minnesota.

PREFACE

Having ready access to timely, complete, accurate, legible, and relevant information is critical to health care organizations, providers, and the patients they serve. Whether it is a nurse administering medication to a comatose patient, a physician advising a patient on the latest research findings for a specific cancer treatment, a billing clerk filing an electronic claim, a chief executive officer justifying to the board the need for building a new emergency department, or a health policy analyst reporting on the cost effectiveness of a new prevention program to the state's Medicaid program, each individual needs access to high-quality information with which to effectively perform his or her job. The need for quality information in health care has never been greater, particularly as this sector of our society strives to provide quality care, contain costs, and ensure adequate access. At the same time as the demand for information has increased, we have seen advances in information technology—such advances have the potential to radically change how health care services are accessed and delivered in the future.

To not only survive but thrive in this new environment, health care executives must have the knowledge, skills, and abilities to effectively manage both clinical and administrative information within their organizations and across the health care sector. Within the next decade or two the predominant model for maintaining health care information will shift from the current, largely paper-based medical record system, in which information is often incomplete, illegible, or unavailable where and when it is needed, to a system in which the patient's clinical information is integrated, complete, stored electronically, and available to the patient and authorized persons anywhere, anytime—regardless of the setting in which services are provided or the health insurance or coverage the patient carries. Patients and other consumers of health care services will also have a much greater role in the content of and access to their personal health information. Comparative data will be publicly available to consumers on the quality and cost of health care services available within the community. Providers involved in patient care will have immediate access to electronic decision-support tools, the latest relevant research findings on a given topic, and patient-specific reminders and alerts. Moreover health care executives will be able to devise strategic initiatives that take advantage of access to real-time, relevant administrative and clinical information.

PURPOSE AND ORGANIZATION OF THIS BOOK

The purpose of this book is to prepare future health care executives with the knowledge and skills they need to manage information and information systems technology effectively in this new environment. We wrote this book with the graduate student (or upper-level undergraduate student) enrolled in a health care management program in mind. Our definition of health care management is fairly broad and includes a range of academic programs from health administration, health information management, and public health programs to master of business administration (MBA) programs with an emphasis in health to nursing administration and physician executive educational programs. This book may also serve as an introductory text in health informatics programs. The first edition was published in 2005 and has been widely used by a variety of health care management and health information systems programs throughout the United States and abroad. We maintain the first edition's organizational structure and chapter order in this second edition, but we have thoroughly revised and updated the content to reflect changes in the health care industry and the renewed focus on health information technology initiatives. We have also added a new chapter that presents sixteen case studies of organizations experiencing management-related information system challenges. These reality-based cases are designed to stimulate discussion among students and enable them to apply concepts in the book to real-life scenarios.

The chapters in this book are organized into four major sections:

Part One: "Health Care Information" (Chapters One through Three)

Part Two: "Health Care Information Systems" (Chapters Four through Seven)

Part Three: "Information Technology" (Chapters Eight through Ten)

Part Four: "Senior Management IT Challenges" (Chapters Eleven through Sixteen)

Part One, "Health Care Information," is designed to be a health information primer for future health care executives. Often health information system textbooks begin by discussing the technology; they assume that the reader understands the basic clinical and administrative information found in a health care organization and the processes that create and use this information. So they jump into health information system or technology solutions without first examining the fundamental characteristics of the information and processes such solutions are designed to support (Chapter One), data quality (Chapter Two), or the laws, regulations, and standards that govern the management of information (Chapter Three) in health care organizations. It has been our experience that many students aspiring to be health care executives do not have a clinical background and therefore have a limited understanding of patient care processes and the information that is created and used during these processes. The three chapters we have included in Part One are designed to set the stage and provide the requisite background knowledge for the remainder of the book. Students with extensive clinical or health information management backgrounds may choose to skim this section as a refresher.

Part Two, "Health Care Information Systems," provides the reader with an understanding of how health care information systems have evolved and the major clinical and administrative applications in use today (Chapter Four). Special attention is given to the use of clinical information systems, with a focus on electronic medical record (EMR) systems. Chapter Five has been entirely revised from the first edition. It provides up-to-date information on the adoption and use of a range of clinical information systems, including systems for electronic medical records and health records, computerized provider order entry (CPOE), medication administration using bar coding, telemedicine, and telehealth. It also includes a section on the personal health record (PHR).

The last two chapters in Part Two describe the process that a health care organization typically goes through in selecting (Chapter Six) and implementing (Chapter Seven) a health care information system. Because most health care organizations are not equipped to develop their own applications, we focus on vendor-acquired systems and describe the pros and cons of contracting with an application service provider (ASP). Despite the best-made plans, things can and do go wrong when an organization is selecting or implementing a health care information system. Chapter Six concludes with a discussion of the issues that can arise during the system acquisition process and strategies for addressing them. We devote a substantial section of Chapter Seven to the organizational and cultural aspects of incorporating information technology (IT) systems into the health care organization. Chapter Seven ends with a discussion of issues that can arise during system implementation and strategies for addressing them.

Part Two focuses on health care information systems and the value they can bring to health care organizations and providers and to the patients they serve. Part Three, "Information Technology," turns to the technology underlying these systems, that is, how they work. The chapters in Part Three are designed to provide a basic understanding of information technology concepts such as architectures and of the core technologies needed to support health care information systems in terms of databases and networks (Chapter Eight), standards (Chapter Nine), and security (Chapter Ten). The intent is to provide the reader with enough IT knowledge that he or she could carry on a fairly intelligent conversation with a chief information officer (CIO) or a technically savvy clinician, understand the reasons why it is important to have a sound technical infrastructure to support systems, and appreciate the benefits of ensuring system security.

Part Four, "Senior Management IT Challenges," provides a top-level view of what it takes to effectively manage, budget, govern, and evaluate information technology services in a health care organization. Chapter Eleven introduces the reader to the IT function, the services typically found in an IT department in a large health care organization, and the types of professionals and staff generally employed there.

We believe it is critical for health care executives to become involved in discussions and decisions that influence their organization's use of IT. These discussions typically cover such topics as the organization's IT strategy (Chapter Twelve), IT budgeting and governance (Chapter Thirteen), management's role in major IT initiatives (Chapter Fourteen), and methods for evaluating return on investment or the value of health care information systems to the organization, the provider, and the patient (Chapter Fifteen). This part concludes with a series of management-related case studies designed to stimulate discussion and problem solving (Chapter Sixteen). Most of the cases are based on actual events or management situations.

Each chapter in the book (except Chapter Sixteen) begins with a set of chapter learning objectives and an overview and concludes with a summary of the material presented and a set of learning activities. These activities are designed to give students an opportunity to explore more fully the concepts introduced in the chapter and to gain hands-on experience by visiting and talking with IT professionals in a variety of health care settings.

Two appendixes offer supplemental information. Appendix A presents an updated overview of the health care IT industry, the companies that provide IT hardware, software, and a wide range of services to health care organizations. Appendix B contains an example of a project charter.

IT CHALLENGES IN HEALTH CARE

The health care industry is one of the most information intensive and technologically advanced in our society. Yet if you asked a roomful of health care executives and providers from a typical health care organization if they have easy access to timely, complete, accurate, reliable, and relevant information when making important strategic or patient-care decisions, most would respond with a resounding no. Despite the need for administrative and clinical information to facilitate the delivery of high-quality, cost-effective services, most organizations still function using paper-based or otherwise insufficient information systems. There are many reasons why this situation exists, not the least of which is that the health care industry is complex, both overall and in many of its functions. This complexity poses challenges for both the purchasers and vendors of health care information systems and related IT products and services.

Health care is often accused of being "behind" other industries in applying IT. Statistics, such as percentage of revenue spent on IT, are often used to indict health care for underinvesting in IT. The health care industry spends an average of 2.7 percent of its revenue on IT. Although this percentage is the same as the average percentage across all industries, it is low for an industry that is information intense. For example, banks spend 5.1 percent of revenue on IT and insurance companies spend 4.1 percent (Gartner, 2007). The indictment of being behind often carries with it an aspersion that health care executives are not as sharp or "on top of it" as executives in other industries. This is not true.

The complexity and the structure of health care organizations, both singly and considered as a group, make it very challenging to implement health care information systems and IT effectively. We emphasize this fact not to excuse health care organizations from having to make thoughtful investments or to claim that all health care executives are world-class but to make it clear that health care executives need to understand the context.

Large Numbers of Small Organizations

The health care industry includes large numbers of very small organizations. A majority of physicians practice in one- or two-physician offices. Thousands of hospitals have fewer than 100 beds. There are over 7,000 home health agencies. Small organizations often find it difficult to fund information system investments. An investment of $25,000 in an electronic medical record may be more than a solo practitioner can bear. In addition these organizations rarely have IT-trained staff members and hence are challenged when technology misbehaves—for example, when a printer malfunctions or files are inadvertently deleted.

The small size of these organizations also makes it difficult for software and hardware vendors to make money from them. Often these vendors cannot charge much for their applications, making it difficult for them to recover the costs of selling to small organizations and providing support to them. As a result most major vendors often avoid small organizations. Those vendors that do sell to this market are often small themselves, having perhaps four to six customers. This smallness means that if they have even one bad year—if, for example, they lose two customers—it may put them out of business. Hence there is significant turnover among small IT vendors. This turnover clearly places the small provider organization at risk of having the vendor of its IT system go out of business.

Unfortunately, there is no obvious answer to the IT challenges posed by the large number of small organizations in health care.

Incentive Misalignment

Many health care information system applications have the potential to improve the quality of care. CPOE can reduce adverse drug events. Reminder systems in the electronic medical record can improve the management of the chronically ill patient. Improvements in care are worthy goals, and providers may opt to bear the costs of the systems to gain them. In truth, however, the provider does not always reap a reward for such actions. The insurance payment mechanism may not provide a financial reward for the provider who has fewer medical errors. There may be no direct financial reward for better management of the diabetic.

Because of this misalignment that means the bearer of the cost may see no financial gain, providers can, rightfully, be hesitant to invest in IT that has care quality improvement as its goal. For them the IT investment reduces their income—with no corresponding financial upside. This misalignment rarely occurs in other industries. For example, if you are in the banking industry and you make IT investments to improve the quality of your service, you expect to be rewarded by having more customers and by having existing customers do more business with you.

Currently, several payers are experimenting with providing financial rewards for quality of care. In some of these experiments, providers are being given extra money when they use clinical systems. If these experiments do not lead to reimbursement approaches that offer payment for quality or if the payment is too small, the problem of incentive misalignment will continue. And providers' rate of IT adoption will remain slow.

Fragmented Care

Most of us, over the course of our lives, will seek care in several health care organizations. At times this care will also occur in various regions of the country. The data about our care are not routinely shared across the organizations we use. And the organizations do not have to be on different sides of this country for this failure to occur; they may be across the street from each other. This failure to share data means that any given provider may not be fully aware of allergies, history, and clinical findings that were recorded in other settings. Medical errors and inefficiencies—for example, unnecessary repeats of tests—can result.

In the past medical information exchange was to a large degree hindered by a lack of standards for health care data and transactions. This problem is now being resolved. The lack of exchange nevertheless continues. Although this is due in part to the fact that many providers still use paper-based systems that make exchange more expensive and less likely to happen, it occurs primarily because there is no incentive for either the sender or the receiver to make the exchange happen. It may seem odd, perhaps counter to the mission of health care, that organizations need financial incentives to do what is best for the patient. However, it is a harsh reality of health care that organizations do need positive operating margins.

Integrated delivery systems are one approach to reducing fragmentation. These systems attempt to pull together diverse types of health care organizations and use information systems to integrate data from these organizations. They do ease fragmentation, but they do not entirely solve the problem. There are insufficient numbers of integrated delivery systems, they vary widely in the degree to which they try to integrate care, and patients often seek care both inside and outside the system.

The fact that patients seek care outside the integrated delivery system poses significant challenges for these systems. These challenges are also present for an individual hospital. If an organization desires to create a composite clinical picture of a person—through the implementation of a clinical data repository, for example—it faces two fundamental problems (in addition to the lack of incentives and limited data and process standards):

- The clinical data typically reside in multiple care settings, potentially dozens or hundreds of settings. Implementing the IT infrastructure needed to support the resulting "pattern" of system interconnections that could access these data may prove to be too expensive or challenging.

- The desired data are randomly dispersed. The site where the patient is currently receiving care may not know whether other data about this patient exist or whether these other data are relevant. When a patient presents at the emergency room, care providers may not know whether the patient has been seen in other hospitals in the city or elsewhere. There have been efforts to develop prototypes of national master patient indexes able to identify the existence of data for a specific patient across multiple organizations. However, these prototypes have not been shown to work at the scale of a state or the country.

Complexity of the Process of Care

If one views the process of care as a manufacturing process (sick people are inputs, a "bunch of stuff" is done to them, and the outputs are better or well people), it is arguable that medical care is the most complex manufacturing process that exists. This high level of complexity has three major sources: the difficulty of defining the best care, care process variability, and process volatility.

Our current ability to define the best care process for treating a particular disease or problem can be limited. Process algorithms, guidelines, or pathways are often

- Based on heuristics (or rules of thumb), which makes consensus within and between organizations difficult or impossible. Available facts and science are often insufficient to define a consistent, let alone the most effective, approach. As a result, competing guidelines or protocols are being issued by payers, provider organization committees, and provider associations.

- Condition or context specific. The treatment of a particular acute illness, for example, can depend on the severity of the illness and the age and general health of the patient.

- Reliant on outcome measurements with severe limitations. For example, these measures may be insensitive to specific interventions, be proxies for "real" outcomes, or reflect the bias of an organization or researcher.

An organization is unlikely to define or adopt a consistent approach for each type of care. And even a defined approach may permit substantial latitude on the part of the provider. This results in great variability in treatment. In an academic medical center a physician may have at his or her disposal 2,500 medications (each with a range of "allowable" frequencies, doses, and routes of administration), 1,100 clinical laboratory tests, 300 radiology procedures, and large numbers of other tests and procedures. The selection of tests and procedures, their sequence, and the relative timing of their use, along with patient condition and comorbidity, all come together to determine the relative utility of a particular approach to treatment. The variability of approaches to treating a disease is compounded by the diversity of diseases and problems. There are approximately 10,000 diseases, syndromes, and problems, each of which, in theory, requires its own pathway, guideline, or approach, and perhaps multiple approaches.

This variability and opportunity for variability is unparalleled by any other manufacturing process. No automobile manufacturer produces 10,000 models of cars or provides for each model 2,500 different types of paint, 300 different arrangements of wheels, and 1,100 different locations for the driver's seat.

These challenges are exacerbated by the volatility of the medical process. In an average year, over 400,000 articles are added to the base of refereed medical literature, articles that may require us to continually revisit our treatment consensus. In addition, medical technology often induces changes in practice before the studies that measure practice efficacy can be completed.

The complexity of the medical process places unique and tough demands on the design of clinical information systems, the ability to support provider and patient decision making, and the ability to measure the quality of the care that providers deliver.

Complexity of Health and Medical Data

A patient's health status and medical condition are difficult to describe using comprehensive, coded data. Several factors contribute to this problem:

- Although research is ongoing, well-accepted methods to formally decompose many key components of the patient record—for example, admission history and physical status—into coded concepts have not yet been developed.

- When data models are developed, vocabularies of standardized terms to use in these models are difficult to compile. The condition of a patient is often complex and probabilistic, requiring a nuanced description. Multifactorial and temporal relationships can exist between pieces of data. This complexity makes it inherently difficult to develop codes for medical data.

- Even when a data model is developed and coded terms are defined, the entry of coded data is cumbersome and constraining for the provider compared to using ordinary text.

- Finally, no single way exists to organize automated medical data, the relational model does not serve the medical domain particularly well, and single sites and groups of sites have developed many idiosyncratic ways to code data. These coding methods have often been devised for good reasons and significant investments have been made to define and implement them, so change will not happen unless the need for it is compelling.

Nature of Provider Organizations

Health care organizations, particularly providers, have attributes that can hinder information system adoption. Provider organizations are unusual in that they have two parallel power structures: the administrative staff and the medical staff. The medical staff side is often loosely organized and lacks an organizational chart with clear lines of authority. This two-part structure leads to a great deal of negotiating and coalition building. Negotiation is an aspect of any major decision within a provider organization, including decisions about health care information systems. This can result in very long decision-making cycles; reaching an agreement on an IT vendor can take months or years.

RISING TO THE CHALLENGES

We do not intend this discussion of complexity and structure to lead the reader to the edge of inconsolable despair, only to an understanding of the landscape. Despite the complexity described here, significant progress may be made. Health care is carried out by many small organizations, but advances are being made in developing IT applications that are both inexpensive and robust. Efforts are under way to address the problem of misaligned incentives. The care process is complex, but the appropriate way to manage many diseases (diabetes, for example) is well understood. Medical data are complex, but there are established data standards for diseases, procedures, and laboratory tests.

Care crosses boundaries, but an electronic medical record that has most of a patient's data is better than a paper record that has most of a patient's data.

Both the consumers and suppliers of health care information system products and services struggle to develop and implement systems that improve care and organizational performance. And their efforts are often successful. These efforts confront the health care industry's core challenges—size, fragmentation, misaligned incentives, and complexity of care processes and medical data.

Health care consumers, payers, and purchasers are demanding that more be done to ensure that health care providers are equipped with the information needed to decrease administrative costs, improve access to care, and improve patient safety, in spite of the significant industry challenges. We hope you will find this book to be a useful resource in ensuring that your health care organization and its information systems are well equipped to handle patients', providers', administrators', and all other stakeholders' health care information needs.

PART

1

HEALTH CARE
INFORMATION

CHAPTER

INTRODUCTION TO HEALTH CARE INFORMATION

LEARNING OBJECTIVES

- To be able to compare and contrast the various definitions of health care information.
- To be able to describe the major types of health care information (internal and external) that are captured or used or both in health care organizations.
- To be able to cite specific examples of the major types of health care information.
- To be able to understand the content and uses of patient records.
- To be able to follow a patient's or client's health information throughout a typical encounter or process.

Although it may seem self-evident, it is worth stating: *health care information is the reason we need health care information systems.* No study of information systems in health care would be complete without an examination of the data and information they are designed to support. The focus of this chapter will be on the data and information that are unique to health care, such as the clinical information created during patients' health care encounters, the administrative information related to those encounters, and the external information used to improve the clinical care and administrative functions associated with those encounters.

We begin the chapter with a brief discussion of some common definitions of health care information. Then we introduce the framework that will be used for exploring various types of health care information. The first major section of the chapter looks at data and information created internally by health care organizations, discussing this information at both the individual client level and the aggregate level. This section also examines some core processes involved in an inpatient and an ambulatory care clinical encounter to further explain how and when internal health care data and information originate and how they are used. The final section examines health care data and information created, at least in part, externally to the health care organization, and addresses both comparative and knowledge-based data and information.

TYPES OF HEALTH CARE INFORMATION

Different texts and articles define *health care information*, or *health information*, differently. Often it is the use or setting of the health information that drives the definition. For example, the government or an insurance company may have a certain definition of health care information, and the hospital, nursing home, or physician's office may have other definitions. In this book we are primarily interested in the *information generated or used by health care organizations*, such as hospitals, nursing homes, physicians' offices, and other ambulatory care settings. Of course this same information may be used by governmental agencies or insurance companies as well.

Definitions of Health Care Information

Health Insurance Portability and Accountability Act Definition   The Health Insurance Portability and Accountability Act (HIPAA), the federal legislation that includes provisions to protect patients' health information from unauthorized disclosure, defines *health information* as

any information, whether oral or recorded in any form or medium, that—
(A) is created or received by a health care provider, health plan, public health authority, employer, life insurer, school or university, or health care clearinghouse; and

(B) relates to the past, present, or future physical or mental health or condition of an individual, the provision of health care to an individual, or the past, present, or future payment for the provision of health care to an individual.

HIPAA refers to this type of information as *protected health information*, or PHI. To meet the definition of PHI, information must first of all be *identifiable*, that is, it must have an individual patient perspective and the patient's identity must be known. HIPAA-defined PHI may exist outside a traditional health care institution and is therefore not an appropriate definition for an organizational view of information such as ours. HIPAA is certainly an important piece of legislation, and it has a direct impact on how health care organizations create and maintain health information (HIPAA is discussed further in Chapter Three). However, not all the information that must be managed in a health care organization is protected health information. Much of the information used by health care providers and executives is neither patient specific nor identifiable in the HIPAA sense.

National Alliance for Health Information Technology Definitions   In an attempt to provide consensus definitions of key health care information terms, the National Alliance for Health Information Technology ("Alliance") released a report "on defining key health information technology terms" in April 2008. Although the terms defined in this report are specific to health records, the definitions contain descriptions of the health information that is maintained by each type of record. The following are the Alliance definitions of *electronic medical record, electronic health record*, and *personal health record*. Each of these definitions refers to patient-specific, identifiable health care information that would meet the HIPAA definition of PHI.

Electronic medical record: An electronic record of health-related information on an individual that can be created, gathered, managed, and consulted by authorized clinicians and staff within one healthcare organization.

Electronic health record: An electronic record of health-related information on an individual that conforms to nationally recognized interoperability standards and that can be created, managed, and consulted by authorized clinicians and staff across more than one healthcare organization.

Personal health record: An electronic record of health-related information on an individual that conforms to nationally recognized interoperability standards and that can be drawn from multiple sources while being managed, shared, and controlled by the individual [Alliance, 2008].

(The Alliance report also contains definitions of *health information exchange, health information organization*, and *regional health information organization*. These definitions will be discussed in subsequent chapters.)

The Joint Commission Definitions   The Joint Commission, the major accrediting agency for health care organizations in the United States, offers a broader framework for examining health care information within health care organizations. It defines not only patient-specific, identifiable health care information but also information that is aggregate, knowledge-based, and comparative.

The Joint Commission accreditation standards have been developed over the years to, among other things, measure the quality of the different types of health care information found in and used with health care organizations. The Joint Commission (2004) urges health care leaders to take "responsibility for managing information, just as they do for . . . human, material, and financial resources." The Joint Commission clearly acknowledges the vital role that information plays in ensuring the provision of quality health care.

The Joint Commission (2004) divides health care information into four categories:

- Patient-specific data and information

- Aggregate data and information

- Knowledge-based information

- Comparative data and information

Health Care Data Framework

Our framework for looking at data and information created, maintained, manipulated, stored, and used within health care organizations is shown in Figure 1.1. The first level of categorization divides data and information into two categories: *internal* and *external*.

FIGURE 1.1.   *Types of Health Care Information Framework*

Internal Data and Information

- Patient encounter
  - Patient-specific
  - Aggregate
  - Comparative
- General operations

External Data and Information

- Comparative
- Expert or knowledge-based

Within the broad category of data and information created *internally* by the health care organization, we will focus on clinical and administrative information directly related to the activities surrounding the *patient encounter*, both the individual encounter and the collective encounter. We break information related to the patient encounter into the subcategories of *patient specific, aggregate*, and *comparative*. Our focus is on the clinical and administrative individual and aggregate health care information that is associated with a patient encounter. Table 1.1 lists the various types of data and information that fall into the patient encounter subcategories of patient-specific and aggregate. Information typically found in a patient medical record is shown in italics. (The comparative data and information subcategory is found in both the internal and external categories; we will discuss it when we discuss external data and information.)

The second major component of internal health care information in our framework is *general operations*. Data and information needed for the health care organization's general operations are not a focus of this text. Health care executives do, however, need to be concerned not only with information directly related to the patient encounter

TABLE 1.1. Examples of Types of Patient Encounter Data and Information

	Primary Purpose	
Type	**Clinical**	**Administrative**
Patient-specific *(items generally included in the patient medical record are in italics)*	*Identification sheet*	*Identification sheet*
	Problem list	*Consents*
	Medication record	*Authorizations*
	History	*Preauthorization*
	Physical	*Scheduling*
	Progress notes	*Admission or registration*
	Consultations	*Insurance eligibility*
	Physicians' orders	*Billing*
	Imaging and X-ray results	*Diagnoses codes*
	Lab results	*Procedure codes*
	Immunization record	
	Operative report	
	Pathology report	
	Discharge summary	
	Diagnoses codes	
	Procedure codes	
Aggregate	Disease indexes	Cost reports
	Specialized registers	Claims denial analysis
	Outcomes data	Staffing analysis
	Statistical reports	Referral analysis
	Trend analysis	Statistical reports
	Ad hoc reports	Trend analysis
		Ad hoc reports

but also with information about the organization's general operations. Health care organizations are, after all, businesses that must have revenues exceeding costs to remain viable. The standard administrative activities of any viable organization also take place in health care settings. Health care executives interact with information and information systems in such areas as general accounting, financial planning, personnel administration, and facility planning on a regular if not daily basis. Our decision to focus on the information that is unique to health care and not a part of general business operations is not intended to diminish the importance of general operations but rather is an acknowledgment that a wealth of resources for general business information and information systems already exists.

In addition to using internally generated patient encounter and general operations data and information, health care organizations use information generated *externally* (Figure 1.1). *Comparative data*, as we will explain, combine internal and external data to aid organizations in evaluating their performance. The other major category of external information used in health care organizations is *expert* or *knowledge-based information*, which is generally collected or created by experts who are not part of the organization. Health care providers and executives use this type of information in decision making, both clinical and administrative. A classic example of knowledge-based clinical information is the information contained in a professional health care journal. Other examples are regional or national databases and informational Web sites related to health or management issues.

INTERNAL DATA AND INFORMATION: PATIENT SPECIFIC—CLINICAL

The majority of clinical, patient-specific information created and used in health care organizations can be found in or has originated in patients' medical records. This section will introduce some basic components of the patient medical record. It will also examine an inpatient and an ambulatory care patient encounter to show how the patient medical record is typically created. All types of health care organizations—inpatient, outpatient, long-term care, and so forth—have patient medical records. These records may be in electronic or paper format, but the purpose and basic content are similar regardless of record or organizational type.

Purpose of Patient Records

Health care organizations maintain medical records for several key purposes. As we move into the discussion of clinical information systems in subsequent chapters, it will be important to remember these purposes. These purposes remain constant whether the record is part of a state-of-the-art electronic system or part of a basic, paper-based manual system.

1. *Patient care.* Patient records provide the documented basis for planning patient care and treatment. This purpose is considered the number one reason for maintaining patient records. Health care executives need to keep this primary purpose

in mind when examining health care information systems. Too often other purposes, particularly billing and reimbursement, may seem to take precedence over patient care.

2. *Communication.* Patient records are an important means by which physicians, nurses, and others can communicate with one another about patient needs. The members of the health care team generally interact with patients at different times during the day, week, or even month. The patient record may be the only means of communication between various providers.

3. *Legal documentation.* Patient records, because they describe and document care and treatment, can also become legal records. In the event of a lawsuit or other legal action involving patient care, the record becomes the primary evidence for what actually took place during the episode of care. An old but absolutely true adage about the legal importance of patient records says, "If it was not documented, it was not done."

4. *Billing and reimbursement.* Patient records provide the documentation patients and payers use to verify billed services. Insurance companies and other third-party payers insist on clear documentation to support any claims submitted. The federal programs Medicare and Medicaid have oversight and review processes in place that use patient records to confirm the accuracy of claims filed. Filing a claim for a service that is not clearly documented in the patient record could be construed as fraud.

5. *Research and quality management.* Patient records are used in many facilities for research purposes and for monitoring the quality of care provided. Patient records can serve as source documents from which information about certain diseases or procedures can be taken, for example. Although research is most prevalent in large academic medical centers, studies are conducted in other types of health care organizations as well.

The importance of maintaining complete and accurate patient records cannot be underestimated. They serve not only as a basis for planning patient care but also as the legal record documenting the care that was provided to patients by the organization. Patient medical records provide much of the source data for health care information that is generated within and across health care organizations. The data captured in a patient medical record become a permanent record of that patient's diagnoses, treatments, and response to treatments.

Content of Patient Records

The American Health Information Management Association (AHIMA) maintains the Web site www.myPHR.com, which lists the following components as being common to most patient records, regardless of facility type or medical record system (electronic or paper based) (AHIMA, 2008). Medical record content is determined to a large extent by external requirements, standards, and regulations (discussed in Chapter Three). This is not an exhaustive list, but with our expanded definitions it provides a general overview of this content and of the person or persons responsible for the content. It reveals that the patient record is a repository for a variety of clinical data and information that is produced by many different individuals involved in the care of the patient.

- *Identification sheet.* Information found on the identification sheet (sometimes called a *face sheet* or *admission* or *discharge record*) originates at the time of registration or admission. The identification sheet is generally the first report or screen a user will encounter when accessing a patient record. It lists at least the patient name, address, telephone number, insurance carrier, and policy number, as well as the patient's diagnoses and disposition at discharge. These diagnoses are recorded by the physicians and coded by administrative personnel. (Diagnosis coding is discussed later in this chapter.) The identification sheet is used as both a clinical and an administrative document. It provides a quick view of the diagnoses that required care during the encounter. The codes and other demographic information are used for reimbursement and planning purposes.

- *Problem list.* Patient records frequently contain a comprehensive problem list, which lists significant illnesses and operations the patient has experienced. This list is generally maintained over time. It is not specific to a single episode of care and may be maintained by the attending or primary care physician or collectively by all the health care providers involved in the patient's care.

- *Medication record.* Sometimes called a *medication administration record* (MAR), this record lists medicines prescribed for and subsequently administered to the patient. It often also lists any medication allergies the patient may have. Nursing personnel are generally responsible for documenting and maintaining medication information. In an inpatient setting, nurses are responsible for administering medications according to physicians' written or verbal orders.

- *History and physical.* The history component of this report describes any major illnesses and surgeries the patient has had, any significant family history of disease, patient health habits, and current medications. The information for the history is provided by the patient (or someone acting on his or her behalf) and is documented by the attending physician at the beginning of or immediately prior to an encounter or treatment episode. The physical component of this report states what the physician found when he or she performed a hands-on examination of the patient. The history and physical together document the initial assessment of the patient and provide the basis for diagnosis and subsequent treatment. They also provide a framework within which physicians and other care providers can document significant findings. Although obtaining the initial history and physical is a one-time activity during an episode of care, continued reassessment and documentation of that reassessment during the patient's course of treatment is critical. Results of reassessments are generally recorded in progress notes.

- *Progress notes.* Progress notes are made by the physicians, nurses, therapists, social workers, and other clinical staff caring for the patient. Each provider is responsible for the content of his or her notes. Progress notes should reflect the patient's response to treatment along with the provider's observations and plans for continued treatment. There are many formats for progress notes. In some organizations all care providers use the same note format; in others each provider type uses a customized format.

- *Consultation.* A consultation note or report records opinions about the patient's condition made by a health care provider other than the attending physician or primary care provider. Consultation reports may come from physicians and others inside or outside a particular health care organization, but copies are maintained as part of the patient record.

- *Physician's orders.* Physician's orders are a physician's directions, instructions, or prescriptions given to other members of the health care team regarding the patient's medications, tests, diets, treatments, and so forth. In the current U.S. health care system, procedures and treatments must be ordered by the appropriate licensed practitioner; in most cases this will be a physician.

- *Imaging and X-ray reports.* The radiologist is responsible for interpreting images produced through X-rays, mammograms, ultrasounds, scans, and the like and for documenting his or her interpretations or findings in the patient's medical record. These findings should be documented in a timely manner so they are available to the appropriate physician(s) to facilitate the appropriate treatment. The actual films or images are generally maintained in the radiology or imaging departments as hard copies or in a specialized computer system. These images are typically not considered part of the patient medical record, but like other reports, they are stored according to state laws and clinical practice guidelines and are important documentation of patient care.

- *Laboratory reports.* Laboratory reports contain the results of tests conducted on body fluids, cells, and tissues. For example, a medical lab might perform a throat culture, urinalysis, cholesterol level, or complete blood count. There are hundreds of specific lab tests that can be run by health care organizations or specialized labs. Lab personnel are responsible for documenting the lab results. Results of the lab work become part of the permanent patient record. However, lab results must also be available during treatment. Health care providers rely on accurate lab results in making clinical decisions, so there is a need for timely reporting of lab results and a system for ensuring that physicians and other appropriate care providers receive the results. Physicians are responsible for documenting any findings and treatment plans based on the lab results.

- *Consent and authorization forms.* Copies of consents to admission, treatment, surgery, and release of information are an important component of the medical record and related to its use as a legal document. The practitioner who actually provides the treatment must obtain informed consent for the treatment. Patients must sign informed consent documents before treatment takes place. Forms authorizing release of information must also be signed by patients before any patient-specific health care information is released to parties not directly involved in the care of the patient.

■ *Operative report.* Operative reports describe any surgery performed and list the names of surgeons and assistants. The surgeon is responsible for the operative report.

■ *Pathology report.* Pathology reports describe tissue removed during any surgical procedure and the diagnosis based on examination of that tissue. The pathologist is responsible for the pathology report.

■ *Discharge summary.* Each hospital medical record contains a discharge summary. The discharge summary summarizes the hospital stay, including the reason for admission, significant findings from tests, procedures performed, therapies provided, responses to treatments, condition at discharge, and instructions for medications, activity, diet, and follow-up care. The attending physician is responsible for documenting the discharge summary at the conclusion of the patient's stay in the hospital.

Figure 1.2 displays a screen from an electronic medical record. A patient record may contain some or all of the documentation just listed. Depending on the patient's illness or injury and the type of treatment facility, he or she may need specialized health care services. These services may require specific documentation. For example, long-term

FIGURE 1.2. *Sample EMR Screen*

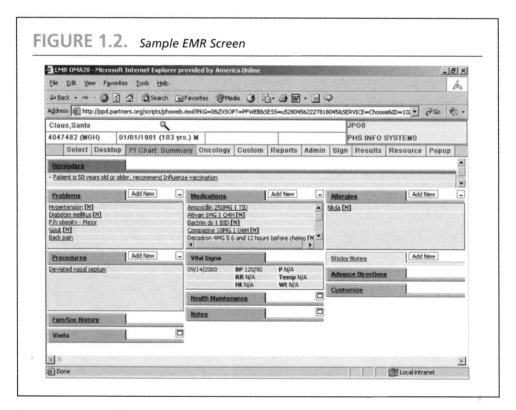

Source: Partners HealthCare

care facilities and behavioral health facilities have special documentation requirements. Our list is intended to introduce the common components of patient records, not to provide a comprehensive list of all possible components. As stated before, the patient record components listed here will exist whether the health care organization uses electronic records, paper records, or a combination of both.

Overview of a Patient Encounter

Where do medical record data and information come from? How do they originate? In this section we will walk through an inpatient encounter and also take a brief look at a physician's office patient encounter. Along the way we will point out how medical record information is created and used. Figure 1.3 diagrams a reasonably typical non-surgical inpatient admission. The middle column represents the basic patient flow in an inpatient episode of care. It shows some of the core activities and processes the patient will undergo during a hospital stay. The left-hand column lists some of the points along the patient flow process where basic medical record information is added to the medical record database or file. The right-hand column lists the hospital personnel who are generally responsible for a patient flow activity or specific medical record documentation or both. Using Figure 1.3 as a guide we will follow a patient, Marcus Low, through his admission to the hospital for radiation treatments.

CASE STUDY

Marcus Low's Admission Mr. Low's admission to the hospital is scheduled by his oncologist, Dr. Good, who serves as the admitting and attending physician during Mr. Low's two-day hospital stay. This process involves the administrative staff in Dr. Good's office calling the Admissions Department of the hospital and arranging a time for Mr. Low to be admitted. The preadmission process involves the hospital corresponding or talking with Mr. Low and with Dr. Good's office to gather the demographic and insurance information that will be needed to file a claim with Mr. Low's insurance company. Generally, hospital personnel contact the patient's insurance company to precertify his or her hospital admission, and in this case the hospital checks that the insurance company agrees that Mr. Low's planned admission is medically necessary and will be approved for payment. The patient medical record is started during the preadmission phase. The Admissions Department must check whether Mr. Low has had a previous stay at the hospital and whether he has an existing medical record number or unique identifier. The *identification sheet* is started at this stage. Mr. Low's hospital has an electronic medical record system, so the demographic information needed is put into the computer system.

On the scheduled day of admission, Mr. Low arrives at the hospital's Admissions Department. There he verifies his demographic and insurance information. He is issued an identification (ID) bracelet and escorted to his assigned room by the hospital staff. Bed assignment is an important activity for the Admissions Department. It involves a great deal of coordination among the Admissions Department, nursing staff, and housekeeping staff. Efficient patient

(Continued)

CASE STUDY (*Continued*)

flow within a hospital relies on this first step of bed assignment. Clean rooms with adequate staff need to be available not only for elective admissions like Mr. Low's but also for emergency admissions. Because this hospital has an electronic medical record, there is no paper chart to go to the nursing floor with Mr. Low, but the admissions staff verify that all pertinent information is recorded in the system. The admissions staff also have Mr. Low sign a general *consent to treatment* and the *authorization* that allows the hospital to share his health information with the insurance company.

Once on the nursing floor, Mr. Low receives a nursing assessment and a visit from the attending physician. The nursing assessment results in a nursing care plan for Mr. Low while he is in the hospital. Because Mr. Low saw Dr. Good in his office during the previous week, the *history and physical* is already stored in the electronic medical record system. Dr. Good records his *orders* in the physician order entry component of the electronic medical record. The nursing staff respond to these orders by giving Mr. Low a mild sedative. The Radiology Department responds to these orders by preparing for Mr. Low's visit to that department later in the day. During his two-day stay Mr. Low receives several medications and three radiation treatments. He receives blood work to monitor his progress. All these treatments are made in response to orders given by Dr. Good and are recorded in the medical record, along with the *progress notes* from each provider. The medical record serves as a primary form of communication among all the providers of care. They check the electronic medical record system regularly to look for new orders and to review the updated results of treatments and tests.

When Mr. Low is ready to be discharged, he is once again assessed by the nursing staff. A member of the nursing staff reviews his discharge orders from the physician and goes over instructions that Mr. Low should follow at home. Shortly after discharge, Dr. Good must dictate or record a *discharge summary* that outlines the course of treatment Mr. Low received. Once the record is flagged to indicate that Mr. Low has been discharged, the personnel in the Health Information Management Department assign codes to the diagnoses and procedures. These codes will be used by the Billing Department to file insurance claims.

When the Billing Department receives the final codes for the records, it will submit the appropriate claims to the insurance companies. It is the Billing Department, or Patient Accounting Department, that manages the patient revenue cycle that begins with scheduling and ends when payments are posted. This department works closely with third-party payers and patients in collecting reimbursement for services provided.

Even in this extremely brief outline of a two-day hospital stay, you can see that patient care and the reimbursement for that care involve many individuals who need access to timely and accurate patient information. The coordination of care is essential to quality, and this coordination relies on the availability of information. Other hospital stays are longer; some are emergency admissions; some involve surgery. These stays will need information additional to that discussed in this section. However, the basic components will be essentially the same as those just described.

FIGURE 1.3. *Inpatient Encounter Flow*

Sample Medical Record Information	Inpatient Encounter	Responsible Party
	Scheduling	
	Determine reason for admission	Physician's office staff
	Determine availability of bed and so forth	Hospital scheduling staff
	Preadmission	
Identification sheet	*Collect demographic and insurance information*	Hospital admission staff
	Determine insurance eligibility	
	Precertify inpatient stay	
	Obtain consents, authorizations	
	Admission or Registration	
Identification sheet	*Verify demographic information*	Hospital admission staff
Consent and authorizations	*Verify insurance*	
	Make bed assignment	
	Issue identification bracelet	
	Treatment	
Problem list	*Coordinate care*	Attending physician
	Medical—	
History and physical	*Initial assessment*	Physicians
Physician orders	*Treatment planning*	
Progress notes	*Orders for treatment, lab, and other*	
Consultations	*diagnostic testing, medications*	
and so forth	*Reassessment*	
	Discharge planning	
	Nursing—	
Nursing notes	*Initial assessment*	Nurses
Medication administration	*Treatment planning*	
record	*Administration of tests, treatment,*	
and so forth	*medication*	
	Discharge planning	
	Ancillary Services (Radiology, Lab, Pharmacy & so forth)—	
X-ray reports	*Assessment*	Lab technicians
Lab results	*Administration of tests, treatment,*	Radiologist and radiology
Pathology	*medication*	technicians
Pharmacy		Pharmacists and so forth
and so forth	**Discharge**	
Identification sheet	*Code diagnoses and procedures*	Medical record
Discharge instructions	*Prepare instructions for continued care*	personnel and coders
Discharge summary	*and follow-up*	Nurses
	Summarize of hospital course	Attending physician

FIGURE 1.4. *Physician's Office Visit Patient Flow*

Check-In
Verify appointment   Front office staff
Update insurance information
Update demographic information
Pull medical record

Move to Exam Room
Take vital signs   Nursing staff
Review reason for admission
Document in medical record

Examination
Discussion of hospital stay   Physician
Discussion of disease course and
next steps

Check out
Set next appointment   Front office staff
Receive payment on bill

Later
Dictate notes   Physician

Code visit   Billing clerk
File insurance

An ambulatory care encounter is somewhat different from a hospital stay. Let's follow Mr. Low again. This time we will describe his follow-up office visit with Dr. Good two weeks after his discharge from the hospital. Figure 1.4 is an outline of the process that Mr. Low followed during his office visit and the individuals who were responsible for each step in the process.

CASE STUDY

Mr. Low's Physician's Office Visit   Dr. Good also maintains a medical record for Mr. Low, but his records are still mainly paper based. There is no direct link between Dr. Good's and the hospital's medical record systems. Fortunately, Dr. Good can access the hospital's electronic medical record system from his office. He can view all the lab results, radiology reports, and discharge summaries for his hospitalized patients. He chooses to print out these reports and file them in the patients' paper medical records. Each medical record in Dr. Good's office contains the general patient demographic and insurance information, an ongoing problem list, a summary of visits, and individual visit notes. These notes include entries by both the nursing staff and Dr. Good. The nursing staff record all their notes by hand. Dr. Good dictates his notes, which are subsequently transcribed by a professional medical transcriber. All phone calls and prescription information are also recorded in the record.

One significant difference between an ambulatory care visit, such as a physician's office visit, and a hospital stay is the scope of the episode of care. During an inpatient stay patients usually receive a course of treatment, with a definite admission point and discharge point. In an ambulatory care setting, particularly primary care physician visits, patients may have multiple problems and treatments that are ongoing. There may not be a definite beginning or end to any one course of treatment. There are likely to be fewer care providers interacting with the patient at any given ambulatory care visit. There may, however, be more consultations over time and a need to coordinate care across organizations. All these characteristics make the clinical information needs of the inpatient setting and the ambulatory care setting somewhat different, but in each setting, this information is equally important to the provision of high-quality care.

Health care information systems and health care processes are closely entwined with one another. Health care processes require the use of data and information and they also produce or create information. Care providers must communicate with one another and often need to share patient information across organizations. The information produced by any one health care process may in turn be used by others. A true web of information sharing is needed.

INTERNAL DATA AND INFORMATION: PATIENT SPECIFIC—ADMINISTRATIVE

As we have seen in the previous section, patient-specific clinical information is captured and stored as a part of the patient medical record. However, there is more to the story—health care organizations need to get paid for the care they provide and to plan for the efficient provision of services to ensure that their operations remain viable. In this section we will examine individual patient data and information used specifically for administrative purposes. Health care organizations need data to effectively perform the tasks associated with the patient revenue cycle, tasks such as scheduling, precertification and insurance eligibility determination, billing, and payment verification. To determine what data are needed, we can look, first, at two standard billing documents, the UB-04 (CMS-1450) and the CMS-1500. In addition, we will discuss the concept of a uniform data set and introduce the Uniform Hospital Discharge Data Set, the Uniform Ambulatory Care Data Set, and the Minimum Data Set for long-term care.

Data Needed to Process Reimbursement Claims

Generally, the health care organization's accounting or billing department is responsible for processing claims, an activity that includes verifying insurance coverage, billing third-party payers (private insurance companies, Medicare, or Medicaid), and processing the payments as they are received. Depending on the type of service provided to the patient, one of two standard billing forms will be submitted to the third-party payer. The UB-04, or CMS-1450, is submitted for inpatient, hospital-based outpatient, home health care, and long-term care services. The CMS-1500 is submitted for health care provider services, such as those provided by a physician's office.

UB-04   In 1975, the American Hospital Association (AHA) formed the National Uniform Billing Committee (NUBC, 1999), bringing the major national provider and payer organizations together for the purpose of developing a single billing form and standard data set that could be used for processing health care claims by institutions nationwide. The first *uniform bill* was the UB-82. It has since been modified and improved upon, resulting, first, in the UB-92 data set and now in the currently used UB-04 (see Exhibit 1.1). UB-04 is the de facto hospital and other institution claim standard. It is required by the federal government and state governments in their role as third-party payers and has been adopted across the United States by private third-party payers as well. One important change implemented with the transition from the UB-92 to the UB-04 is the requirement that each claim include a valid National Provider Identifier (NPI) (Centers for Medicare and Medicaid [CMS], 2006). The NPI is a unique identification number for each HIPAA-covered health care provider. Covered health care providers and all health plans and health care clearinghouses use NPIs in the administrative and financial transactions adopted under HIPAA. The NPI is a ten-position, "intelligence-free" numeric identifier, meaning that this ten-digit number does not carry any additional information about the health care provider to which it is assigned, such as the state in which the provider works or the provider's medical specialty (CMS, 2008).

CMS-1500   The National Uniform Claim Committee (NUCC, 2008) was created by the American Medical Association (AMA) to develop a standardized data set for the noninstitutional health care community to use in the submission of claims (much as the NUBC has done for institutional providers). Members of this committee represent key provider and payer organizations, with the AMA appointing the committee chair. The standardized claim form developed and overseen by NUCC is the CMS-1500. This claim form has been adopted by the federal government, and like the UB-04 for institutional care, has become the de facto standard for all types of noninstitutional provider claims, such as those for physician services (see Exhibit 1.2).

It is important to recognize that both the UB-04 and the CMS-1500 claim forms incorporate standardized data sets. Regardless of a health care organization's location or a patient's insurance coverage, the same data elements are collected. In many states UB-04 data and CMS-1500 data must be reported to a central state agency responsible for aggregating and analyzing the state's health data. At the federal level the Centers for

EXHIBIT 1.1. *Uniform Bill: UB-04*

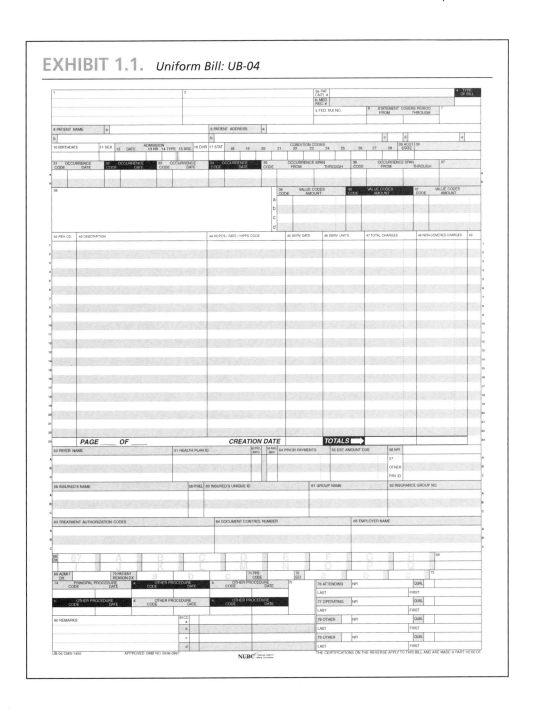

EXHIBIT 1.1. (Continued)

UB-04 NOTICE: THE SUBMITTER OF THIS FORM UNDERSTANDS THAT MISREPRESENTATION OR FALSIFICATION OF ESSENTIAL INFORMATION AS REQUESTED BY THIS FORM, MAY SERVE AS THE BASIS FOR CIVIL MONETARTY PENALTIES AND ASSESSMENTS AND MAY UPON CONVICTION INCLUDE FINES AND/OR IMPRISONMENT UNDER FEDERAL AND/OR STATE LAW(S).

Submission of this claim constitutes certification that the billing information as shown on the face hereof is true, accurate and complete. That the submitter did not knowingly or recklessly disregard or misrepresent or conceal material facts. The following certifications or verifications apply where pertinent to this Bill:

1. If third party benefits are indicated, the appropriate assignments by the insured /beneficiary and signature of the patient or parent or a legal guardian covering authorization to release information are on file. Determinations as to the release of medical and financial information should be guided by the patient or the patient's legal representative.

2. If patient occupied a private room or required private nursing for medical necessity, any required certifications are on file.

3. Physician's certifications and re-certifications, if required by contract or Federal regulations, are on file.

4. For Religious Non-Medical facilities, verifications and if necessary re-certifications of the patient's need for services are on file.

5. Signature of patient or his representative on certifications, authorization to release information, and payment request, as required by Federal Law and Regulations (42 USC 1935f, 42 CFR 424.36, 10 USC 1071 through 1086, 32 CFR 199) and any other applicable contract regulations, is on file.

6. The provider of care submitter acknowledges that the bill is in conformance with the Civil Rights Act of 1964 as amended. Records adequately describing services will be maintained and necessary information will be furnished to such governmental agencies as required by applicable law.

7. For Medicare Purposes: If the patient has indicated that other health insurance or a state medical assistance agency will pay part of his/her medical expenses and he/she wants information about his/her claim released to them upon request, necessary authorization is on file. The patient's signature on the provider's request to bill Medicare medical and non-medical information, including employment status, and whether the person has employer group health insurance which is responsible to pay for the services for which this Medicare claim is made.

8. For Medicaid purposes: The submitter understands that because payment and satisfaction of this claim will be from Federal and State funds, any false statements, documents, or concealment of a material fact are subject to prosecution under applicable Federal or State Laws.

9. For TRICARE Purposes:

(a) The information on the face of this claim is true, accurate and complete to the best of the submitter's knowledge and belief, and services were medically necessary and appropriate for the health of the patient;

(b) The patient has represented that by a reported residential address outside a military medical treatment facility catchment area he or she does not live within the catchment area of a U.S. military medical treatment facility, or if the patient resides within a catchment area of such a facility, a copy of Non-Availability Statement (DD Form 1251) is on file, or the physician has certified to a medical emergency in any instance where a copy of a Non-Availability Statement is not on file;

(c) The patient or the patient's parent or guardian has responded directly to the provider's request to identify all health insurance coverage, and that all such coverage is identified on the face of the claim except that coverage which is exclusively supplemental payments to TRICARE-determined benefits;

(d) The amount billed to TRICARE has been billed after all such coverage have been billed and paid excluding Medicaid, and the amount billed to TRICARE is that remaining claimed against TRICARE benefits;

(e) The beneficiary's cost share has not been waived by consent or failure to exercise generally accepted billing and collection efforts; and,

(f) Any hospital-based physician under contract, the cost of whose services are allocated in the charges included in this bill, is not an employee or member of the Uniformed Services. For purposes of this certification, an employee of the Uniformed Services is an employee, appointed in civil service (refer to 5 USC 2105), including part-time or intermittent employees, but excluding contract surgeons or other personal service contracts. Similarly, member of the Uniformed Services does not apply to reserve members of the Uniformed Services not on active duty.

(g) Based on 42 United States Code 1395cc(a)(1)(j) all providers participating in Medicare must also participate in TRICARE for inpatient hospital services provided pursuant to admissions to hospitals occurring on or after January 1, 1987; and

(h) If TRICARE benefits are to be paid in a participating status, the submitter of this claim agrees to submit this claim to the appropriate TRICARE claims processor. The provider of care submitter also agrees to accept the TRICARE determined reasonable charge as the total charge for the medical services or supplies listed on the claim form. The provider of care will accept the TRICARE-determined reasonable charge even if it is less than the billed amount, and also agrees to accept the amount paid by TRICARE combined with the cost-share amount and deductible amount, if any, paid by or on behalf of the patient as full payment for the listed medical services or supplies. The provider of care submitter will not attempt to collect from the patient (or his or her parent or guardian) amounts over the TRICARE determined reasonable charge. TRICARE will make any benefits payable directly to the provider of care, if the provider of care is a participating provider.

SEE http://www.nubc.org/ FOR MORE INFORMATION ON UB-04 DATA ELEMENT AND PRINTING SPECIFICATIONS

Medicare and Medicaid Services (CMS) aggregates the data from these claims forms for analyzing national health care reimbursement, clinical, and population trends. Having uniform data sets means that data can be compared not only within organizations but within states and across the country.

EXHIBIT 1.2. *Claim Form: CMS-1500*

1500
HEALTH INSURANCE CLAIM FORM
APPROVED BY NATIONAL UNIFORM CLAIM COMMITTEE 08/05

PICA · · · PICA

1. MEDICARE   MEDICAID   TRICARE CHAMPUS   CHAMPVA   GROUP HEALTH PLAN   FECA BLK LUNG   OTHER
   (Medicare #) (Medicaid #) (Sponsor's SSN) (Member ID#) (SSN or ID) (SSN) (ID)
1a. INSURED'S I.D. NUMBER   (For Program in Item 1)

2. PATIENT'S NAME (Last Name, First Name, Middle Initial)
3. PATIENT'S BIRTH DATE   MM DD YY   SEX M F
4. INSURED'S NAME (Last Name, First Name, Middle Initial)

5. PATIENT'S ADDRESS (No., Street)
6. PATIENT RELATIONSHIP TO INSURED   Self Spouse Child Other
7. INSURED'S ADDRESS (No., Street)

CITY   STATE
8. PATIENT STATUS   Single Married Other
CITY   STATE

ZIP CODE   TELEPHONE (Include Area Code) ( )
   Employed Full-Time Student Part-Time Student
ZIP CODE   TELEPHONE (Include Area Code) ( )

9. OTHER INSURED'S NAME (Last Name, First Name, Middle Initial)
10. IS PATIENT'S CONDITION RELATED TO:
11. INSURED'S POLICY GROUP OR FECA NUMBER

a. OTHER INSURED'S POLICY OR GROUP NUMBER
a. EMPLOYMENT? (Current or Previous)   YES NO
a. INSURED'S DATE OF BIRTH   MM DD YY   SEX M F

b. OTHER INSURED'S DATE OF BIRTH   MM DD YY   SEX M F
b. AUTO ACCIDENT?   YES NO   PLACE (State)
b. EMPLOYER'S NAME OR SCHOOL NAME

c. EMPLOYER'S NAME OR SCHOOL NAME
c. OTHER ACCIDENT?   YES NO
c. INSURANCE PLAN NAME OR PROGRAM NAME

d. INSURANCE PLAN NAME OR PROGRAM NAME
10d. RESERVED FOR LOCAL USE
d. IS THERE ANOTHER HEALTH BENEFIT PLAN?   YES NO   *If yes,* return to and complete item 9 a-d.

READ BACK OF FORM BEFORE COMPLETING & SIGNING THIS FORM.
12. PATIENT'S OR AUTHORIZED PERSON'S SIGNATURE I authorize the release of any medical or other information necessary to process this claim. I also request payment of government benefits either to myself or to the party who accepts assignment below.
SIGNED   DATE
13. INSURED'S OR AUTHORIZED PERSON'S SIGNATURE I authorize payment of medical benefits to the undersigned physician or supplier for services described below.
SIGNED

14. DATE OF CURRENT: MM DD YY   ILLNESS (First symptom) OR INJURY (Accident) OR PREGNANCY(LMP)
15. IF PATIENT HAS HAD SAME OR SIMILAR ILLNESS. GIVE FIRST DATE MM DD YY
16. DATES PATIENT UNABLE TO WORK IN CURRENT OCCUPATION   FROM MM DD YY   TO MM DD YY

17. NAME OF REFERRING PROVIDER OR OTHER SOURCE
17a.
17b. NPI
18. HOSPITALIZATION DATES RELATED TO CURRENT SERVICES   FROM MM DD YY   TO MM DD YY

19. RESERVED FOR LOCAL USE
20. OUTSIDE LAB?   YES NO $ CHARGES

21. DIAGNOSIS OR NATURE OF ILLNESS OR INJURY (Relate Items 1, 2, 3 or 4 to Item 24E by Line)
1. ___ 3. ___
2. ___ 4. ___
22. MEDICAID RESUBMISSION CODE   ORIGINAL REF. NO.

23. PRIOR AUTHORIZATION NUMBER

24. A. DATE(S) OF SERVICE   From MM DD YY   To MM DD YY | B. PLACE OF SERVICE | C. EMG | D. PROCEDURES, SERVICES, OR SUPPLIES (Explain Unusual Circumstances) CPT/HCPCS   MODIFIER | E. DIAGNOSIS POINTER | F. $ CHARGES | G. DAYS OR UNITS | H. EPSDT Family Plan | I. ID. QUAL. | J. RENDERING PROVIDER ID. #
1   NPI
2   NPI
3   NPI
4   NPI
5   NPI
6   NPI

25. FEDERAL TAX I.D. NUMBER   SSN EIN
26. PATIENT'S ACCOUNT NO.
27. ACCEPT ASSIGNMENT? (For govt. claims, see back)   YES NO
28. TOTAL CHARGE $
29. AMOUNT PAID $
30. BALANCE DUE $

31. SIGNATURE OF PHYSICIAN OR SUPPLIER INCLUDING DEGREES OR CREDENTIALS (I certify that the statements on the reverse apply to this bill and are made a part thereof.)
SIGNED   DATE
32. SERVICE FACILITY LOCATION INFORMATION
a. NPI   b.
33. BILLING PROVIDER INFO & PH # ( )
a. NPI   b.

NUCC Instruction Manual available at: www.nucc.org   **PLEASE PRINT OR TYPE**   APPROVED OMB-0938-0999 FORM CMS-1500 (08-05)

CARRIER

PATIENT AND INSURED INFORMATION

PHYSICIAN OR SUPPLIER INFORMATION

EXHIBIT 1.2. *(Continued)*

BECAUSE THIS FORM IS USED BY VARIOUS GOVERNMENT AND PRIVATE HEALTH PROGRAMS, SEE SEPARATE INSTRUCTIONS ISSUED BY APPLICABLE PROGRAMS.

NOTICE: Any person who knowingly files a statement of claim containing any misrepresentation or any false, incomplete or misleading information may be guilty of a criminal act punishable under law and may be subject to civil penalties.

REFERS TO GOVERNMENT PROGRAMS ONLY

MEDICARE AND CHAMPUS PAYMENTS: A patient's signature requests that payment be made and authorizes release of any information necessary to process the claim and certifies that the information provided in Blocks 1 through 12 is true, accurate and complete. In the case of a Medicare claim, the patient's signature authorizes any entity to release to Medicare medical and nonmedical information, including employment status, and whether the person has employer group health insurance, liability, no-fault, worker's compensation or other insurance which is responsible to pay for the services for which the Medicare claim is made. See 42 CFR 411.24(a). If item 9 is completed, the patient's signature authorizes release of the information to the health plan or agency shown. In Medicare assigned or CHAMPUS participation cases, the physician agrees to accept the charge determination of the Medicare carrier or CHAMPUS fiscal intermediary as the full charge, and the patient is responsible only for the deductible, coinsurance and noncovered services. Coinsurance and the deductible are based upon the charge determination of the Medicare carrier or CHAMPUS fiscal intermediary if this is less than the charge submitted. CHAMPUS is not a health insurance program but makes payment for health benefits provided through certain affiliations with the Uniformed Services. Information on the patient's sponsor should be provided in those items captioned in "Insured"; i.e., items 1a, 4, 6, 7, 9, and 11.

BLACK LUNG AND FECA CLAIMS

The provider agrees to accept the amount paid by the Government as payment in full. See Black Lung and FECA instructions regarding required procedure and diagnosis coding systems.

SIGNATURE OF PHYSICIAN OR SUPPLIER (MEDICARE, CHAMPUS, FECA AND BLACK LUNG)

I certify that the services shown on this form were medically indicated and necessary for the health of the patient and were personally furnished by me or were furnished incident to my professional service by my employee under my immediate personal supervision, except as otherwise expressly permitted by Medicare or CHAMPUS regulations.

For services to be considered as "incident" to a physician's professional service, 1) they must be rendered under the physician's immediate personal supervision by his/her employee, 2) they must be an integral, although incidental part of a covered physician's service, 3) they must be of kinds commonly furnished in physician's offices, and 4) the services of nonphysicians must be included on the physician's bills.

For CHAMPUS claims, I further certify that I (or any employee) who rendered services am not an active duty member of the Uniformed Services or a civilian employee of the United States Government or a contract employee of the United States Government, either civilian or military (refer to 5 USC 5536). For Black-Lung claims, I further certify that the services performed were for a Black Lung-related disorder.

No Part B Medicare benefits may be paid unless this form is received as required by existing law and regulations (42 CFR 424.32).

NOTICE: Any one who misrepresents or falsifies essential information to receive payment from Federal funds requested by this form may upon conviction be subject to fine and imprisonment under applicable Federal laws.

NOTICE TO PATIENT ABOUT THE COLLECTION AND USE OF MEDICARE, CHAMPUS, FECA, AND BLACK LUNG INFORMATION
(PRIVACY ACT STATEMENT)

We are authorized by CMS, CHAMPUS and OWCP to ask you for information needed in the administration of the Medicare, CHAMPUS, FECA, and Black Lung programs. Authority to collect information is in section 205(a), 1862, 1872 and 1874 of the Social Security Act as amended, 42 CFR 411.24(a) and 424.5(a) (6), and 44 USC 3101;41 CFR 101 et seq and 10 USC 1079 and 1086; 5 USC 8101 et seq; and 30 USC 901 et seq; 38 USC 613; E.O. 9397.

The information we obtain to complete claims under these programs is used to identify you and to determine your eligibility. It is also used to decide if the services and supplies you received are covered by these programs and to insure that proper payment is made.

The information may also be given to other providers of services, carriers, intermediaries, medical review boards, health plans, and other organizations or Federal agencies, for the effective administration of Federal provisions that require other third parties payers to pay primary to Federal program, and as otherwise necessary to administer these programs. For example, it may be necessary to disclose information about the benefits you have used to a hospital or doctor. Additional disclosures are made through routine uses for information contained in systems of records.

FOR MEDICARE CLAIMS: See the notice modifying system No. 09-70-0501, titled, 'Carrier Medicare Claims Record,' published in the Federal Register, Vol. 55 No. 177, page 37549, Wed. Sept 12, 1990, or as updated and republished.

FOR OWCP CLAIMS: Department of Labor, Privacy Act of 1974, "Republication of Notice of Systems of Records," Federal Register Vol. 55 No. 40. Wed Feb. 28, 1990. See ESA-5, ESA-6, ESA-12, ESA-13, ESA-30, or as updated and republished.

FOR CHAMPUS CLAIMS: PRINCIPLE PURPOSE(S): To evaluate eligibility for medical care provided by civilian sources and to issue payment upon establishment of eligibility and determination that the services/supplies received are authorized by law.

ROUTINE USE(S): Information from claims and related documents may be given to the Dept. of Veterans Affairs, the Dept. of Health and Human Services and/or the Dept. of Transportation consistent with their statutory administrative responsibilities under CHAMPUS/CHAMPVA; to the Dept. of Justice for representation of the Secretary of Defense in civil actions; to the Internal Revenue Service, private collection agencies, and consumer reporting agencies in connection with recoupment claims; and to Congressional Offices in response to inquiries made at the request of the person to whom a record pertains. Appropriate disclosures may be made to other federal, state, local, foreign government agencies, private business entities, and individual providers of care, on matters relating to entitlement, claims adjudication, fraud, program abuse, utilization review, quality assurance, peer review, program integrity, third-party liability, coordination of benefits, and civil and criminal litigation related to the operation of CHAMPUS.

DISCLOSURES: Voluntary; however, failure to provide information will result in delay in payment or may result in denial of claim. With the one exception discussed below, there are no penalties under these programs for refusing to supply information. However, failure to furnish information regarding the medical services rendered or the amount charged would prevent payment of claims under these programs. Failure to furnish any other information, such as name or claim number, would delay payment of the claim. Failure to provide medical information under FECA could be deemed an obstruction.

It is mandatory that you tell us if you know that another party is responsible for paying for your treatment. Section 1128B of the Social Security Act and 31 USC 3801-3812 provide penalties for withholding this information.

You should be aware that P.L. 100-503, the "Computer Matching and Privacy Protection Act of 1988", permits the government to verify information by way of computer matches.

MEDICAID PAYMENTS (PROVIDER CERTIFICATION)

I hereby agree to keep such records as are necessary to disclose fully the extent of services provided to individuals under the State's Title XIX plan and to furnish information regarding any payments claimed for providing such services as the State Agency or Dept. of Health and Human Services may request.

I further agree to accept, as payment in full, the amount paid by the Medicaid program for those claims submitted for payment under that program, with the exception of authorized deductible, coinsurance, co-payment or similar cost-sharing charge.

SIGNATURE OF PHYSICIAN (OR SUPPLIER): I certify that the services listed above were medically indicated and necessary to the health of this patient and were personally furnished by me or my employee under my personal direction.

NOTICE: This is to certify that the foregoing information is true, accurate and complete. I understand that payment and satisfaction of this claim will be from Federal and State funds, and that any false claims, statements, or documents, or concealment of a material fact, may be prosecuted under applicable Federal or State laws.

According to the Paperwork Reduction Act of 1995, no persons are required to respond to a collection of information unless it displays a valid OMB control number. The valid OMB control number for this information collection is 0938-0999. The time required to complete this information collection is estimated to average 10 minutes per response, including the time to review instructions, search existing data resources, gather the data needed, and complete and review the information collection. If you have any comments concerning the accuracy of the time estimate(s) or suggestions for improving this form, please write to: CMS, Attn. PRA Reports Clearance Officer, 7500 Security Boulevard, Baltimore, Maryland 21244-1850. This address is for comments and/or suggestions only. DO NOT MAIL COMPLETED CLAIM FORMS TO THIS ADDRESS.

Other Uniform Data Sets

Other uniform data sets have been developed for use in the United States. Three examples are the Uniform Hospital Discharge Data Set (UHDDS), the Uniform Ambulatory Care Data Set (ACDS), and the Minimum Data Set (MDS) used for long-term care. These data sets share two purposes:

1. To identify the data elements that should be collected for each patient, and

2. To provide uniform definitions for common terms and data elements [LaTour, 2002, p. 123].

The UHDDS is the oldest uniform data set used in the United States. The earliest version was developed in 1969 by the National Center for Health Statistics. In 1974, the federal government adopted the UHDDS definitions as the standard for the Medicare and Medicaid programs. The UHDDS has been revised several times. The current version includes the data elements listed in Exhibit 1.3.

The ACDS was approved by the National Committee on Vital and Health Statistics in 1989. The goal of the ACDS is to improve the data collected in ambulatory and outpatient settings. The ACDS has not, however, been incorporated into federal rules or regulations. It remains a recommended rather than a required data set.

The MDS for long-term care is a federally mandated standard assessment tool that is used to collect demographic and clinical information about long-term care facility residents. It is an extensive data set with detailed data elements in twenty major categories. The MDS provides a structured way to organize resident information so that an effective care plan can be developed (LaTour, 2002).

INTERNAL DATA AND INFORMATION: PATIENT SPECIFIC—COMBINING CLINICAL AND ADMINISTRATIVE

As we have discussed in earlier sections of this chapter, diagnostic and procedural information is captured during the patient encounter to track clinical progress and to document care for reimbursement and other administrative purposes. This diagnostic and procedural information is initially captured in narrative form through physicians' and other health care providers' documentation in the patient record. This documentation is subsequently translated into numerical codes. Coding facilitates the classification of

---

EXHIBIT 1.3. *UHDDS Elements and Definitions*

UHDDS elements as adopted in 1986 are:

1. **Personal identification:** the unique number assigned to each patient within a hospital that distinguishes the patient and his or her hospital record from all others in that institution.

2. **Sex:** male or female.

3. **Race:** White, Black, Asian or Pacific Islander, American Indian/Eskimo/Aleut, or other.

4. **Ethnicity:** Spanish origin/Hispanic, Non-Spanish origin/Non-Hispanic

5. **Residence:** zip code, code for foreign residence.

6. **Hospital identification**: a unique institutional number within a data collection system.

7–8. **Admission and discharge dates:** month, day, and year of both admission and discharge. An inpatient admission begins with the formal acceptance by a hospital of a patient who is to receive physician, dentist, or allied services while receiving room, board, and continuous nursing services. An inpatient discharge occurs with the termination of the room, board, and continuous nursing services, and the formal release of an inpatient by the hospital.

9–10. **Attending physician and operating physician:** each physician must have a unique identification number within the hospital. The attending physician and the operating physician (if applicable) are to be identified.

Attending physician: the clinician who is primarily and largely responsible for the care of the patient from the beginning of the hospital episode.

Operating physician: the clinician who performed the principal procedure (see item 12 for definition of a principal procedure).

11. **Diagnoses:** all diagnoses that affect the current hospital stay.

Principal diagnosis is designated and defined as the condition established after study to be chiefly responsible for occasioning the admission of the patient to the hospital for care. **Other diagnoses** are designated and defined as all conditions that coexist at the time of admission, that develop subsequently, or that affect the treatment received or length of stay. Diagnoses that relate to an earlier episode that have no bearing on the current hospital stay are to be excluded.

12. **Procedure and date:** all significant procedures are to be reported. A significant procedure is one that is surgical in nature, or carries a procedural risk, or carries an anesthetic risk, or requires specialized training. For significant procedures, the identity (by unique number within the hospital) of the person performing the procedure and the data must be reported. When more than one procedure is reported, the principal procedure is to be designated. In determining which of several procedures is principal, the following criteria apply:

> The principal procedure is one that was performed for **definitive treatment** rather than one performed for diagnostic or exploratory purposes, or was necessary to take care of a complication. If there appear to be two procedures that are principal, then the one most related to the principal diagnosis should be selected as the principal procedure. For reporting purposes, the following definition should be used: surgery includes incision, excision, amputation, introduction, endoscopy, repair, destruction, suture, and manipulation.
>
> 13. **Disposition of patient:** discharged to home (routine discharge); left against medical advice; discharged to another short-term hospital; discharged to a long-term institution; died, or other.
>
> 14. **Expected payer** for most of this bill (anticipated financial guarantor for services): this refers to the single major source that the patient expects will pay for his or her bill, such as Blue Cross, other insurance companies, Medicare, Medicaid, Workers' Compensation, other government payers, self-pay, no-charge (free, charity, special research, or teaching), or other.

Source: Dougherty, 2001, p. 72.

diagnoses and procedures not only for reimbursement purposes but also for clinical research and comparative studies.

Two major coding systems are employed by health care providers today:

- ICD-9-CM (International Classification of Diseases, Ninth Revision, Clinical Modification—modified for use in the United States), published by the National Center for Health Statistics

- CPT (Current Procedural Terminology), published by the American Medical Association

Use of these systems is required by the federal government for reimbursement, and they are recognized by health care agencies both nationally and internationally.

ICD-9-CM

The ICD-9-CM classification system is derived from the International Classification of Diseases, Ninth Revision, which was developed by the World Health Organization to capture disease data. ICD-9-CM is used in the United States to code not only disease information but also procedure information. An update to the ICD-9-CM is published each year. This publication is considered a federal government document whose contents may be used freely by others. However, multiple companies republish this government document in easier-to-use, annotated, formally copyrighted versions. The precursors to the current ICD system were developed to allow morbidity (illness) and mortality (death) statistics to be compared across nations. ICD-9-CM coding, however, has come to play a major role in reimbursement to hospitals. Since 1983, it has been used for determining

---

EXHIBIT 1.4. *Excerpt from the ICD-9-CM Disease Index*

ARTHROPATHIES AND RELATED DISORDERS (710-719)
Excludes: disorders of spine (720.0-724.9)

710	Diffuse diseases of connective tissue

Includes: all collagen diseases whose effects are not mainly confined to a single system
Excludes: those affecting mainly the cardiovascular system, i.e., polyarteritis nodosa and allied
conditions (446.0-446.7)
   710.0   Systemic lupus erythematosus
           Disseminated lupus erythematosus
           Libman-Sacks disease
Use additional code to identify manifestation, as:
           endocarditis (424.91)
           nephritis (583.81)
           chronic (582.81)
           nephrotic syndrome (581.81)
Excludes: lupus erythematosus (discoid) NOS (695.4)
   710.1   Systemic sclerosis
           Acrosclerosis
           CRST syndrome
           Progressive systemic sclerosis
           Scleroderma
Use additional code to identify manifestation, as:
           lung involvement (517.2)
           myopathy (359.6)
Excludes: circumscribed scleroderma (701.0)
   710.2   Sicca syndrome
           Keratoconjunctivitis sicca
           Sjögren's disease
   710.3   Dermatomyositis
           Poikilodermatomyositis
           Polymyositis with skin involvement
   710.4   Polymyositis
   710.5   Eosinophilia myalgia syndrome
           Toxic oil syndrome
Use additional E to identify drug, if drug induced
   710.8   Other specified diffuse diseases of connective tissue
           Multifocal fibrosclerosis (idiopathic) NEC
           Systemic fibrosclerosing syndrome
   710.9   Unspecified diffuse connective tissue disease
           Collagen disease NOS

Source: National Center for Health Statistics, 2004.

the *diagnosis related group* (*DRG*) into which a patient is assigned. DRGs are the basis for determining appropriate inpatient reimbursements for Medicare, Medicaid, and many other health care insurance beneficiaries. Accurate ICD-9-CM coding has as a consequence become vital to accurate institutional reimbursement. Exhibit 1.4 is an excerpt from the ICD-9-CM classification system. It shows the system in its text form, but large health care organizations generally use encoders, computer applications that facilitate accurate coding. Whether a book or text file or encoder is used, the classification system is the same.

It should be noted that a tenth revision of the ICD has been published by the World Health Organization and is widely used in countries other than the United States. The U.S. government has published draft modifications of ICD-10, but these have not yet been finalized and adopted for use in this country. The original adoption date for ICD-10-CM was to be late 2001, but as of this writing it has not been released. The conversion from ICD-9-CM to ICD-10-CM will be a tremendous undertaking for health care organizations. ICD-10 includes substantial increases in content and many structural changes. When the U.S. modification is released, all health care providers will need to adjust their systems to handle the conversion from ICD-9-CM to ICD-10-CM.

CPT

The American Medical Association (AMA) publishes an updated Current Procedural Terminology each year. Unlike ICD-9-CM, CPT is copyrighted, with all rights to publication and distribution held by the AMA. CPT was first developed and published in 1966. The stated purpose for developing CPT was to provide a uniform language for describing medical and surgical services. In 1983, however, the government adopted CPT, in its entirety, as the major component (known as Level 1) of the Healthcare Common Procedure Coding System (HCPCS). Since then CPT has become the standard for physician's office, outpatient, and ambulatory care coding for reimbursement purposes. Exhibit 1.5 is a patient encounter form with examples of HCPCS/CPT codes.

Coding Standards

As coding has become intimately linked to reimbursement, directly determining the amount of money a health care organization can receive for a claim from insurers, the government has increased its scrutiny of coding practices. There are official guidelines for accurate coding, and health care facilities that do not adhere to these guidelines are liable to charges of fraudulent coding practices. In addition the Office of Inspector General of the Department of Health and Human Services (HHS OIG) publishes compliance guidelines to facilitate health care organizations' adherence to ethical and legal coding practices. The OIG is responsible for (among other duties) investigating fraud involving government health insurance programs. More specific information about compliance guidelines can be found on the OIG Web site (www.oig.hhs.gov) (HHS OIG, 2004).

INTERNAL DATA AND INFORMATION: AGGREGATE—CLINICAL

In the previous section we examined different sets of clinical and administrative data that are collected during or in the time closely surrounding the patient encounter. Patient records, uniform billing information, and discharge data sets are the main sources of the data that go into the literally hundreds of aggregate reports or queries that are developed and used by providers and executives in health care organizations. Think of these source data as one or more data repositories, with each data element available to health care providers and executives. What can these data tell you about the organization and the

EXHIBIT 1.5. *Patient Encounter Form*

Pediatric Associates P.A. 123 Children's Avenue Anytown, USA

Office Visits

99211 Estab Pt—minimal
99212 Estab Pt—focused
99213 Estab Pt—expanded
99214 Estab Pt—detailed
99215 Estab Pt—high complexity

99201 New Pt—problem focused
99202 New Pt—expanded
99203 New Pt—detailed
99204 New Pt—moderate complexity
99205 New Pt—high complexity

99050 After Hours
99052 After Hours—after 10 pm
99054 After Hours—Sundays and Holidays

Outpatient Consult
99241 99242 99243 99244 99245

Preventive Medicine—New
99381 Prev Med 0–1 years
99382 Prev Med 1–4 years
99383 Prev Med 5–11 years
99384 Prev Med 12–17 years
99385 Prev Med 18–39 years

Preventive Medicine—Established
99391 Prev Med 0–1 years
99392 Prev Med 1–4 years
99393 Prev Med 5–11 years
99394 Prev Med 12–17 years
99395 Prev Med 18–39 years

99070 10 Arm Sling
99070 11 Sterile Dressing
99070 45 Cervical Cap

Immunizations, Injections, and Office Laboratory Services

90471 Adm of Vaccine 1
90472 Adm of Vaccine >1
90648 HIB
90658 Influenza
90669 Prevnar
90701 DTP
90702 DT
90707 MMR
90713 Polio Injection
90720 DTP/HIB
90700 DTaP
90730 Hepatitis A
90733 Meningococcal
90744 Hepatitis B 0–11
90746 Hepatitis B 18+ years

81000 Urinalysis w/ micro
81002 Urinalysis w/o micro
82270 Hemoccult Stool
82948 Dextrostix
83655 Lead Level
84030 PKU
85018 Hemoglobin
87086 Urine Culture
87081 Throat Culture
87205 Gram Stain
87208 Ova Smear (pin worm)
87210 Wet Prep
87880 Rapid Strep

Diagnosis

Patient Name
No.
Date
Time
Address
DOB
Name of Insured   ID
Insurance Company
Return Appointment _____

care provided to patients? How can you process these data into meaningful information? The number of aggregate reports that could be developed from patient records or patient accounting information is practically limitless, but there are some common categories of clinical, administrative, and combined reports that the health care executive will likely encounter. We will discuss a few of these in this and the following sections.

On the clinical side, disease indexes and specialized registers are often used.

Disease and Procedure Indexes

Health care organization management often wants to know summary information about a particular disease or treatment. Examples of questions that might be asked are: What is the most common diagnosis in the facility? What percentage of diabetes patients are African American? What is the most common procedure performed on patients admitted with gastritis (or heart attack or any other diagnosis)? Traditionally, such questions have been answered by looking in disease and procedure indexes. Prior to the widespread use of databases and computers, disease and procedure indexes were large card catalogues or books that kept track of the numbers of diseases treated and procedures occurring in a facility by disease and procedure ICD codes. Now that databases and computers are common, the disease and procedure index function is generally handled as a component of the patient medical record system or the registration and discharge system. The retrieval of information related to diseases and procedures is still based on ICD-9-CM and CPT codes, but the queries are limitless. Users can search the disease and procedure

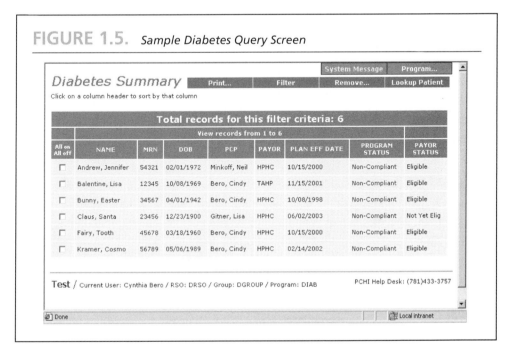

FIGURE 1.5. *Sample Diabetes Query Screen*

Source: Partners HealthCare

database for general frequency statistics for any number of combinations of data. Figure 1.5 is an example of a screen resulting from a query for a list of diabetes patients.

Specialized Registers

Another type of aggregate information that has benefited tremendously from the use of computerized databases is the specialized register. Registers are lists that generally contain the names, and sometimes other identifying information, of patients seen in a particular area of the health care facility. A health facility might want an accounting of patients seen in the emergency department or operating room, for example. In general a register allows data retrieval in a particular area of the organization. With the increased availability of large databases, many of these registers can be created on an ad hoc basis.

Trauma and tumor registries are specialized registries that often involve data collection beyond that done for the patient medical record and patient billing process. These registries may be found in facilities with high-level trauma or cancer centers. They are used to track information about patients over time and to collect detailed information for research purposes.

Many other types of aggregate clinical reports are used by health care providers and executives. The easy-to-use, ad hoc reporting that is available with databases today gives providers and executives access to any number of summary reports based on the data elements collected during the patient encounter.

INTERNAL DATA AND INFORMATION: AGGREGATE—ADMINISTRATIVE

Just as with clinical aggregate reports, a limitless number of reports can be created for administrative functions from today's databases and data repositories. Commonly used administrative aggregate reports include basic health care statistical reports, claims denial reports, and cost reports. (In keeping with our focus on information unique to health care we will not discuss traditional income statements, cash flow statements, or other general accounting reports.) Two basic types are described in this section: Medicare cost reports and basic health care statistical reports.

Medicare Cost Reports

Exhibit 1.6 is a portion of a Medicare cost report for a skilled nursing facility (CMS-2552-96). Medicare cost reports are filed annually by all hospitals, home health agencies, skilled nursing facilities, and hospices that accept Medicare or Medicaid. These reports must be filed within a specified time after the end of the fiscal year and are subject to scrutiny via compliance audits. The cost report contains such provider information as facility characteristics, utilization data, costs and charges by cost center (in total and for Medicare), Medicare settlement data, and financial statement data. Preparation instructions and the actual forms can be found on the CMS Web site (www.cms.gov). Medicare cost reports are used by CMS not only to determine portions of an individual facility's reimbursement but also to determine Medicare rate adjustments, cost limits, and various wage indexes.

EXHIBIT 1.6. *Section of a Medicare Cost Report for a Skilled Nursing Facility*

3690 (Cont.)	CMS FORM-2552-96				06-03
COMPUTATION OF INPATIENT OPERATING COST		PROVIDER NO.:	COMPONENT NO.:	PERIOD: FROM _____ TO	WORKSHEET D-1, PARTS III & IV

Check applicable boxes	[ ] Title V - I/P [ ] Title XVIII, Part A [ ] Title XIX - I/P	[ ] Hospital [ ] NF [ ] Subprovider [ ] ICF/MR [ ] SNF	[ ] PPS [ ] TEFRA [ ] Other

PART III - SKILLED NURSING FACILITY, OTHER NURSING FACILITY, AND ICF/MR ONLY

66	Skilled nursing facility/other nursing facility/ICF/MR routine service cost (line 37)		66
67	Adjusted general inpatient routine service cost per diem (line 66 ÷ line 2)		67
68	Program routine service cost (line 9 x line 67)		68
69	Medically necessary private room cost applicable to Program (line 14 x line 35)		69
70	Total Program general inpatient routine service costs (line 68 + line 69)		70
71	Capital-related cost allocated to inpatient routine service costs (from Worksheet B, sum of Parts II and III, column 27)		71
72	Per diem capital-related costs (line 71 ÷ line 2)		72
73	Program capital-related costs (line 9 x line 72)		73
74	Inpatient routine service cost (line 70 minus line 73)		74
75	Aggregate charges to beneficiaries for excess costs (from provider records)		75
76	Total Program routine service costs for comparison to the cost limitation (line 74 minus line 75)		76
77	Inpatient routine service cost per diem limitation		77
78	Inpatient routine service cost limitation (line 9 x line 77)		78
79	Reasonable inpatient routine service costs (see instructions)		79
80	Program inpatient ancillary services (see instructions)		80
81	Utilization review - physician compensation		81
82	Total Program inpatient operating costs (sum of lines 79 through 81)		82

PART IV - COMPUTATION OF OBSERVATION BED PASS THROUGH COST

83	Total observation bed days (see instructions)		83
84	Adjusted general inpatient routine cost per diem (line 27 ÷ line 2)		84
85	Observation bed cost (line 83 x line 84) (see instructions)		85

COMPUTATION OF OBSERVATION BED PASS THROUGH COST

		Cost 1	Routine Cost (from line 27) 2	col. 1 + col. 2 3	Total Observation Bed Cost (from line 85) 4	Observation Bed Pass Through Cost (col. 3 x col. 4) (see instructions) 5	
86	Old capital-related cost						86
87	New capital-related cost						87
88	Non Physician Anesthetist						88
89	Medical Education						89

FORM CMS-2552-96 (11/98) (INSTRUCTIONS FOR THIS WORKSHEET ARE PUBLISHED IN CMS PUB. 15-II, SECTIONS 3622.3-3622.4)

Health Care Statistics

The categories of statistics that are routinely gathered for health care executives or others include

■ *Census statistics.* These data reveal the number of patients present at any one time in a facility. Several commonly computed rates are based on this census data, including the average daily census and bed occupancy rates.

■ *Discharge statistics.* This group of statistics is calculated from data accumulated when patients are discharged. Some commonly computed rates based on discharge statistics are average length of stay, death rates, autopsy rates, infection rates, and consultation rates.

General health care statistics are frequently used to describe the characteristics of the patients within an organization. They may also provide a basis for planning and monitoring patient services.

INTERNAL DATA AND INFORMATION: AGGREGATE—COMBINING CLINICAL AND ADMINISTRATIVE

Health care executives are often interested in aggregate reports that combine clinical and administrative data. Ad hoc statistical reports and trend analyses may draw from both clinical and administrative data sources, for example. These reports may be used for the purpose of improving customer service, quality of patient care, or overall operational efficiency. Examples of aggregate data that relate to customer service are the average time it takes to get an appointment at a clinic and the average referral volume by physician. Quality of care aggregate data take many forms, revealing such things as infection rates and unplanned returns to the operating room. Cost per case, average reimbursement by DRG, and staffing levels by patient acuity are examples of aggregate data that could be used to improve efficiency. These examples represent only a few uses for combined aggregate data. Again, with today's computerized clinical and administrative databases, any number of ad hoc queries, statistical reports, and trend analyses should be readily available to health care executives. Health care executives need to know what source data are collected and must be able to trust in data accuracy. Executives should be creative in designing aggregate reports to meet their decision-making needs.

EXTERNAL DATA AND INFORMATION: COMPARATIVE

Comparative data and information, gathered internally and externally, are used for both clinical and administrative purposes by health care organizations.

Outcome Measures and Balanced Scorecards

Comparative data and information are often aligned with organizations' quality improvement efforts. For example, an organization might collect data on specific outcome measures and then use this information in a benchmarking process. *Outcome measures* are the measurable results of a process. This could be a clinical process, such as a particular treatment, or an administrative process, such as a claim filing. Outcome measures can be applied to individuals or groups. An example of a simple clinical outcome measure is the percentage of similar lab results that occur within a month for a particular medical group. An example of an administrative outcome measure is the percentage of claims denied by Medicare during one month. Implicit in the idea of measuring outcomes is that they can be usefully compared over time or against a set standard. The process of comparing one or more outcome measures against a standard is called *benchmarking*. Outcome measures and benchmarking may be limited to internally set standards; however, frequently they are involved in comparisons with externally generated benchmarks or standards.

Balanced scorecards are another method for measuring performance in health care organizations. The concept of the balanced scorecard meets executives' need to design measurement systems aligned with their organization's strategy goals (Kelly, 2007). Balanced scorecard systems examine multiple measures, rather than the single set of measures common in traditional benchmarking. Suppose a health care organization uses "lowest-cost service in the region" as an outcome measure for benchmarking its performance against that of like facilities in the region. The organization does very well over time on this measure. However, you can see that it may be ignoring some other important performance indicators. What about patient satisfaction? Employee morale? Patient health outcomes? Balanced scorecards employ multiple measures along several dimensions to ensure that the organization is performing well across the board. The *clinical value compass* is a similar method for measuring clinical process across multiple dimensions (Kelly, 2007).

Comparative Health Care Data Sets

Organizations may select from many publicly and privately available health care data sets for benchmarking. A few of the more commonly accessed data sets are listed in Exhibit 1.7 (along with Web site addresses). These data sets are divided into five categories: patient satisfaction, practice patterns, health plans, clinical indicators, and population measures. Many of the listed Web sites provide examples of the data sets, along with detailed information about their origins and potential uses.

Patient Satisfaction   Patient satisfaction data generally come from survey data. The three organizations listed in Exhibit 1.7, NRC+Picker, Press Ganey, and the health care division of Gallup, provide extensive consulting services to health care organizations across the country. One of these services is to conduct patient satisfaction surveys. There are other organizations that provide similar services, and some health care organizations undertake patient satisfaction surveys on their own. The advantage of using a national organization is the comparative database it offers, which organizations can use for benchmarking purposes.

Practice Patterns   The Commonwealth Fund Quality Chartbook series and the Dartmouth Atlas of Health Care allow health care organizations to view practice patterns across the United States. The Dartmouth Atlas provides an online interactive tool that allows organizations to customize comparative reports based primarily on Medicare data (Figure 1.6).

Health Plans   The mission of the National Committee for Quality Assurance (NCQA) is "to improve the quality of health care." NCQA's efforts are organized around two major activities, accreditation and performance measurement. (We will discuss the accreditation activity in Chapter Three.) To facilitate these activities NCQA developed the Health Plan Employer Data and Information Set (HEDIS) in the late 1980s. HEDIS currently consists of seventy-one measures across eight domains of

---

EXHIBIT 1.7. *Sources of Comparative Data for Health Care Managers*

Patient Satisfaction

NRC+Picker (National Research Corporation and the Picker Institute): nrcpicker.com

Press Gainey Associates: www. pressganey.com

The Gallup Organization: healthcare.gallup.com

Practice Patterns

Leatherman, S., and D. McCarthy. 2002. Quality of Healthcare in the United States: A Chartbook. New York: The Commonwealth Fund. http://www.commonwealthfund.org/publications/publications_show.htm?doc_id=221238

The Center for the Evaluative Clinical Sciences, Dartmouth Medical School. 2008. The Dartmouth Atlas of Healthcare. Chicago: The American Hospital Publishing Company. www.dartmouthatlas.org.

Health Plans

National Committee for Quality: www.ncqa.org

Clinical Indicators

Joint Commission on Accreditation of Healthcare Organizations

- Quality Check: www. qualitycheck.org

Centers for Medicare and Medicaid Services Medicare Clinical Indicators

- Hospital Compare: www.hospitalcompare.hhs.gov

- Nursing Home Compare: http://www.medicare.gov/NHCompare/

- Home Health Compare: http://www.medicare.gov/HHCompare/

- Physician Focused Quality Initiative: http://www.cms.hhs.gov/pqri/

Population Measures

State and Local Health Departments

Centers for Disease Control and Prevention, National Center of Health Statistics: www.cdc.gov/nchs

AHRQ—Health Care Innovations Exchange (including Quality and Disparities Reports): http://www.innovations.ahrq.gov

Source: Used with permission from *Applying Quality Management in Healthcare*, 2nd Edition, by Diane Kelly (Chicago: Health Administration Press, 2007), p. 185.

care and is used by more than 90 percent of America's health plans. A few of the health issues measured by HEDIS are (NCQA, 2008d)

- Asthma medication use
- Persistence of beta-blocker treatment after a heart attack
- Controlling high blood pressure
- Comprehensive diabetes care

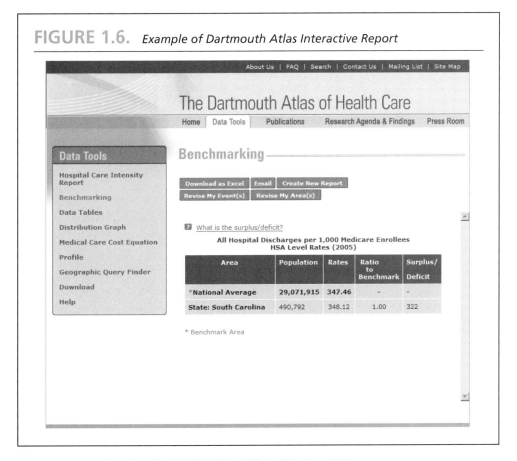

FIGURE 1.6. *Example of Dartmouth Atlas Interactive Report*

Source: Dartmouth Institute for Health Policy & Clinical Practice, 2008.

- Breast cancer screening
- Antidepressant medication management
- Childhood and adolescent immunization status
- Advising smokers to quit

The NCQA Web site offers an interactive tool for obtaining *report cards* on specific health plans that have undergone NCQA accreditation. Multiple health plans can be compared to each other and against national averages. The comparison of two South Carolina health plans in Figure 1.7 is an example of an NCQA report card.

Clinical Indicators   Both The Joint Commission and CMS are committed to the improvement of clinical outcomes. The Joint Commission's Quality Check has evolved since its introduction in 1994 to become a comprehensive guide to health care organizations in the United States. Visitors to www.qualitycheck.org can search for health care organizations by a variety of parameters, identify accreditation status, and download hospital performance measures. In addition the Joint Commission-accredited organizations

FIGURE 1.7. *Example of NCQA Report Card*

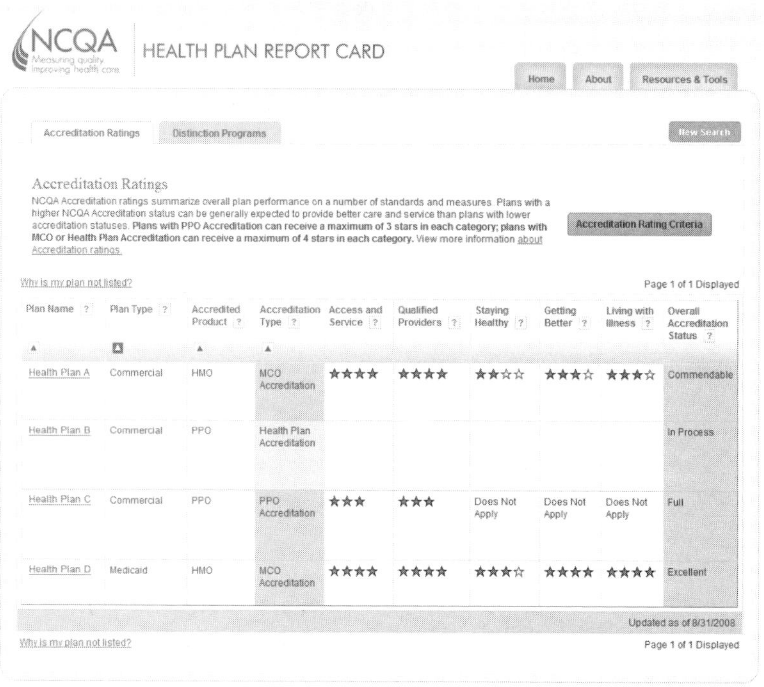

Source: NCQA, 2008c.

can get a summary of their performance measured in terms of the Joint Commission's National Patient Safety Goals and Quality Improvement Goals (The Joint Commission, 2008a).

The CMS quality programs are aimed at hospitals, nursing homes, home care, and physicians' practices. The Hospital Compare Web site (www.hospitalcompare.hhs.gov) and interactive comparison tool was developed in collaboration with other public and private organizational members of the Hospital Quality Alliance. Comparison reports for hospitals can be created based on location and on specific medical conditions or surgical procedures. The resulting reports provide information on process of care measures, outcome of care measures, surveys of patient experiences, and medical payment information (HHS, 2008c).

Population Measures   Other comparative data sources that could be useful for the health care manager are those that provide population measures. Most state health departments collect statewide morbidity and mortality data. These data generally come from a variety of sources, including hospital and provider bills. At the national level both the Centers for Disease Control and Prevention (CDC) and the Agency for Healthcare Research and Quality (AHRQ) provide a wealth of population-based health care data.

EXTERNAL DATA AND INFORMATION: EXPERT OR KNOWLEDGE BASED

The Joint Commission (2004) defines knowledge-based information as, "A collection of stored facts, models, and information that can be used for designing and redesigning processes and for problem solving. In the context of the [The Joint Commission accreditation] manual, knowledge-based information is found in the clinical, scientific, and management literature." Health care executives and health care providers rely on knowledge-based information to maintain their professional competence and to discover the latest techniques and procedures. The content of any professional journal falls into the category of knowledge-based information. Other providers of knowledge-based information are the many online health care and health care management references and resources. With the development of rule-based computer systems, the Internet, and push technologies, health care executives and providers are finding that they often have access to vast quantities of expert or knowledge-based information at the time they need it, even at the patient bedside. Most clinical and administrative professional organizations not only publish print journals but also maintain up-to-date Web sites where members or other subscribers can get knowledge-based information. Several organizations also provide daily, weekly, or other periodic e-mail notifications of important events that are pushed onto subscribers' personal computers.

Knowledge-based information can also be incorporated into electronic medical records or health care organization Web sites. Figure 1.8 is a sample of the knowledge-based information resources available through an electronic medical record interface.

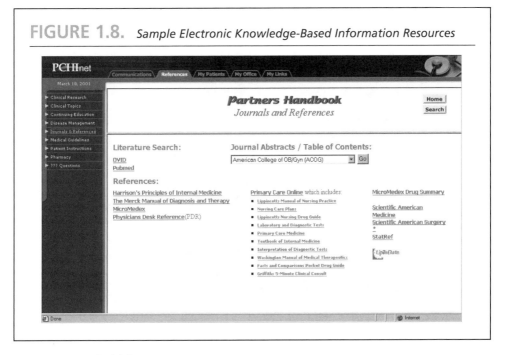

FIGURE 1.8.   *Sample Electronic Knowledge-Based Information Resources*

Source: Partners HealthCare

SUMMARY

Without health care data and information there would be no need for health care information systems. Health care information is a valuable asset in health care organizations, and it must be managed like other assets. To manage information effectively, health care executives should have an understanding of the sources and uses of health care data and information. In this chapter we introduced a framework for discussing types of health care information, looked at a wide range of internal data and information whose creation and use must be managed in health care organizations, and also discussed a few associated processes that are typically part of patient encounters. We examined not only patient-specific (individual) internal information but also aggregate information. We addressed both clinical and administrative data and information in our discussions. In addition we examined several types of external data and information that are available for use by health care organizations, including comparative and knowledge-based data and information. Throughout, our view of data and information was organizational and the focus was on that information that is unique to health care.

KEY TERMS

Aggregate data and information
American Health Information
   Management Association (AHIMA)
American Hospital Association
American Medical Association (AMA)
Balanced scorecards
Benchmarking
Centers for Disease Control and
   Prevention (CDC)
Centers for Medicare and Medicaid
CMS-1500
Comparative data and information
Current Procedural Terminology (CPT)
Electronic health record
Electronic medical record
External data and information
Health care information
Health information
Health Insurance Portability and
   Accountability Act (HIPAA)
Health Plan Employer Data and
   Information Set (HEDIS)

Internal data and information
International Classification of Diseases,
   Clinical Modification, 9th edition
   (ICD-9-CM)
The Joint Commission
Knowledge-based data and information
Minimum Data Set (MDS)
National Provider Identifier (NPI)
Office of the Inspector General (OIG)
Outcomes measures
Patient records
Patient-specific data and information
Personal health record
Protected health information
Quality Check
UB-04
Uniform Ambulatory Care Data Set
   (ACDS)
Uniform Bill
Uniform Hospital Discharge Data Set
   (UHDDS)

LEARNING ACTIVITIES

1.   Contact a health care facility (hospital, nursing home, physician's office, or other organization) to ask permission to view a sample of the health records they maintain. These records may be in paper or electronic form. Answer the following questions for each record:

   a.   What is the primary reason (or condition) for which the patient was admitted to the hospital?

   b.   How long has the patient had this condition?

   c.   Did the patient have surgery during this admission? If so, what procedure(s) was (were) done?

   d.   Did the patient experience any complications during this admission? If so, what were they?

   e.   How does the physician's initial assessment of the patient compare with the nurse's initial assessment? Where in the record would you find this information?

   f.   To where was the patient discharged?

   g.   What were the patient's discharge orders or instructions? Where in the record should you find this information?

2.   Make an appointment to meet with the business manager at a physician's office or health care clinic. Discuss the importance of ICD-9-CM coding or CPT coding (or both) for that office. Ask to view the books or encoders that the office uses to assign diagnostic and procedure codes. After the visit, write a brief summary of your findings and impressions.

3.   Visit www.oig.hhs.gov. What are the major responsibilities of the Office of Inspector General as they relate to coded health care data? What other responsibilities related to health care fraud and abuse does this office have?

4.   List and briefly describe several types of aggregate health care reports that you believe would be commonly used by health care executives in a hospital or other health care setting.

5.   Using the Internet sites identified in this chapter or found during your own searches, find a report card for one or more local hospitals. If you were trying to make a decision about which hospital to use for health care for yourself or for a family member, would you find this information useful? Why or why not?

CHAPTER

2

HEALTH CARE DATA QUALITY

LEARNING OBJECTIVES

- To be able to discuss the relationship between health care data and health care information.
- To be able to identify problems associated with poor quality health care data.
- To be able to define the characteristics of data quality.
- To be able to discuss the challenges associated with measuring and ensuring health care data quality.

Chapter One provided an overview of the various types of health care data and information that are generated and used by health care organizations. We established the importance of understanding health care data and information in order to reach the goal of having effective health care information systems. There is another fundamental aspect of health care data and information that is central to developing effective health care information systems—data quality. Consider for a moment an organization with sophisticated health care information systems that affect every type of health care information, from patient specific to knowledge based. What if the quality of the documentation going into the systems is poor? What if there is no assurance that the reports generated from the systems are accurate or timely? How would the users of the systems react? Are those information systems beneficial or detrimental to the organization in achieving its goals?

In this chapter we will examine several aspects of data quality. We begin by distinguishing between health care data and health care information. We then look at some problems associated with poor-quality health care data, both at an organizational level and across organizations. The discussion continues with a presentation of two sets of guidelines that can be used in evaluating data quality and ends with an examination of the major types of health care data errors.

DATA VERSUS INFORMATION

What is the difference between data and information? The simple answer is that *information* is *processed data*. Therefore we can say that *health care information* is *processed health care data*. (We interpret *processing* broadly to cover everything from formal analysis to explanations supplied by the individual decision maker's brain.) Health care data are raw health care facts, generally stored as characters, words, symbols, measurements, or statistics. One thing apparent about health care data is that they are generally not very useful for decision making. Health care data may describe a particular event, but alone and unprocessed they are not particularly helpful. Take for example this figure: 79 percent. By itself, what does it mean? If we process this datum further by indicating that it represents the average bed occupancy for a hospital for the month of January, it takes on more meaning. With the additional facts attached, is this figure now information? That depends. If all a health care executive wants or needs to know is the bed occupancy rate for January, this could be considered information. However, for the hospital executive who is interested in knowing the trend of the bed occupancy rate over time or how the facility's bed occupancy rate compares to that of other, similar facilities, this is not yet information.

Knowledge is seen by some as the highest level in a hierarchy with data at the bottom and information in the middle (Figure 2.1). *Knowledge* is defined by Johns (1997) as "a combination of rules, relationships, ideas, and experience." Another way of thinking about knowledge is that it is information applied to rules, experiences, and relationships, with the result that it can be used for decision making. A journal article that describes the use of bed occupancy rates in decision making or one health care facility's experience with improving its occupancy rates might be an example of knowledge.

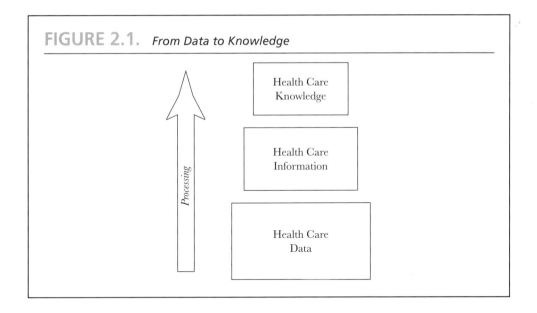

FIGURE 2.1. *From Data to Knowledge*

Where do health care data end and where does health care information begin? Information is an *extremely* valuable asset at *all* levels of the health care organization. Health care executives, clinical staff, and others rely on information to get their jobs accomplished. An interesting point to think about is that the same data may provide different information to different users. One person's data may be another person's information. Think back to our bed occupancy example. The health care executive needing verification of the rate for January has found her information. The health care executive needing trend analysis that includes this rate has not. In the second case the rate for January is data needing to be processed further. The goal of this discussion is not to pinpoint where data end and information begins but rather to further an understanding of the relationship between health care data and information—health care data are the beginnings of health care information. You cannot create information without data (Lee, 2002).

PROBLEMS WITH POOR-QUALITY DATA

Now that we have established the relationship between health care data and health care information, we can look at some of the problems associated with having poor-quality data. Health care data are the source of health care information, so it stands to reason that a health care organization cannot have high-quality health care information without first establishing that it has high-quality health care data. Data quality must be established at the most *granular* level. Much health care information is gathered through patient care documentation by clinical providers and administrative staff. As was discussed in Chapter One, the patient record is the source for most of the clinical information generated by the health care organization. This clinical information is in turn coded for purposes of reimbursement and research. We also saw that medical record information is shared across many providers and payers, aggregated, and used to make comparisons relevant to health care and related issues.

Poor-quality data collection and reporting can affect each of the purposes for which we maintain patient records. At the organizational level a health care organization may find diminished quality in patient care, poor communication among providers and patients, problems with documentation, reduced revenue generation due to problems with reimbursement, and a diminished capacity to effectively evaluate outcomes or participate in research activities. Sharon Schott (2003) has summarized some of the common problems associated with poor-quality medical record documentation (see the following Perspective). She focuses on the medical record used as evidence in court, but the same problems can lead to poor quality of care, poor communication, and poor documentation. As we will see in later chapters, some of the problems presented may actually be reduced with the implementation of effective information technology (IT) solutions.

PERSPECTIVE

DOCUMENTATION

In pointing out the serious consequences of documentation problems when records (especially paper-based records) are called into evidence in court cases, Sharon Schott cites several specific examples, including these three:

> Simple things such as misspelled names of common drugs or procedures can have a major effect on jurors' impression of the competency of the clinician documenting in the record. In one recent case, a nurse administered 5,000 units of Heparin when the order was for 2,500 units. The patient became critically ill as a result. When the documentation was reviewed, it was discovered that the nurse committing the error had misspelled Heparin as "Hepirin." This spelling error was presented to the jury as an additional demonstration of incompetence. The plaintiff's attorney argued that Heparin is a commonly used drug and obviously this nurse had no knowledge of it, because she couldn't spell it correctly. Juries will also doubt the competence of a nurse who writes "The wound on the left heal is healed."

> The nurse who documented an assessment with a post date was called as a witness. She was asked to explain how she could perform an assessment two days after the patient died. The nurse explained that Friday was the actual due date for the assessment but because she had some extra time on Tuesday, she decided to do it early and put Friday's date on it to be compliant with the due date. The plaintiff's attorney then asked, "Is that the

only place in the chart that you lied?" Then the jury was suspicious of the integrity of the entire medical record and the nurse.

The continuity of the record also needs special scrutiny on a regular basis. Some institutions allow the record to be "split," which means placing the progress notes at the bedside while maintaining the rest of the chart documentation at the nurses' station. To avoid having to go back to the bedside to document, a nurse might take a new progress note sheet, document findings, and then put the page in the chart at the nurses' station. This documentation will not be in proper sequence with the progress notes from the bedside when they are entered into the chart.

As you read these vignettes, think about ways that information systems could assist in preventing these problems.

Source: Examples from Schott, 2003, pp. 22-23.

The problems with poor-quality patient care data are not limited to the patient medical record or other data collected and used at the organizational level. In a recent report the Medical Records Institute (MRI), a professional organization dedicated to the improvement of patient records through technology, has identified five major functions that are negatively affected by poor-quality documentation (MRI, 2004). These problems are found not only at the organizational level but also across organizations and throughout the overall health care environment.

- *Patient safety* is affected by inadequate information, illegible entries, misinterpretations, and insufficient interoperability.
- *Public safety*, a major component of public health, is diminished by the inability to collect information in a coordinated, timely manner at the provider level in response to epidemics and the threat of terrorism.
- *Continuity of patient care* is adversely affected by the lack of shareable information among patient care providers.
- *Health care economics* are adversely affected, with information capture and report generation costs currently estimated to be well over $50 billion annually.
- *Clinical research and outcomes analysis* is adversely affected by a lack of uniform information capture that is needed to facilitate the derivation of data from routine patient care documentation [MRI, 2004, p. 2].

This same report identifies health care documentation as having two parts: information capture and report generation. *Information capture* is "the process of recording representations of human thought, perceptions, or actions in documenting patient care, as well as device-generated information that is gathered and/or computed about a patient as part of health care" (MRI, 2004, p. 2). Some means of information capture in health care organizations are handwriting, speaking, typing, touching a screen or pointing and clicking on words or phrases, videotaping, audio recording, and generating images through X-rays and scans. *Report generation* "consists of the formatting and/or structuring of captured information. It is the process of analyzing, organizing, and presenting recorded patient information for authentication and inclusion in the patient's healthcare record" (MRI, 2004, p. 2). In order to have high-quality documentation resulting in high-quality data both information capture and report generation must be considered.

ENSURING DATA AND INFORMATION QUALITY

The importance of having quality health care information available to providers and heath care executives cannot be overstated. Health care decision makers rely on high-quality information. The issue is not whether quality information is important but rather how it can be achieved. Before an organization can measure the quality of the information it produces and uses, it must establish data standards. That is, data can be identified as high quality only when they conform to a recognized standard. Ensuring this conformance is not as easy as it might seem because, unfortunately, there is no universally recognized set of health care data quality standards in existence today. One reason for this is that the quality of the data needed in any situation is driven by the use to which the data or the information that comes from the data will be put. For example, in a patient care setting the margin of error for critical lab tests must be zero or patient safety is in jeopardy. However, a larger margin of error may be acceptable in census counts or discharge statistics. Health care organizations must establish data quality standards specific to the intended use of the data or resulting information.

Although we have no nationally recognized data quality standards, two organizations have published guidance that can assist a health care organization in establishing its own data quality standards: the Medical Records Institute (MRI) has published a set of "essential principles of healthcare documentation," and the American Health Information Management Association (AHIMA) has published a data quality management tool. These two guides are summarized in the following sections.

MRI Principles of Health Care Documentation

The MRI argues that there are many steps that must be taken to create systems that ensure quality health care documentation. It has developed the following key principles that should be adhered to as these systems (and their accompanying policies) are established:

- Unique patient identification must be assured within and across healthcare documentation systems.

- Healthcare documentation must be

   Accurate and consistent.

   Complete.

   Timely.

   Interoperable across types of documentation systems.

   Accessible at any time and at any place where patient care is needed.

   Auditable.

- Confidential and secure authentication and accountability must be provided [MRI, 2004, p. 3].

The MRI takes the position that when practitioners interact with electronic resources they have an increased ability to meet these guidelines (MRI, 2004).

AHIMA Data Quality Model

AHIMA has published a generic data quality management model and an accompanying set of general data characteristics. There are similarities between these characteristics and the MRI principles. AHIMA strives to include all health care data, however, and does limit the characteristics of clinical documentation. The AHIMA model is reprinted in Figure 2.2 and Table 2.1.

The AHIMA data quality characteristics listed in Table 2.1 can serve as the basis for establishing data quality standards because they represent common dimensions of health care data that should always be present, regardless of the use of the data or resulting information. Here's a further review of these common dimensions:

- *Data accuracy.* Data that reflect correct, valid values are accurate. Typographical errors in discharge summaries and misspelled names are examples of inaccurate data.

- *Data accessibility.* Data that are not available to the decision makers needing them are of no use.

- *Data comprehensiveness.* *All* of the data required for a particular use must be present and available to the user. Even relevant data may not be useful when they are incomplete.

- *Data consistency.* Quality data are consistent. Use of an abbreviation that has two different meanings provides a good example of how lack of consistency can lead to

---

FIGURE 2.2. *AHIMA Data Quality Management Model*

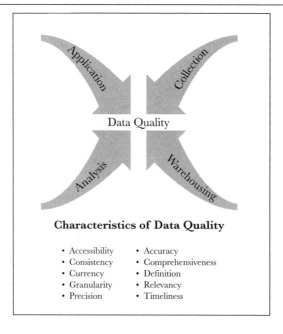

Characteristics of Data Quality

- Accessibility
- Consistency
- Currency
- Granularity
- Precision

- Accuracy
- Comprehensiveness
- Definition
- Relevancy
- Timeliness

Application – The purpose for which the data are collected.

Collection – The processes by which data elements are accumulated.

Warehousing – Processes and systems used to archive data and data journals.

Analysis – The process of translating data into information utilized for an application.

Source: AHIMA, Data Quality Management Task Force, 1998.

---

problems. For example, a nurse may use the abbreviation CPR to mean *cardiopulmonary resuscitation* at one time and use it to mean *computer-based patient record* at another time, leading to confusion.

■ *Data currency.* Many types of health care data become obsolete after a period of time. A patient's admitting diagnosis is often not the same as the diagnosis recorded upon discharge. If a health care executive needs a report on the diagnoses treated during a particular time frame, which of these two diagnoses should be included?

■ *Data definition.* Clear definitions of data elements must be provided so that both current and future data users will understand what the data mean. One way to supply clear data definitions is to use data dictionaries. A case described by A. M. Shakir (1999) offers an excellent example of the need for clear data definitions.

TABLE 2.1. **AHIMA Data Quality Management Characteristics**

Characteristic	Application	Collection	Warehousing	Analysis
Data accuracy Data are the correct values and are valid.	To facilitate accuracy, determine the application's purpose, the question to be answered, or the aim for collecting the data element.	Ensuring accuracy involves appropriate education and training and timely and appropriate communication of data definitions to those who collect data. For example, data accuracy will help ensure that if a patient's sex is female, it is accurately recorded as female and not male.	To warehouse data, appropriate edits should be in place to ensure accuracy. For example, error reports should be generated for inconsistent values such as a diagnosis inappropriate for age or gender. Exception or error reports should be generated and corrections should be made.	To accurately analyze data, ensure that the algorithms, formulas, and translation systems are correct. For example, ensure that the encoder assigns correct codes and that the appropriate DRG is assigned for the codes entered. Also, ensure that each record or entry within the database is correct.
Data accessibility Data items should be easily obtainable and legal to collect.	The application and legal, financial, process, and other boundaries determine which data to collect. Ensure that collected data are legal to collect for the application. For example, recording the age and race in medical records may be appropriate. However, it may be illegal to collect this information in human resources departments.	When developing the data collection instrument, explore methods to access needed data and ensure that the best, least costly method is selected. The amount of accessible data may be increased through system interfaces and integration of systems. For example, the best and easiest method to obtain demographic information may be to obtain it from an existing system. Another method may be to assign data collection by the expertise of each team member. For example, the admission staff collects demographic data, the nursing staff collects symptoms, and the HIM [health information management] staff assigns codes. Team members should be assigned accordingly.	Technology and hardware impact accessibility. Establish data ownership and guidelines for who may access data and/or systems. Inventory data to facilitate access.	Access to complete, current data will better ensure accurate analysis. Otherwise results and conclusions may be inaccurate or inappropriate. For example, use of the Medicare case mix index (CMI) alone does not accurately reflect total hospital CMI. Consequently, strategic planning based solely on Medicare CMI may not be appropriate.

(Continued)

TABLE 2.1. *(Continued)*

Characteristic	Application	Collection	Warehousing	Analysis
Data comprehensiveness All required data items are included. Ensure that the entire scope of the data is collected and document intentional limitations.	Clarify how the data will be used and identify end-users to ensure complete data are collected for the application. Include a problem statement and cost-benefit or impact study when collected data are increased. For example, in addition to outcome it may be important to gather data that impact outcomes.	Cost-effective comprehensive data collection may be achieved via interface to or download from other automated systems. Data definition and data precision impact comprehensive data collection (see these characteristics below).	Warehousing includes managing relationships of data owners, data collectors, and data end-users to ensure that all are aware of the available data in the inventory and accessible systems. This also helps to reduce redundant data collection.	Ensure that all pertinent data impacting the application are analyzed in concert.
Data consistency The value of the data should be reliable and the same across applications.	Data are consistent when the value of the data is the same across applications and systems, such as the patient's medical record number. In addition, related data items should agree. For example, data are inconsistent when it is documented that a male patient has had a hysterectomy.	The use of data definitions, extensive training, standardized data collection (procedures, rules, edits, and process), and integrated/interfaced systems facilitate consistency.	Warehousing employs edits or conversion tables to ensure consistency. Coordinate edits and tables with data definition changes or data definition differences across systems. Document edits and tables.	Analyze data under reproducible circumstances by using standard formulas, scientific equations, variance calculations, and other methods. Compare "apples to apples."
Data currency The data should be up-to-date. A datum value is up-to-date if it is current for a specific point in time. It is outdated if it was current at some preceding time yet incorrect at a later time.	The appropriateness or value of an application changes over time. For example, traditional quality assurance applications are gradually being replaced by those with the more current application of performance improvement.	Data definitions change or are modified over time. These should be documented so that current and future users know what the data mean. These changes should be communicated in a timely manner to those collecting data and to the end-users.	To ensure current data are available, warehousing involves continually updating systems, tables, and databases. The dates of warehousing events should be documented.	The availability of current data impacts the analysis of data. For example, to study the incidence of diseases or procedures, ICD-9-CM codes may be used. Coding practices or the actual code for a disease or procedure may change over time. This should be taken into consideration when analyzing trends.

Data definition Clear definitions should be provided so that current and future data users will know what the data mean. Each data element should have clear meaning and acceptable values.	The application's purpose, the question to be answered, or the aim for collecting the data element must be clarified to ensure appropriate and complete data definitions.	Clear, concise data definitions facilitate accurate data collection. For example, the definition of patient disposition may be "the patient's anticipated location or status following release or discharge." Acceptable values for this data element should also be defined. The instrument of collection should include data definitions and ensure that data integrity characteristics are managed.	Warehousing includes archiving documentation and data. Consequently, data ownership documentation and definitions should be maintained over time. Inventory maintenance activities (purging, updates, and others), purpose for collecting data, collection policies, information management policies, and data sources should be maintained over time also.	For appropriate analysis, display data need to reflect the purpose for which the data were collected. This is defined by the application. Appropriate comparisons, relationships, and linkages need to be shown.
Data granularity The attributes and values of data should be defined at the correct level of detail.	A single application may require varying levels of detail or granularity. For example, census statistics may be utilized daily, weekly, or monthly depending upon the application. Census is needed daily to ensure adequate staffing and food service. However, the monthly trend is needed for long-range planning.	Collect data at the appropriate level of detail or granularity. For example, the temperature of 100° may be recorded. The granularity for recording outdoor temperatures is different from recording patient temperatures. If patient Jane Doe's temperature is 100°, does that mean 99.6° or 100.4°? Appropriate granularity for this application dictates that the data need to be recorded to the first decimal point while appropriate granularity for recording outdoor temperatures may not require it.	Warehouse data at the appropriate level of detail or granularity. For example, exception or error reports reflect granularity based on the application. A spike (exception) in the daily census may show little or no impact on the month-to-date or monthly reports.	Appropriate analysis reflects the level of detail or granularity of the data collected. For example, a spike (exception) in the daily census resulting in immediate action to ensure adequate food service and staffing may have had no impact on analysis of the census for long-range planning.
Data precision Data values should be just large enough to support the application or process.	The application's purpose, the question to be answered, or the aim for collecting the data element must be clarified to ensure data precision.	To collect data precise enough for the application, define acceptable values or value ranges for each data item. For example, limit values for gender to male, female, and unknown; or collect information by age ranges.		

(Continued)

TABLE 2.1. (Continued)

Characteristic	Application	Collection	Warehousing	Analysis
Data relevancy The data are meaningful to the performance of the process or application for which they are collected.	The application's purpose, the question to be answered, or the aim for collecting the data element must be clarified to ensure relevant data.	To better ensure relevancy, complete a pilot of the data collection instrument to validate its use. A "parallel" test may also be appropriate, completing the new or revised instrument and the current process simultaneously. Communicate results to those collecting data and to the end-users. Facilitate or negotiate changes as needed across disciplines or users.	Establish appropriate retention schedules to ensure availability of relevant data. Relevancy is defined by the application.	For appropriate analysis, display data to reflect the purpose for which the data were collected. This is defined by the application. Show appropriate comparisons, relationships, and linkages.
Data timeliness Timeliness is determined by how the data are being used and their context.	Timeliness is defined by the application. For example, patient census is needed daily to provide sufficient day-to-day operations staffing, such as nursing and food service. However, annual or monthly patient census data are needed for the facility's strategic planning.	Timely data collection is a function of the process and collection instrument.	Warehousing ensures that data are available per information management policy and retention schedules.	Timely data analysis allows for the initiation of action to avoid adverse impacts. For some applications, timely may be seconds. For others, it may be years.

Note: The terms *data dictionary* and *data warehouse* will be discussed in Chapter Eight. Basically, a data dictionary lists the terms used in an organization's systems. A data warehouse is a specific type of database, used primarily for decision support.

Source: AHIMA, Data Quality Management Task Force, 1998.

PERSPECTIVE

DATA DEFINITIONS

A large national health maintenance organization (HMO) was planning to create a disease management program for pediatric care. As part of the planning effort, the HMO decided to conduct a survey of its regional sites to determine the utilization pattern for pediatric care. It sent a questionnaire to each of the 12 regional offices asking these two questions:

1.   How many pediatric members were enrolled as of year-end 1990?

2.   How many pediatric visits took place in 1990?

On the surface, the questions seemed quite simple and appropriate. The HMO would determine the number of pediatric members and the number of pediatric visits by region. It could then compute pediatric utilization by region—and across the program as a whole. This data would then be used to determine a baseline for development of utilization management programs and would assist in comparative analysis of pediatric utilization across regions.

There was only one problem—the absence of common data definitions. Each of the regions operated somewhat autonomously and interpreted the request for information differently. As a result, the regional offices raised a number of questions and revealed numerous discrepancies in their interpretations of data definitions:

What is a pediatric member?

A dependent member under the age of 18

A dependent member under the age of 21

A dependent child member, regardless of age

A patient under the age of 18

What is a pediatric visit?

A visit by a pediatric member

A visit by a patient under the age of 18

Any visit to the pediatric department

A visit with a pediatrician

Attempts to answer these questions only raised more questions. What is a member? What does it mean to be enrolled? What is a dependent? How is patient/member age calculated? What is a visit? What is a patient and how does

(Continued)

PERSPECTIVE (*Continued*)

one differ from a member? What is a department? What are the department types? What is a pediatrician?

. . . This story shows us how important it is that suppliers and consumers of data agree on data definitions before exchanging information. Had the regions not revealed their assumptions, the discrepancies in their interpretations of the data definitions might never have been recognized, and the organization would have unknowingly compared apples to oranges. In the long term, a business strategy with significant implications would have been based upon invalid information.

Source: Shakir, 1999, pp. 48-49.

- *Data granularity.* Data granularity is sometimes referred to as *data atomicity.* That is, individual data elements are "atomic" in the sense that they cannot be further subdivided. For example, a typical patient's name should generally be stored as three data elements (last name, first name, middle name—"Smith" and "John" and "Allen") not as a single data element ("John Allen Smith"). Again, granularity is related to the purpose for which the data are collected. Although it is possible to subdivide a person's birth date into separate fields for the month, the date, and the year, this is usually not desirable. The birth date is at its lowest practical level of granularity when used as a patient identifier. Values for data should be defined at the correct level for their use.

- *Data precision.* Precision often relates to numerical data. Precision denotes how close to an actual size, weight, or other standard a particular measurement is. Some health care data must be very precise. For example, in figuring a drug dosage it is not all right to round up to the nearest gram when the drug is to be dosed in milligrams.

- *Data relevancy.* Data must be relevant to the purpose for which they are collected. We could collect very accurate, timely data about a patient's color preferences or choice of hairdresser, but is this relevant to the care of the patient?

- *Data timeliness.* Timeliness is a critical dimension in the quality of many types of health care data. For example, critical lab values must be available to the health care provider in a timely manner. Producing accurate results after the patient has been discharged may be of little or no value to the patient's care.

Types and Causes of Data Errors

Failures of data to meet established quality standards are called data errors. A data error will have a negative impact on one or more of the characteristics of quality data. For example, if a final diagnosis is coded incorrectly, that datum is no longer accurate. If the same diagnosis is coded in several different ways, those data are not consistent.

Both examples represent data errors. Data errors are often discussed in terms of two types of underlying cause, systematic errors and random errors (Table 2.2). *Systematic errors* are errors that can be attributed to a flaw or discrepancy in adherence to standard operating procedures or systems. The diagnosis coding errors just described would be systematic errors if they resulted from incorrect programming of the encoding software or improper training of the individuals assigning the codes. Systematic health care data errors can also be caused by unclear data definitions or a failure to comply with the established data collection protocols, such as leaving out required information. If the diagnosis coding errors were the result of poor handwriting or transcription errors, they would be considered *random errors*. Carelessness rather than lack of training leads to random errors (Arts, DeKeizer, & Scheffer, 2002).

Preventing, Detecting, and Fixing Data Errors

Both systematic and random errors lead to poor-quality data and information. Both types need to be prevented to the extent possible. Errors that are not preventable need to be detected so that they can be corrected. There are multiple points during data collection and processing where system design can reduce data errors. Arts, DeKeizer, and Scheffer (2002) have published a useful framework for ensuring data quality in a centralized health care database (or *medical registry*, as these authors call it). Although the entire framework is not reproduced here, several key aspects are outlined in Figure 2.3. This framework illustrates that there are multiple reasons for data errors and multiple approaches to preventing and correcting these errors. The following Perspective describes some issues with using IT to improve data quality.

TABLE 2.2. **Some Causes of Poor Health Care Data Quality**

Systematic	Random
Unclear data definitions	Illegible handwriting in data source
Unclear data collection guidelines	Typing errors
Poor interface design	Lack of motivation
Programming errors	Frequent personnel turnover
Incomplete data source	Calculation errors (not built into the
Unsuitable data format in the source	system)
Data dictionary is lacking or not available	
Data dictionary is not adhered to	
Guidelines or protocols are not adhered to	
Lack of sufficient data checks	
No system for correcting detected data errors	
No control over adherence to guidelines and data definitions	

Source: Arts, DeKeizer, & Scheffer, 2002, p. 604.

PERSPECTIVE

TESTING THE USE OF IT

In April 2007, the U.S. Government Accountability Office (GOA) published a report on the findings from eight hospital case studies that examined the impact of information technology on the collection and submission of required Centers for Medicare and Medicaid (CMS) health care quality data. The study hospitals used six steps to collect and submit the required data:

1. Identify the patients.

2. Locate information in their medical records.

3. Determine appropriate values for the data elements.

4. Transmit the data to CMS.

5. Ensure that the data have been accepted by CMS.

6. Supply copies of medical records to CMS to validate the data.

The case studies demonstrated that the hospitals' existing IT systems helped the data abstractors to gather some of the data but fell short of allowing the hospitals to automate that process. The IT systems improved accessibility to and legibility of the patient medical records. However, multiple limitations were noted:

■ Hospitals had a mix of paper and electronic records, requiring abstractors to look in multiple locations for required data elements.

■ Most data were recorded as unstructured or narrative text, which made locating information within records time consuming.

■ Hospitals had IT systems that were not integrated, requiring abstractors to access multiple IT systems to obtain related data.

The GOA report recommends that the secretary of the U.S. Department of Health and Human Services identify specific plans to promote the use of IT for the collection and submission of data to CMS.

Source: Adapted from GAO, 2007.

Using IT to Improve Data Quality

Information technology has tremendous potential as a tool for improving health care data quality. To date some of this potential has been realized, but many opportunities remain that are not commonly employed by health care organizations. Clearly, electronic medical records (EMRs) improve legibility and accessibility of health care

---

FIGURE 2.3. *Activities for Improving Data Quality*

Data Error Prevention

Compose a minimum set of necessary data items

Define data and data characteristics in a data dictionary

Develop a data collection protocol

Create user friendly data entry forms or interface

Compose data checks

Create a quality assurance plan

Train and motivate users

Data Error Detection

Perform automatic data checks

Perform data quality audits

Review data collection protocols and procedures

Check inter- and intraobserver variability (if appropriate)

Visually inspect completed forms (online or otherwise)

Routinely check completeness of data entry

Actions for Data Quality Improvement

Provide data quality reports to users

Correct inaccurate data and fill in incomplete data detected

Control user correction of data errors

Give feedback of data quality results and recommendations

Resolve identified causes of data errors

Implement identified system changes

Communicate with users

Source: Arts, DeKeizer, & Scheffer, 2002, p. 605.

data and information. But what about the remaining dimensions of health care data quality? As noted earlier, a recent GAO report (2007) found that many of the data in existing EMR systems were recorded in an unstructured format—"in narrative form or other text, rather than in data fields designated to contain specific pieces of information." Physician notes and discharge summaries are often dictated and transcribed. This lack of structure limits the ability of an EMR to be a data quality improvement tool. In systems requiring structured data input, data comprehensiveness, relevance, and consistency can be improved. When health care providers respond to a series of prompts, rather than dictating a free-form narrative, they are reminded to include all necessary elements of a health record entry. Data precision and accuracy are improved when these systems also incorporate error checking. A clear example of data improvement achieved through information technology is the result seen from incorporating medication administration systems designed to prevent medication error (see Chapter Five). With structured data input and sophisticated error prevention, these systems can significantly reduce medication errors.

SUMMARY

Without health care data and information there would be no need for health care information systems. Health care information is a valuable asset in health care organizations and it must be managed like other assets. To manage information effectively, health care executives should have an understanding of health care data and information and recognize the importance of ensuring data quality. Health care decisions, both clinical and administrative, are driven by data and information. Data and information are used to provide patient care and to monitor facility performance. It is critical that the data and information be of high quality. After all, the most sophisticated of information systems cannot overcome the inherent problems associated with poor-quality source data and data collection or entry errors. The data characteristics and frameworks presented here can be useful tools in the establishment of mechanisms for ensuring the quality of health care data.

The challenge of health care organizations today is to implement information technology solutions that work to improve the quality of their health care data.

KEY TERMS

Data
Data accessibility
Data accuracy
Data comprehensiveness
Data consistency
Data currency
Data definition
Data errors
Documentation

Government Accountability Office
  (GAO)
Information
Information capture
Knowledge
Random errors
Report generation
Systematic errors
Unique patient identifier

 ## LEARNING ACTIVITIES

1. Contact a health care facility (hospital, nursing home, physicians' office, or other facility) to ask permission to view a sample of the health records they maintain. These records may be in paper or electronic form. For each record, answer the following questions about data quality:

    a. How would you assess the quality of the data in the patient's record? Use the MRI's key principles and AHIMA's data characteristics as guides.

    b. What proportion of the data in the patient's medical record is captured electronically? What information is recorded manually? Do you think the method of capture affects the quality of the information?

    c. How does the data quality compare with what you expected?

2.   Visit a health care organization to explore the ways in which the facility monitors or evaluates data quality.

3.   Consider the following scenarios and the questions they raise about data quality. What should an organization do? How does one create an environment that promotes data quality? What are some of the problems associated with having poor-quality data?

A late entry is written to supply information that was omitted at the time of the original entry. It should be done only if the person completing it has total recall of the omission. For example, a nurse completed her charting on December 12, 2002, and forgot to note that the physician had talked with the patient. When she returned to work on December 13, she wrote a late entry for the day before and documented the physician visit. The clinician must enter the current date and the documentation must be identified as a late entry including the date of the omission. Additionally, a late entry should be added as soon as possible.

A late entry cannot be used to supplement a record because of a negative clinical outcome that occurs after the original entry. For example, while a patient received an antibiotic for two days, the nurse charted nothing unusual. Yet, on the third day, the patient had an acute episode of shortness of breath and chest pain and died later that same day. At the time of death, documentation revealed that the patient had a dark red rash on his chest.

An investigation into the cause of death was conducted and all the nurses who provided care during the three days were interviewed and asked whether they had seen the rash prior to the patient's death. None of the nurses remembered the rash. However, one nurse wrote a late entry for each of the first two days that the patient was receiving the antibiotic stating that there was no rash on those days. This is an incorrect late entry. Her statement is part of the investigation conducted after the fact and was not an omission from her original entry [Schott, 2003, 23-24].

CHAPTER

3

HEALTH CARE INFORMATION REGULATIONS, LAWS, AND STANDARDS

LEARNING OBJECTIVES

- To be able to discuss how accreditation, facility licensure, and certification influence the information needs of health care facilities.
- To be able to identify and differentiate among major health care accrediting bodies.
- To be able to understand and manage the impact of the health record as a legal document.
- To be able to discuss the HIPAA privacy regulations and their relevance to health care organizations and consumers.
- To be able to describe the laws, regulations, and standards that govern patient confidentiality.

Chapters One and Two focused on the health care information and data that are available to, used by, and managed by health care organizations. We mentioned that there are external drivers that affect and in some cases dictate the types of health care information that health care organizations maintain and to a certain extent the ways in which those types are maintained. These external forces take the form of laws and regulations mandated at both the state and federal levels. Voluntary accreditation standards are additional external forces. In this chapter we will examine more closely the most important of these laws, regulations, and standards and the external organizations that promulgate them. We will do this under two main headings.

In the section titled "Licensure, Certification, and Accreditation," we define these processes and examine some of the missions and general functions of two of the major accrediting organizations in the United States, The Joint Commission and the National Committee for Quality Assurance (NCQA), and introduce several other accrediting bodies. These discussions focus on how the licensure, certification, and accreditation processes affect health care information and, as a consequence, health care information systems.

Then, in the section titled "Legal Aspects of Managing Health Information," we look at state and federal laws that address the use of the patient medical record as a legal document, and current laws and regulations that govern patient privacy and confidentiality. These legal requirements have a significant impact on how patient-specific health care information is maintained and secured in health care information systems.

LICENSURE, CERTIFICATION, AND ACCREDITATION

Health care organizations, such as hospitals, nursing homes, home health agencies, and the like, must be licensed to operate. If they wish to file Medicare or Medicaid claims they must also be certified, and if they wish to demonstrate excellence they will undergo an accreditation process. What are these processes, and how are they related? If a health care organization is licensed, certified, and accredited how will this affect the health care information that it creates, uses, and maintains? In this section we will examine each of these processes and their impact on the health care organizations. We will also discuss their relationships with one another.

Licensure

Licensure is the process that gives a facility legal approval to operate. As a rule, state governments oversee the licensure of health care facilities, and each state sets its own licensure laws and regulations. All facilities must have a license to operate, and it is generally the state department of health or a similar agency that carries out the licensure function. Licensure regulations tend to emphasize areas such as physical plant standards, fire safety, space allocations, and sanitation. They may also contain minimum standards for equipment and personnel. A few states tie licensure to professional standards and quality of care. In their licensure regulations, most states set minimum standards for the content, retention, and authentication of patient medical records. Exhibit 3.1 is an excerpt from the South Carolina licensure regulations for hospitals. This excerpt governs

EXHIBIT 3.1. *Medical Record Content: Excerpt from South Carolina Standards for Licensing Hospitals and Institutional General Infirmaries*

601.5 Contents:

A. Adequate and complete medical records shall be written for all patients admitted to the hospital and newborns delivered in the hospital. All notes shall be legibly written or typed and signed. Although use of initials in lieu of licensed nurses' signatures is not encouraged, initials will be accepted provided such initials can be readily identified within the medical record. A minimum medical record shall include the following information:

1. Admission Record: An admission record must be prepared for each patient and must contain the following information, when obtainable: Name; address, including county; occupation; age; date of birth; sex; marital status; religion; county of birth; father's name; mother's maiden name; husband's or wife's name; dates of military service; health insurance number; provisional diagnosis; case number; days of care; social security number; the name of the person providing information; name, address and telephone number of person or persons to be notified in the event of emergency; name and address of referring physician; name and address and telephone number of attending physician; date and hour of admission;

2. History and physical within 48 hours after admission;

3. Provisional or working diagnosis;

4. Pre-operative diagnosis;

5. Medical treatment;

6. Complete surgical record, if any, including technique of operation and findings, statement of tissue and organs removed and post-operative diagnosis;

7. Report of anesthesia;

8. Nurses' notes;

9. Progress notes;

10. Gross pathological findings and microscopic;

11. Temperature chart, including pulse and respiration;

12. Medication Administration Record or similar document for recording of medications, treatments and other pertinent data. Nurses shall sign this record after each medication administered or treatment rendered;

13. Final diagnosis and discharge summary;

14. Date and hour of discharge summary;

15. In case of death, cause and autopsy findings, if autopsy is performed;

16. Special examinations, if any, e.g., consultations, clinical laboratory, x-ray and other examinations.

Source: South Carolina Department of Health and Environmental Control, Standards for Licensing Hospitals and Institutional General Infirmaries, Regulation 61-16 § 601.5 (2003).

patient medical record content (with the exception of newborn patient records, which are addressed in a separate section of the regulations). Although each state has its own set of licensure standards, these are fairly typical in scope and content.

An initial license is required before a facility opens its doors, and this license to operate must generally be renewed annually. Some states allow organizations with the Joint Commission accreditation to forgo a formal licensure survey conducted by the state; others require the state survey regardless of accreditation status. As we will see in the section on accreditation, the Joint Commission standards are more detailed and generally more stringent than the state licensure regulations. Also, the Joint Commission standards are updated annually; most licensure standards are not.

Certification

Certification gives a health care organization the authority to participate in the federal Medicare and Medicaid programs. In other words, an organization must be certified to receive reimbursement from the Centers for Medicare and Medicaid Services (CMS). Legislation passed in 1972 mandated that hospitals had to be reviewed and certified in order to participate in the Medicare and Medicaid programs. At that time the Health Care Financing Administration (now the Centers for Medicare and Medicaid Services) developed a set of minimum standards known as the Conditions of Participation (CoPs). The federal government is required to inspect facilities to make sure they meet these minimum standards; however, this survey process is generally contracted out to the states to perform. In the case of hospitals, those accredited by The Joint Commission are *deemed* to have met the federal certification standards. One interesting historical fact is that the original CoPs were essentially the same as the then existing The Joint Commission standards. The Joint Commission standards, however, have undergone tremendous change over the past forty years whereas the CoPs have not. Exhibit 3.2 displays the section of the current Medicare and Medicaid Conditions of Participation for Hospitals that governs the content of hospital medical records.

Accreditation

Accreditation is an external review process that an organization elects to undergo. The accrediting agency grants recognition to organizations that meet its predetermined performance and outcome standards. The review process and standards are devised and regulated by the accrediting agency. By far the best-known health care accrediting agency in the United States is The Joint Commission. A few other notable accrediting agencies are the National Committee for Quality Assurance (NCQA), the Commission on Accreditation of Rehabilitation Facilities (CARF), and the Accreditation Association for Ambulatory Health Care (AAAHC).

Although accreditation is voluntary, there are financial and legal incentives for health care organizations to seek accreditation. As we stated earlier, the Joint Commission accreditation can lead to deemed status for CMS programs, and many states recognize accreditation in lieu of their own licensure surveys. Other benefits for an organization are that accreditation

- Is required for reimbursement from certain payers
- Validates the quality of care within the organization
- May favorably influence liability insurance premiums
- May enhance access to managed care contracts
- Gives the organization a competitive edge over nonaccredited organizations

---

EXHIBIT 3.2. *Medical Record Content: Excerpt from the Conditions of Participation for Hospitals*

Sec. 482.24 Condition of participation: Medical record services.

(**c**) Standard: Content of record. The medical record must contain information to justify admission and continued hospitalization, support the diagnosis, and describe the patient's progress and response to medications and services.

(1) All entries must be legible and complete, and must be authenticated and dated promptly by the person (identified by name and discipline) who is responsible for ordering, providing, or evaluating the service furnished.

(i) The author of each entry must be identified and must authenticate his or her entry.

(ii) Authentication may include signatures, written initials or computer entry.

(2) All records must document the following, as appropriate:

(i) Evidence of a physical examination, including a health history, performed no more than 7 days prior to admission or within 48 hours after admission.

(ii) Admitting diagnosis.

(iii) Results of all consultative evaluations of the patient and appropriate findings by clinical and other staff involved in the care of the patient.

(iv) Documentation of complications, hospital acquired infections, and unfavorable reactions to drugs and anesthesia.

(v) Properly executed informed consent forms for procedures and treatments specified by the medical staff, or by Federal or State law if applicable, to require written patient consent.

(vi) All practitioners' orders, nursing notes, reports of treatment, medication records, radiology, and laboratory reports, and vital signs and other information necessary to monitor the patient's condition.

(vii) Discharge summary with outcome of hospitalization, disposition of case, and provisions for follow-up care.

(viii) Final diagnosis with completion of medical records within 30 days following discharge.

Source: Conditions of Participation: Medical Record Services, 42 C.F.R. §§ 482.24c et seq. (2007).

Joint Commission on Accreditation of Healthcare Organizations   The Joint Commission's stated mission is "to continuously improve the safety and quality of care provided to the public through the provision of health care accreditation and related services that support performance improvement in health care organizations" (The Joint Commission, 2008c).

The Joint Commission on Accreditation of Hospitals (as The Joint Commission was first called) was formed as an independent, not-for-profit organization in 1951, as a joint effort of the American College of Surgeons, American College of Physicians, American Medical Association, and American Hospital Association. The Joint Commission has grown and evolved to set standards for and accredit more than 15,000 health care organizations and programs in the United State. Today The Joint Commission has accreditation programs not only for hospitals but also for organizations that offer ambulatory care, assisted living, long-term care, behavioral health care, home care, laboratory services, managed care, and office-based surgery.

In order to maintain accreditation a health care organization must undergo an on-site survey by a The Joint Commission survey team every three years. This survey is conducted to ensure that the organization continues to meet the established standards. The standards themselves are a result of an ongoing, dynamic process that incorporates the experience and perspectives of health care professionals and others throughout the country. New standards manuals are published annually, and health care organizations are responsible for knowing and incorporating any changes as they occur.

A the Joint Commission survey results in one of six official accreditation decisions:

- *Accreditation:* for organizations in full compliance.

- *Provisional accreditation:* for organizations that fail to address all requirements for improvement within 90 days following a survey.

- *Conditional accreditation:* for organizations that are not in substantial compliance with the standards. These organizations must remedy the problem areas and undergo an additional follow-up survey.

- *Preliminary denial of accreditation:* for organizations for which there is justification for denying accreditation. This decision is subject to appeal.

- *Denial of accreditation:* for organizations that fail to meet standards and that have exhausted all appeals.

- *Preliminary accreditation:* for organizations that demonstrate compliance with selected standards under a special early survey option.

In addition The Joint Commission may place an organization on *accreditation watch*. This designation can be publicly disclosed when a *sentinel event* has occurred and the organization fails to make adequate plans to prevent similar events in the future (The Joint Commission, 2008c). A sentinel event is one that occurs unexpectedly and either leads to or presents a significant risk of death or serious injury.

One clear The Joint Commission focus is the quality of care provided in health care facilities. This focus on quality dates back to the early 1900s when the American College of Surgeons began surveying hospitals and established a hospital standardization program. With the program came the question, How is quality of care measured? One of the early concerns of the standardization program was the lack of documentation in patient records. The early surveyors found that documentation was so poor they had no way to judge the quality of care provided. The Joint Commission's emphasis on health care information and the documentation of care has continued to the present. For example, as the outline of the Joint Commission's information management (IM) standards for hospitals, shown in Exhibit 3.3, suggests, the content of patient records is greatly influenced, if not determined, by these standards. Health care information and patient records remain a major focus for the Joint Commission accreditation; 150 of the Joint Commission hospital standards are scored on the patient medical record alone (The Joint Commission, 2008d).

The Joint Commission Information Management Standards   The Joint Commission hospital accreditation standards include an entire section devoted to the management of information. These standards were developed under the basic premise that a

---

EXHIBIT 3.3. *Management of Information Standards*

IM 1.10   The organization plans and designs information management processes to meet internal and external information needs.

IM 2.10   Information privacy and confidentiality are maintained.

IM 2.20   Information security, including data integrity, is maintained.

IM 2.30   Continuity of information is maintained.

IM 3.10   The organization has processes in place to effectively manage information, including the capturing, reporting, processing, storing, retrieving, disseminating, and displaying of clinical/service and nonclinical data and information.

IM 4.10   The information management system provides information for use in decision making.

IM 5.10   Knowledge-based information resources are readily available, current, and authoritative.

IM 6.10   The organization has a complete and accurate medical record for every patient assessed, cared for, treated, or served.

IM 6.20   Records contain patient-specific information, as appropriate to the care, treatment, and services provided.

IM 6.30   The medical record thoroughly documents operative or other procedures and the use of moderate or deep sedation or anesthesia. (See also standards PC.13.30 and PC.13.40)

IM 6.40   For patients receiving continuing ambulatory care services, the medical record contains a summary list(s) of all significant diagnoses, procedures, drug allergies, and medications.

IM 6.50   Designated qualified staff accept and transcribe verbal orders from authorized individuals.

IM 6.60   The organization provides access to all relevant information from a patient's record when needed for use in patient care, treatment, and services.

Source: Adapted from The Joint Commission, 2008d.

hospital's provision of care, treatment, and services is highly dependent on information and that information is a resource that must be managed like any other resource within a health care facility. The goal of the information management function is "to support decision making to improve patient outcomes, improve health care documentation, assure patient safety, and improve performance in patient care, treatment, and services, governance, management, and support processes" (The Joint Commission, 2004d). Although The Joint Commission acknowledges that "efficiency, effectiveness, patient safety, and the quality of patient care, treatment, and services can be improved by computerization and other technologies," the standards apply whether information systems are paper based or electronic. The last section of the IM overview demonstrates The Joint Commission's strong belief that quality information management influences quality care that continues as we move from paper-based systems to electronic ones:

"The quality of care, treatment, and services is affected by the many transitions in information management that are currently in progress in health care, such as the transition from handwriting and traditional paper-based documentation to electronic information management, as well as the transition from free text to structured and interactive text" (The Joint Commission, 2004d).

Hospitals are expected to undertake an assessment process to be in compliance with the Joint Commission IM standards. They must base their information management processes on an analysis of both internal and external information needs.

National Committee for Quality Assurance   The National Committee for Quality Assurance (NCQA) was discussed in Chapter One as the developer and overseer of the Health Plan Employer Data and Information Set (HEDIS) and for its work in providing quality measures for health plans. In addition to these programs, the NCQA also serves as an accrediting body for health plans and managed care organizations (MCOs).

NCQA began accrediting MCOs in 1991 in response to the need for "standardized, objective information about the quality of these organizations" (NCQA, 2008a). Although the NCQA accreditation process is voluntary, many large employers, including American Airlines, IBM, AT&T, and Federal Express, will not do business with a health plan that is not NCQA accredited. More than half of all states recognize NCQA accreditation, eliminating the need for accredited plans to undergo separate state review.

The NCQA accreditation process includes a survey to ensure the organization meets NCQA published standards. There are over sixty specific standards, grouped into five categories:

- *Access and Service*—Do health plan members have access to the care and services they need? Does the health plan resolve grievances quickly and fairly?

- *Qualified Providers*—Does the health plan thoroughly check the credentials of all of its providers?

- *Staying Healthy*—Does the health plan help people maintain good health and avoid illness?

- *Getting Better*—How well does the plan care for members when they become sick?

- *Living with Illness*—How well does the plan help people manage chronic illness? [NCQA, 2008e, p. 2].

NCQA accreditation surveys are conducted by teams of physicians and other health care providers. These surveys rely heavily on health care data and information, including the HEDIS measures. The results of the surveys are evaluated by a national oversight committee that assigns one of five accreditation levels:

- Excellent
- Commendable
- Accredited
- Provisional
- Denied

The NCQA accreditation process is viewed as rigorous. A health plan must be aggressively managing quality in order to achieve accreditation at the excellent level. NCQA provides a free, online *health plan report card* that shows the accreditation status of all plans that it has surveyed (NCQA, 2008b).

Other Accrediting Organizations   Although The Joint Commission and NCQA are arguably the most visible and well-known accrediting bodies in the U.S. health care system, there are others. The Commission on Accreditation of Rehabilitation Facilities (CARF) accredits rehabilitative services and programs (CARF, 2004). The Accreditation Association for Ambulatory Health Care (AAAHC) accredits HMOs and ambulatory care organizations (AAAHC, 2003). These accreditation processes have several features in common. They are based on preestablished standards aimed at improving the quality of health care, they require an on-site survey, they make health care information and documentation critical components of the process, and they award a level of accreditation or approval. All have standards that affect organizations' health care information and health care information systems.

In the first half of this chapter, we have taken a brief overview of the licensure, certification, and accreditation processes and of the laws, standards, and regulations that affect health care information and information systems. These processes and the laws, standards, and regulations provide guidance to organizations for the development of information planning, retention, and retrieval and to a great extent determine the content of patient records. Health care executives must be familiar with the laws, standards, and regulations that apply to their health care organizations to ensure that their information management plans and information systems will facilitate compliance.

LEGAL ASPECTS OF MANAGING HEALTH INFORMATION

Health care information, particularly patient-specific information, is governed by multiple state and federal laws and regulations in addition to those for licensure and certification. Laws and regulations governing the privacy and confidentiality of patient information and also record retention and authentication have existed for many years. When all patient records were on paper, it was fairly easy to identify what constituted a patient record and what did not. Authentication was a signature on a document, and destruction of records involved burning or shredding. As patient records are increasingly stored in electronic form and involve multiple types of media from paper to digital images, implementation of the regulations governing health care information has had to change. In some cases the laws and regulations themselves have been rewritten.

At this juncture it is worth emphasizing that laws governing patient information and medical records vary from state to state and a full discussion of them is beyond the scope of this text. The complexity of the U.S. legal system makes it very important for health care organizations to employ personnel who are knowledgeable about all state and federal laws and regulations that govern their patients' information and to have legal counsel available who can provide specific guidance. With that caveat, in this section we will look at several legal aspects of managing health care information, including a brief discussion of some of the significant laws and regulations related to each aspect and a discussion of legal compliance in an increasingly multimedia environment. Specifically, we will address the medical record as a legal document, including the issues of retention and authentication of health care information, and the privacy and confidentiality of patient information, including an overview of the Health Insurance Portability and Accountability Act (HIPAA) and the HIPAA Privacy Rule.

The Health Record as a Legal Document

When the patient medical record is a file folder full of paper housed in the health information management department of the hospital, identifying the *legal* record is fairly straightforward. Records kept in the normal course of business (in this case, providing care to patients) represent an exception to the hearsay rule, are generally admissible in a court, and therefore can be subpoenaed—they are legal documentation of the care provided to the patients. The health care organization might struggle with which documents to file in an individual's medical record, because of varying and changing state and federal laws and regulations, but once those decisions are made, the entire legal record for any given patient can be found on the file shelf when it is needed. Only one "official," original copy exits.

When the patient record is a hybrid of electronic and paper documents or when it is totally computer based, how does that change the definition of the legal record? There is no simple, one-paragraph answer to this question, as state governments and the federal government are modifying laws and regulations to reflect the change from paper to digital documentation. However, some general guidelines have been proposed (Amatayakul et al., 2001). Exhibit 3.4 reprints the "Guidelines for Defining the Health Record for Legal Purposes" of the American Health Information Management Association (AHIMA). These guidelines define the *legal health record* (LHR) as "the documentation of the healthcare services provided to an individual in any aspect of healthcare delivery by a healthcare provider organization." They also recommend that patient-identifiable source data, such as photographs, diagnostic images, tracings, and monitoring strips, be considered a part of the LHR. Administrative data and derived data, however, are not considered part of the LHR.

Each health care organization must conduct a thorough review and assessment of how and where patient-identifiable information is stored. Data and information that can be classified as part of the LHR must be identified and included in any resulting LHR definition. The organization should document its definition of the content of the LHR and clearly state in what forms the content originated and is stored.

EXHIBIT 3.4. *AHIMA Guidelines for Defining the Health Record for Legal Purposes*

Legal Health Record

The legal business record generated at or for a healthcare organization. This record would be released upon request.

The LHR is the documentation of the healthcare services provided to an individual in any aspect of healthcare delivery by a healthcare provider organization. The LHR is individually identifiable data, in any medium, collected and directly used in and/or documenting healthcare or health status. The term includes records of care in any health-related setting used by healthcare professionals while providing patient care services, for reviewing patient data, or documenting observations, actions, or instructions. Some types of documentation that comprise the legal health record may physically exist in separate and multiple paper-based or electronic/computer-based databases (see examples listed below).

The LHR *excludes* health records that are *not* official business records of a healthcare provider organization (even though copies of the documentation of the healthcare services provided to an individual by a healthcare provider organization are provided to and shared with the individual). Thus, records such as personal health records (PHRs) that are patient controlled, managed, and populated would not be part of the LHR.

Copies of PHRs that are patient owned, managed, and populated by the individual but are provided to a healthcare provider organization(s) may be considered part of the LHR, if such records are used by healthcare provider organizations to provide patient care services, review patient data, or document observations, actions, or instructions. This includes patient owned, managed, and populated "tracking" records, such as medication tracking records and glucose/insulin tracking records.

Examples of documentation found in the LHR:

- advance directives
- anesthesia records
- care plan
- consent for treatment forms
- consultation reports
- discharge instructions
- discharge summary
- e-mail containing patient-provider or provider-provider communication

(Continued)

EXHIBIT 3.4. *(Continued)*

- emergency department record
- functional status assessment
- graphic records
- immunization record
- intake/output records
- medication orders
- medication profile
- minimum data sets (MDS, OASIS, etc.)
- multidisciplinary progress notes/documentation
- nursing assessment
- operative and procedure reports
- orders for diagnostic tests and diagnostic study results (e.g., laboratory, radiology, etc.)
- patient-submitted documentation
- pathology reports
- practice guidelines or protocols/clinical pathways that imbed patient data
- problem list
- records of history and physical examination
- respiratory therapy, physical therapy, speech therapy, and occupational therapy records
- selected waveforms for special documentation purposes
- telephone consultations
- telephone orders

Patient-Identifiable Source Data

An adjunct component of the legal business record as defined by the organization. Often maintained in a separate location or database, these records are provided the same level of confidentiality as the legal business record. The information is usually retrievable upon request. In the absence of documentation (e.g., interpretations, summarization, etc.), the source data should be considered part of the LHR.

Patient-identifiable source data are data from which interpretations, summaries, notes, etc., are derived. Source data should be accorded the same level of confidentiality as the LHR. These data are increasingly captured in multimedia form. For example, in a telehealth encounter, the videotape recording of the encounter would not represent the LHR but rather would be considered source data.

Examples of patient-identifiable source data:

- analog and digital patient photographs for identification purposes only
- audio of dictation
- audio of patient telephone call

- diagnostic films and other diagnostic images from which interpretations are derived
- electrocardiogram tracings from which interpretations are derived
- fetal monitoring strips from which interpretations are derived
- videos of office visits
- videos of procedure
- videos of telemedicine consultations

Administrative Data

While it should be provided the same level of confidentiality as the LHR, administrative data are not considered part of the LHR (such as in response to a subpoena for the "medical record").

Administrative data are patient-identifiable data used for administrative, regulatory, healthcare operations, and payment (financial) purposes.

Examples of administrative data:

- authorization forms for release of information
- birth and death certificates
- correspondence concerning requests for records
- event history/audit trails
- patient-identifiable claim
- patient-identifiable data reviewed for quality assurance or utilization management
- patient identifiers (e.g., medical record number, biometrics)
- protocols/clinical pathways, practice guidelines, and other knowledge sources that do not imbed patient data.

Derived Data

While it should be provided the same level of confidentiality as the LHR, derived data are not considered part of the LHR (such as in response to a subpoena for the "medical record").

Derived data consists of information aggregated or summarized from patient records so that there are no means to identify patients.

Examples of derived data:

- accreditation reports
- anonymous patient data for research purposes
- best practice guidelines created from aggregate patient data
- MDS report
- OASIS report
- ORYX report
- public health records
- statistical reports

Source: Amatayakul et al., 2001.

Retention of Health Records

The majority of states have specific retention requirements for health care information. These state requirements should be the basis for the health care organization's formal retention policy. (The Joint Commission and other accrediting agencies also address retention but generally refer organizations back to their own state regulations for specifics.) When no specific retention requirement is made by the state, all patient information that is a part of the LHR should be maintained for at least as long as the state's statute of limitations or other regulation requires. In the case of minor children the LHR should be retained until the child reaches the age of majority as defined by state law, usually eighteen or twenty-one. Health care executives should be aware that statutes of limitations may allow a patient to bring a case as long as ten years after the patient learns that his or her care caused an injury (AHIMA, 2002b). In 2002, AHIMA published "recommended retention standards," which state that patient health records for adults should be retained for ten years after the most recent encounter and patient health records for children should be retained until the time the person reaches the age of majority plus the time stated in the relevant statute of limitations.

Although some specific retention requirements and general guidelines exist, it is becoming increasingly popular for health care organizations to keep all LHR information indefinitely, particularly if the information is stored in an electronic format. If an organization does decide to destroy LHR information, this destruction must be carried out in accordance with all applicable laws and regulations. Some states require that health care organizations create an abstract of the patient record prior to its destruction. Others specify methods of destruction that can be used. If specific methods of destruction are not specified, the health care organization can follow general guidelines, such as those in the following list (AHIMA, 2002a). These destruction guidelines apply to any patient-identifiable health care information, whether or not that information is identified as part of the LHR.

- Destroy the records so there is no possibility of reconstruction.

    Burn, shred, pulp, or pulverize paper.

    Recycle or pulverize microfilm or microfiche.

    Pulverize write-once read-many laser disks.

    Degauss computerized data stored on internal or external magnetic media (that is, alter the magnetic alignment of the storage media, making it impossible to recover previously recorded data).

- Document the destruction.

    Date of destruction.

    Method of destruction.

Description of destroyed records.

Inclusive dates of destroyed records.

A statement that the records were destroyed in the normal course of business.

Signatures of individuals supervising and witnessing the destruction.

- Maintain the destruction documentation indefinitely.

Authentication of Health Record Information

The 2008 *The Joint Commission Hospital Accreditation Manual* defines *authentication* as, "The validation of correctness for both the information itself and for the person who is the author or the user of the information" (The Joint Commission, 2008d). State and federal laws and accreditation standards require that medical record entries be authenticated. This is to ensure that the legal document shows the person or persons responsible for the care provided. Generally, authentication of an LHR entry is accomplished when the physician or other health care professional signs it, either with a handwritten signature or an electronic signature.

Electronic signatures are created when the provider enters a unique code, biometric, or password that verifies his or her identity. Often electronic signatures show up on the computer screen or printout in this form: "Electronically authenticated by Jane H. Doe, M.D." (AHIMA, 2003b). Electronic signatures are now accepted by both The Joint Commission and CMS. State laws and regulations vary on the acceptability of electronic signatures, so it is important that health care organizations know what their respective state laws and regulations are before implementing such signatures. Most states do allow for electronic signatures in some fashion or are silent on the subject.

Regardless of the state laws and regulations, policies and procedures must be adopted by the health care organization to ensure that providers do not share any codes or passwords that are used to produce electronic signatures. Generally, a provider is required to sign a statement that he or she is the only person who has possession of the signature "key" and that he or she will be the only one to use it (AHIMA, 2003b).

Privacy and Confidentiality

Privacy is an individual's constitutional right to be left alone, to be free from unwarranted publicity, and to conduct his or her life without its being made public. In the health care environment, *privacy* is the individual's right to limit access to his or her health care information. *Confidentiality* is the expectation that information shared with a health care provider during the course of treatment will be used only for its intended purpose and not disclosed otherwise. Confidentiality relies on trust.

Recent studies indicate that patients do not fully trust that their private health care information is being kept confidential. A 2005 survey by the California

HealthCare Foundation found that two-thirds of Americans were concerned about the confidentiality of personal health information. Most respondents also reported being "largely unaware of their privacy rights." Further findings of the same survey show that one in eight patients "engages in behavior to protect personal privacy, presenting a potential risk to their health." More than half of the survey respondents were concerned about their employers using health information to limit employment opportunities. The Health Privacy Project (2007) reports that one in five American adults believes that a health care provider, insurance plan, government agency, or employer has improperly disclosed personal medical information. Half of these individuals also reported that the disclosure resulted in embarrassment or harm. This lack of trust exists in spite of state and federal laws and regulations designed to protect patient privacy and confidentiality and in spite of the ethical tenets under which health care providers work.

There are many sources for the legal and ethical requirement that health care professionals maintain the confidentiality of patient information and protect patient privacy. Ethical and professional standards, such as those published by the American Medical Association and other organizations, address professional conduct and the need to hold patient information in confidence. Accrediting bodies, such as those mentioned in the previous section (The Joint Commission, NCQA, and so forth), and the CMS CoPs dictate that health care organizations follow standard practice, state, and federal laws to ensure the confidentiality of patient information. State regulations, as a component of state facility licensure or other statutes, also address confidentiality and privacy. However, the regulations and statutes vary widely from state to state. Protections offered by the states also vary according to the holder of the information and the type of information. For example, state regulations may address the confidentiality of AIDS or sexually transmitted disease (STD) information but remain silent on all other types of health care information. Few states specifically address the redisclosure of information, and the lack of uniformity among states causes difficulty when interstate health care transactions are necessary. In today's environment it is not uncommon for a preferred provider of a technical medical procedure to be out of state. Telemedicine also often requires interstate communication of patient information.

In spite of the existing protections, cases of privacy and confidentiality breaches continue to be documented. A few recent violations reported by the Health Privacy Project (2007) are listed in the accompanying Perspective. Part of the problem is that until recently there was no overarching federal law that outlined privacy rules. Several laws addressed some aspects of keeping patient information confidential, but no single law provided guidance to health care organizations and providers. This lack of a clear federal regulation meant that health information might be released for reasons that had nothing to do with treatment or reimbursement. For example, a health plan could pass information to a lender or employer.

PERSPECTIVE

RECENT HEALTH CARE PRIVACY VIOLATIONS

■ A North Carolina resident was fired from her job after being diagnosed with a genetic disorder that required treatment (2000).

■ The medical records of an Illinois woman were posted on the Internet after she was treated for complications of an abortion (2001).

■ An Atlanta truck driver lost his job after his employer was told by the insurance company that the man had sought alcohol abuse treatment (2000).

■ A hospital clerk in Florida stole Social Security numbers from registered patients. These numbers were used to open bank and credit card accounts (2002).

■ A computer that contained the files of people with AIDS and other STDs was put up for sale by the state of Kentucky (2003).

■ Due to a software flaw, individuals who had requested drug and alcohol treatment information had their names and addresses exposed through a government-run Web site (2001).

■ Two health care organizations in Washington State discarded medical records in unlocked dumpsters (2000).

Source: Adapted from Health Privacy Project, 2007.

This situation changed with the passage of the Health Insurance Portability and Accountability Act (HIPAA) and more specifically the HIPAA Privacy Rule, which was first published in 2000, by the U.S. Department of Health and Human Services, and became effective in its current form in 2003. The Privacy Rule establishes a "floor of safeguards" to protect confidentiality and privacy. In following sections we will outline the current federal laws and regulations that pertain to privacy and confidentiality, up to and including HIPAA.

Federal Privacy Laws Predating HIPAA   In 1966, the Freedom of Information Act (FOIA) was passed. This legislation provides the American public with the right to obtain information from federal agencies. The Act covers all records created by the federal government with nine exceptions. The sixth exception is for personnel and medical information "the disclosure of which would constitute a clearly unwarranted invasion of personal privacy." There was, however, concern that this exception to the FOIA was not strong enough to protect federally created patient records and other health information. Consequently, Congress enacted the Privacy Act of 1974. This Act was written specifically to protect patient confidentiality only in *federally operated* health care facilities, such as Veterans Administration hospitals, Indian Health Service facilities, and military health care organizations. Because the protection was limited to those facilities operated by the federal government, most general hospitals and other nongovernment health care organizations did not have to comply. Nevertheless, the Privacy Act of 1974 was an important piece of legislation, not only because it addressed the FOIA exception for patient information but also because it explicitly stated that patients had a right to access and amend their medical records. It also required facilities to maintain documentation of all disclosures. Neither of these things was standard practice at the time.

During the 1970s, people became increasingly aware of the extrasensitive nature of drug and alcohol treatment records. This led to the regulations currently found in 42 C.F.R. (Code of Federal Regulations) Part 2, Confidentiality of Alcohol and Drug Abuse Patient Records. These regulations have been amended twice, with the latest version published in 1999. They offer specific guidance to health care organizations that treat patients with alcohol or drug problems. Not surprisingly, they set stringent release of information standards, designed to protect the confidentiality of patients seeking alcohol or drug treatment.

HIPAA The HIPAA Privacy Rule is an important federal regulation. It is the first comprehensive federal regulation that offers specific protection to private health information. As we discussed, prior to the HIPAA Privacy Rule there was no single federal regulation governing the privacy and confidentiality of patient-specific information. To put the Privacy Rule in context, we will begin our discussion by briefly outlining the content of the entire Act that authorized this regulation. We will then discuss the specifics of the Privacy Rule and its impact on the maintenance, use, and release of health care information.

The Health Insurance Portability and Accountability Act of 1996 has two main parts:

- Title I addresses health care access, portability, and renewability, offering protection for individuals who change jobs or health insurance policies. Although Title I is an important piece of legislation, it does not address health care information specifically and will therefore not be addressed in this chapter.

- Title II includes a section titled Administrative Simplification. It is in a subsection to this section that the requirement to establish privacy regulations for individually identifiable health information is found. Two additional subsections under Administration Simplification are particularly relevant to health care information: Transaction and Code Sets, standards for which were finalized in 2000, and Security, standards for which were finalized in 2002. (HIPAA security regulations are discussed at length in Chapter Ten.)

HIPAA Privacy Rule Although the HIPAA Privacy Rule is a comprehensive set of federal standards, it permits the enforcement of existing state laws that are more protective of individual privacy, and states are also free to pass more stringent laws in the future. Therefore health care organizations must still be familiar with their own state laws and regulations related to privacy and confidentiality.

The HIPAA Privacy Rule defines *covered entities*, that is, those individuals and organizations that must comply. This definition is broad and includes

- Health plans, which pay or provide for the cost of medical care.

- Health care clearinghouses, which process health information (for example, billing services).

- Health care providers who conduct certain financial and administrative transactions electronically. (These transactions are defined broadly, so that the reality of the HIPAA Privacy Rule is that it governs nearly all health care providers who receive any type of third-party reimbursement.)

If any of these covered entities shares information with others, it must establish contracts to protect the shared information.

HIPAA-protected information is also defined broadly under the Privacy Rule. *Protected health information* (PHI) is information that

- Relates to a person's physical or mental health, the provision of health care, or the payment for health care

- Identifies the person who is the subject of the information

- Is created or *received* by a covered entity

- Is transmitted or maintained in *any* form (paper, electronic, or oral)

There are five major components to the HIPAA Privacy Rule:

1. *Boundaries.* PHI may be disclosed for health purposes only, with very limited exceptions.

2. *Security.* PHI should not be distributed without patient authorization, unless there is a clear basis for doing so, and the individuals who receive the information must safeguard it.

3. *Consumer control.* Individuals are entitled to access and control their health records and are to be informed of the purposes for which information is being disclosed and used.

4. *Accountability.* Entities that improperly handle PHI can be charged under criminal law and punished and are subject to civil recourse as well.

5. *Public responsibility.* Individual interests must not override national priorities in public health, medical research, preventing health care fraud, and law enforcement in general (CMS, 2002).

The HIPAA Privacy Rule is relatively new, and as such, it has not been extensively tested by the U.S. legal system. As has occurred with other federal regulations, this rule is likely to undergo some modification or amendment. The tension it sets up inside health care organizations is between the need to *protect* patient information and the need to *use* patient information. Thinking back to Chapter One, remember the purposes for maintaining patient-specific health information. The number one reason is patient care; however, there are other legitimate reasons for sharing or "releasing" identifiable health information.

Release of Information

Because of the various state and federal laws and regulations that exist to protect patient-specific information, health care organizations must have comprehensive release of information policies and procedures in place that ensure compliance. Exhibit 3.5 is a sample of a release of information form used by a hospital, showing the elements that should be present on a valid release form:

- Patient identification (name and date of birth)

- Name of the person or entity to whom the information is being released

- Description of the specific health information authorized for disclosure

- Statement of the reason for or purpose of the disclosure

- Date, event, or condition on which the authorization will expire, unless it is revoked earlier

- Statement that the authorization is subject to revocation by the patient or the patient's legal representative

- Patient's or legal representative's signature

- Signature date, which must be *after the date of the encounter that produced the information to be released*

Health care organizations need clear policies and procedures for releasing patient-identifiable information. There should be a central point of control through which all nonroutine requests for information pass, and all of these disclosures should be well documented.

In some instances patient-specific health care information can be released without the patient's authorization. For example, some state laws require disclosing certain health information. It is always good practice to obtain a patient authorization prior to releasing information when feasible, but in state-mandated cases it is not required. Some examples of situations in which information might need to be disclosed to authorized recipients without the patient's consent are the presence of a communicable disease, such as AIDS and STDs, that must be reported to the state or county department of health; suspected child abuse or adult abuse that must be reported to designated authorities; situations in which there is a legal duty to warn another person of a clear and imminent danger from a patient; bona fide medical emergencies; and the existence of a valid court order.

In addition to situations mandated by law, there are other instances in which patient information can be released without an authorization. In general, health information can be released to another health care provider who is directly involved in the care of the patient, but the regulations governing this may vary from state to state. Information can also be released to other authorized persons within a health care organization to

EXHIBIT 3.5. *Sample Release of Information Form*

MUSC
MEDICAL UNIVERSITY
OF SOUTH CAROLINA

AUTHORIZATION TO DISCLOSE PROTECTED HEALTH INFORMATION

Patient Name: _____   Date of Birth: _____

Medical Record Number: _____   Social Security Number: _____

I authorize MUSC Medical Center and/or Charleston Memorial Hospital to disclose/release information on the above named individual.

The type of information to be disclosed is as follows:
☐ problem list   ☐ medication list   ☐ laboratory results   ☐ physician progress note / visit notes   ☐ consultation reports
☐ list of allergies   ☐ immunization record   ☐ radiology reports   ☐ nurses notes   ☐ entire record
☐ history and physical   ☐ discharge summary   ☐ films / images   ☐ physician orders   ☐ other_____

For dates of service: _____

I understand this information may include reference to (check all that apply):
☐ psychiatric/psychological care   **☐ drug abuse and/or**
☐ sexual assault   **☐ results of tests for all infectious diseases including HIV/AIDS.**
☐ alcohol abuse and/or

I authorize the disclosure of this information via (check preferred method):
☐ mail ☐ fax ☐ e-mail ☐ other_____

The information is to be disclosed to: Name of individual/organization: _____

_____

Street address:_____ City:_____ State:_____ Zip code:_____

Phone number: _____ Fax number:_____ E-mail address:_____

The purpose of the disclosure is: _____

I understand that I have a right to cancel/revoke this authorization at any time. I understand that if I cancel/revoke this authorization I must do so in writing and present my written cancellation/revocation to the Health Information Services Department (Medical Records). I understand that the cancellation/revocation will not apply to information, which has already been released in response to this authorization as stated in the Notice of Privacy Practice. Unless otherwise canceled/revoked this authorization will expire/end 90 days from this date.

I understand that a reasonable, cost-based fee for copies of protected health information and postage fees will be charged.

I understand that authorizing the disclosure of protected health information is voluntary. I can refuse to sign this authorization. I do not need to sign this form to receive treatment. I understand I may review and/or copy the information to be disclosed, as provided in CFR 164.524. I understand that any disclosure of information carries with it the possibility of unauthorized disclosure by the person/organization receiving the information. If I have questions about the disclosure or use of my protected health information, I may contact the MUSC Patient and Family Liaison. The number is (843) 792-5555.

I understand I will be given a copy of this authorization.

I understand that if this information is requested in person I will be asked to provide picture identification (e.g. driver's license). A copy of my identification will be made and attached to this authorization.

_____   _____
Signature of Patient or Legal Guardian/Representative   Date

_____
Printed Name of Patient or Legal Guardian/Representative

_____   _____
Relationship to Patient, if signed by legal guardian/representative   Witness Signature

Description of patient representative's authority: _____
(Why patient not signing)
To contact Health Information Services (Medical Records) in writing the address is: 169 Ashley Avenue / PO Box 250349 / Attention: Release of Information / Charleston, South Carolina 29425; the phone number is (843) 792-3881.

facilitate patient care. Information can also be used by the organization for billing or reimbursement purposes once a patient signs a proper consent form for treatment. It may be released for medical research purposes provided all patient identifiers have been removed.

The HIPAA rule attempts to sort out the routine and nonroutine use of health information by distinguishing between patient *consent* to use PHI and patient *authorization* to release PHI. Health care providers and others must obtain a patient's written consent prior to disclosure of health information for routine uses of treatment, payment, and health care operations. There are some exceptions to this in emergency situations, and the patient has a right to request restrictions on the disclosure. However, health care providers can deny treatment if they feel that limiting the disclosure would be detrimental. Health care providers and others must obtain the patient's written authorization for nonroutine uses or disclosures of PHI. This authorization for release of information has more details than a consent form (see Exhibit 3.5 and the list of necessary elements given earlier), sets an expiration date, and states specifically what, to whom, and for what purpose information is being disclosed (CMS, 2002).

SUMMARY

In this chapter we examined a number of external drivers that dictate not only the types of health care information that health care organizations maintain but also the way in which they are maintained. These external forces include federal and state laws and regulations and voluntary accreditation standards. Specifically, this chapter was divided into two main sections. In the first section we defined licensure, certification, and accreditation and examined some of the

missions and the general functions of several major accrediting organizations. In the second section we looked at legal issues in managing health care information, including state and federal laws that address the use of the patient medical record as a legal document and current laws and regulations that govern patient privacy and confidentiality. This chapter concluded with discussions of the HIPAA Privacy Rule and release of information practices.

KEY TERMS

42 C.F.R. (Code of Federal Regulations) Part 2, Confidentiality of Alcohol and Drug Abuse Patient Records
Accreditation
Accreditation Association for Ambulatory Health Care (AAAHC)
Authentication
Centers for Medicare and Medicaid Services (CMS)
Certification

Commission on Accreditation of Rehabilitation Facilities (CARF)
Conditions of Participation
Confidentiality
Covered entities
Freedom of Information Act (FOIA)
Health Insurance Portability and Accountability Act (HIPAA)
HIPAA Privacy Rule
Laws
Legal health record

Licensure
National Committee for Quality
  Assurance (NCQA)
Privacy
Privacy Act of 1974
Protected health information (PHI)

Record Retention
Regulations
Release of Information
Standards
U.S. Department of Health and Human
  Services (DHHS)

LEARNING ACTIVITIES

1. Visit a health care organization to find out about its current licensure, accreditation, and certification status. How are these processes related to one another in your state?

2. Visit the CMS Web site: www.cms.gov. Find the Conditions of Participation for a particular type of health care facility (hospital, nursing home, and so forth). Review this document and comment on the standards. Are they minimal or optimal standards? Support your answer.

3. Visit the Joint Commission Web site: www.jcaho.org. What accreditation programs other than the Hospital Accreditation Program does The Joint Commission have? List the programs and their respective missions.

4. Visit the NCQA Web site: www.ncqa.org. Look up a health care plan with which you are familiar. What does the report card tell you about this plan?

5. Do an Internet or library search for a recent article discussing the impact of the HIPAA privacy regulations on health care practice. Write a summary of the article.

6. Contact a health care facility (hospital, nursing home, physician's office, or other organization) to talk with the person responsible for maintaining patient records. Ask about the organization's release of information, retention, and destruction policies.

PART

2

HEALTH CARE INFORMATION SYSTEMS

CHAPTER

4

HISTORY AND EVOLUTION OF HEALTH CARE INFORMATION SYSTEMS

LEARNING OBJECTIVES

- To be able to describe the history and evolution of health care information systems from the 1960s to the present.
- To be able to identify the major advances in information technology and significant federal initiatives that influenced the adoption of health care information systems.
- To be able to identify the major types of administrative and clinical information systems used in health care.
- To be able to discuss why information technology (IT) adoption rates are lower in health care compared with other industries.
- To be able to discuss the relationship between incentives and health care IT adoption and use.

After reading Chapters One, Two, and Three (or from your own previous experience), you should have an understanding of the nature of health care information and the processes and regulations that influence the management of information in health care organizations. In this chapter we build upon these fundamental concepts and introduce *health care information systems*, a broad category that includes both administrative and clinical applications. We describe how health care information systems have evolved during the past fifty years. Much of this evolution can be attributed to environmental factors, changes in reimbursement practices, and major advances in information technology. Over the years the health care executive's role and involvement in making information systems–related decisions have also changed considerably. We discuss these changes and conclude by describing the challenges many organizations face as they try to integrate data from various health care applications and to get clinical and administrative applications to interoperate, or "talk," with each other.

DEFINITION OF TERMS

Health care executives interact frequently with professionals from a variety of disciplines and may find the terminology used confusing or intimidating. It's no wonder. Most professional disciplines have their own terminology to describe concepts related to their normal course of business. Even professionals within a single discipline often use different terms to describe the same concepts and the same terms to describe different concepts! Throughout the remainder of this book we will use a variety of terms related to information systems. Our goal is to expose you to many of the information technology–related terms you are likely to encounter in discussions with your organization's chief information officer, information technology (IT) staff, and IT-savvy health care professionals.

An *information system* (IS) is an arrangement of information (data), processes, people, and information technology that interact to collect, process, store, and provide as output the information needed to support the organization (Whitten & Bentley, 2005). Note that information technology is a component of every information system. *Information technology* is a contemporary term that describes the combination of computer technology (hardware and software) with data and telecommunications technology (data, image, and voice networks). Often in current management literature the terms *information system* and *information technology* are used interchangeably.

In health care the *organization* is the hospital, the physician practice, the integrated delivery system, the nursing home, or the rural health clinic. That is, it is any setting where health-related services are provided. Thus a *health care information system* (HCIS) is an arrangement of information (data), processes, people, and information technology that interact to collect, process, store, and provide as output the information needed to support the *health care* organization.

This definition of an HCIS is congruent with the definitions of *data* and *information* provided in Chapter Two. Data are raw facts about people, places, events, and things that are of importance in an organization. Information is data that have been processed or reorganized into a more meaningful form for the user; information can lead to knowledge and facilitate decision making. To simplify, we will assume that the information in a health care information system is made up of both raw and processed data.

There are two primary classes of health care information systems, *administrative* and *clinical*. A simple way to distinguish them is by purpose and the type of data they contain. An *administrative information system* (or an *administrative application*) contains primarily administrative or financial data and is generally used to support the management functions and general operations of the health care organization. For example, an administrative information system might contain information used to manage personnel, finances, materials, supplies, or equipment. It might be a system for human resource management, materials management, patient accounting or billing, or staff scheduling. In contrast a *clinical information system* (or *clinical application*) contains clinical or health-related information used by providers in diagnosing and treating a patient and monitoring that patient's care. Clinical information systems may be departmental systems—such as radiology, pharmacy, or laboratory systems—or clinical decision-support, medication administration, computerized provider order entry, or electronic medical record systems, to name a few. They may be limited in their scope to a single area of clinical information (for example, radiology, pharmacy, or laboratory), or they may be comprehensive and cover virtually all aspects of patient care (as an electronic medical record system does, for example). Clinical information systems will be discussed more fully in Chapter Five. They are presented here in the context of their role in the history and evolution of health care information systems. Table 4.1 lists common types of clinical and administrative health care information systems.

HISTORY AND EVOLUTION

The history of the development and implementation of information systems in health care is most meaningful when considered in the context of a chronology of major health care sector and information technology events. In this section we explore the history and evolution of health care information systems in each of the past four decades and in the present era by asking several key questions:

- What was happening in the health care environment and at the federal level that influenced organizations to adopt or use computerized systems?

- What was the state of information technology at the time?

- How did the environmental factors, coupled with advances in information technology, affect the adoption and use of health care information systems?

We start with the 1960s and move forward to the current day (see Table 4.2).

1960s: Billing Is the Center of the Universe; Managing the Money; Mainframes Roam the Planet

It was in the mid-1960s that President Lyndon Johnson signed into law Medicare and Medicaid. These two federal programs provided, for the first time, guaranteed health care insurance benefits to the elderly and the poor. Initially, Medicare provided health care benefits primarily to individuals sixty-five and older. The program has since been

TABLE 4.1. Common Types of Administrative and Clinical Information Systems

Administrative Applications	Clinical Applications
Patient administration systems	**Ancillary information systems**
Admission, discharge, transfer (ADT): tracks the patient's movement of care in an inpatient setting	*Laboratory information:* supports collection, verification, and reporting of laboratory tests
Registration: may be coupled with ADT system; includes patient demographic and insurance information as well as date of visit(s), provider information	*Radiology information:* supports digital image generation (picture archiving and communication systems [PACS]), image analysis, image management
Scheduling: aids in the scheduling of patient visits; includes information on patients, providers, date and time of visit, rooms, equipment, other resources	*Pharmacy information:* supports medication ordering, dispensing, and inventory control; drug compatibility checks; allergy screening; medication administration
Patient billing or accounts receivable: includes all information needed to submit claims and monitor submission and reimbursement status	**Other clinical information systems**
Utilization management: tracks use and appropriateness of care	*Nursing documentation:* facilitates nursing documentation from assessment to evaluation, patient care decision support (care planning, assessment, flow-sheet charting, patient acuity, patient education)
Other administrative and financial systems	*Electronic medical record (EMR):* facilitates electronic capture and reporting of patient's health history, problem lists, treatment and outcomes; allows clinicians to document clinical findings, progress notes, and other patient information; provides decision-support tools and reminders and alerts
Accounts payable: monitors debts incurred by the organization and status of purchases	
General ledger: monitors general financial management and reporting	*Computerized provider order entry (CPOE):* enables clinicians to directly enter orders electronically and access decision-support tools and clinical care guidelines and protocols
Personnel management: manages human resource information for staff, including salaries, benefits, education, training	
Materials management: monitors ordering and inventory of supplies, equipment needs and maintenance	*Telemedicine and telehealth:* supports remote delivery of care; common features include image capture and transmission, voice and video conferencing, text messaging
Payroll: manages information about staff salaries, payroll deductions, tax withholding, pay status	*Rehabilitation service documentation:* supports the capturing and reporting of occupational therapy, physical therapy, and speech pathology services
Staff scheduling: assists in scheduling and monitoring staffing needs	
Staff time and attendance: tracks employee work schedules and attendance	*Medication administration:* typically used by nurses to document medication given, dose, and time

TABLE 4.2. **Timeline of Major Events + Advances in Information Technology = HCIS**

Decade	Health Care Environment	State of Information Technology	Use of Health Care Information Systems
1960s	Enactment of Medicare and Medicaid Cost-based reimbursement "Building" mode Focus on financial needs and capturing revenues	Large mainframe computers Centralized processing Few vendor-developed products	Administrative or financial information systems used primarily in large hospitals and academic medical centers ■ Developed and maintained in-house ■ Shared systems available to smaller hospitals Centralized data processing
1970s	Still time of growth Medicare and Medicaid expenditures rising Late in decade, recognition of need to contain health care costs	Mainframes still in use Minicomputers become available, smaller, more affordable	Turnkey systems available through vendor community Increased interest in clinical applications (for example, laboratory, radiology, pharmacy) Shared systems still used
1980s	Medicare introduces prospective payment system for hospitals Medicaid and private insurers follow suit Need for financial and clinical information	Microcomputer or personal computer (PC) becomes available—far more powerful, affordable; brings computing power to desktop; revolutionizes how companies process data and do business Advent of local area networks	Distributed data processing Expansion of clinical information systems in hospitals Physician practices introduce billing systems Integrating financial and administrative information becomes important

(Continued)

TABLE 4.2. *(Continued)*

Decade	Health Care Environment	State of Information Technology	Use of Health Care Information Systems
1990s	Medicare changes physician reimbursement to a resource-based relative value scale (RBRVS) Health care reform efforts of Clinton era (HIPAA) Growth of managed care and integrated delivery systems Institute of Medicine (IOM) calls for computer-based patient record (CPR) adoption	Unveiling of the Internet and World Wide Web—revolutionizes how organizations communicate with each other, market services, conduct business	Growth of Internet has profound effect on health care organizations business Vendor community explodes Products more widely available and affordable Enterprise-wide systems Increased interest in clinical application Relatively small percentage of health care organizations adopt CPR
2000+	IOM report on patient safety and medical errors Both President Bush and President Obama call for electronic health record (EHR) adoption HIPAA privacy and security regulations in effect Leapfrog Group Medicare Modernization Act Transparency on quality and price; consumer empowerment Pay for performance	Internet expansion continues Broadband access in rural areas Portable devices become more widespread (including multipurpose cell phones) Bar coding Advances in voice and handwriting recognition Wireless technology Podcasts, wikis, Web 2.0 technologies Standards and connectivity	Focus on EHR systems Vendors promote CCHIT certification Health care organizations invest in information systems that promote safety (for example, CPOE, medication administration, e-prescribing, and other decision-support systems) Personal health record (offered by insurers, Google, and Microsoft) Health information exchange activities promulgated

Decade	Health Care Environment	State of Information Technology	Use of Health Care Information Systems
	Funding for health information technology (HIT) initiatives	Radio-frequency identification devices (RFIDs)	
	Certification Commission for Healthcare Information Technology (CCHIT) certification of EHR products		
	Reimbursement practices changing to include telehealth		
	Physician Quality Report Initiative launched		

expanded to provide health care coverage to individuals with long-term disabilities. Through a combination of federal and state funds, the Medicaid program provides health care coverage to the poor. Initially, both of these programs reimbursed hospitals for services using a cost-based reimbursement methodology. Basically, this meant hospitals were reimbursed for services based on their financial cost reports; in other words, they received a percentage above what they reported it cost them to render the services. Hospitals at that time were also still benefiting from the funds made available through the Hospital Survey and Construction Act (also known as the Hill-Burton Act) of 1946, which had provided them with easier access to capital to build new facilities and expand their services. In these cost-based reimbursement times, the more a hospital built, the more patients it served, and the longer the patients stayed, the more revenue the hospital generated.

Health care executives realized that to capitalize on these sources of funds, their organizations needed information systems that could automate the patient billing process and facilitate accurate cost reporting. Most of the early information systems in health care were therefore administrative applications almost exclusively driven by financial needs. The primary focus was to collect and process patient demographic data and insurance information and merge it with charge data to produce patient bills. The sooner the hospital could bill Medicare or Medicaid, the sooner it could get paid for services. Patient accounting systems also enabled hospitals to keep better records of all activities, reducing the amounts of *lost charges* and *unbilled services*. Revenue reports and volume of service statistics were needed to justify new capital equipment, just as billing, accounts receivable, and general ledger data were needed for reimbursement. Few clinical data were captured by these information systems.

The administrative applications that existed in the 1960s were generally found in large hospitals, such as those affiliated with academic medical centers. These larger facilities were often the only ones with the resources and staff available to develop, implement, and support such systems. These facilities often developed their own administrative or financial information systems in-house, in what were then known as data processing departments. Reflecting its primary purpose, the data processing department was generally under the direction of the finance department or chief financial officer. The data processing department got its name from the fact that the systems were transaction based, with the primary function of processing billing data.

These early administrative and financial applications ran on large *mainframe* computers (Figure 4.1), which had to be housed in large rooms, with sufficient environmental controls and staff to support them. Because the IS focus at the time was on automating manual administrative processes and computers were so expensive, only the largest,

FIGURE 4.1. *Typical Mainframe Computer*

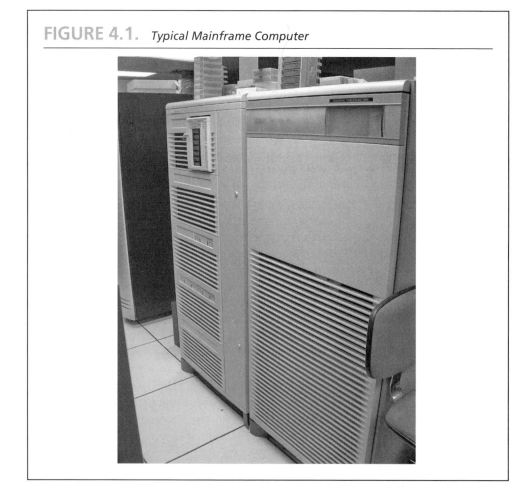

Source: Medical University of South Carolina.

most complex tasks were candidates for mainframe computing. The high cost limited the development of departmental or clinical systems, although there were notable efforts in this direction, such as the Technicon system at El Camino Hospital. The mainframe was also associated with centralized rather than distributed computing. Centralized computing meant that end users entered data through *dumb* terminals, which were connected to a remote computer, the mainframe, where the data were processed. A dumb terminal had no processing power itself but was simply a device for entering data and viewing results.

Recognizing that small, community-based hospitals could not bear the high cost of an in-house, mainframe system, leading vendors began to offer *shared systems*, so called because they allowed hospitals to share the use of a mainframe with other hospitals. A hospital using a shared system captured billing data manually or electronically and sent them in *batch* form to a company that then processed the claims for the hospital. Most shared systems processed data in a central or regional data center. Shared Medical Systems (now known as Siemens), located in Malvern, Pennsylvania, was one of the first vendors to offer data processing services to hospitals. These vendors charged participating hospitals for computer time and storage, for the number of terminals connected, and for reports. Like many of the in-house systems, most shared systems began with financial and patient accounting functions and gradually migrated toward clinical functions, or applications.

1970s: Clinical Departments Wake Up; Debut of the Minicomputer

By the 1970s, health care costs were escalating rapidly, partially due to high Medicare and Medicaid expenditures. Rapid inflation in the economy, expansion of hospital expenses and profits, and changes in medical care, including greater use of technology, medications, and conservative approaches to treatment also contributed to the spiraling health care costs. Health care organizations began to recognize the need for better access to clinical information for specific departments and for the facility as a whole. Departmental systems began to emerge as a way to improve productivity and capture charges and thereby maximize revenues.

The development of departmental systems coincided with the availability of *minicomputers*. Minicomputers were smaller and also more powerful than some mainframe computers and available at a cost that could be justified by a clinical department such as laboratory or pharmacy. At the same time, improvements in handling clinical data and specimens often showed a direct impact on the quality of patient care because of faster turnaround of tests, more accurate results, and a reduction in the number of repeat procedures (Kennedy & Davis, 1992). The increased demand for patient-specific data coupled with the availability of relatively low-cost minicomputers opened a market for a host of new companies that wanted to develop applications for clinical departments, particularly *turnkey systems*. These software systems, which were developed by a vendor and installed on a hospital's computers, were known as turnkey systems because all a health care organization had to do was turn the system on and it was fully operational. Rarely could a turnkey system be modified to meet the unique information needs of an organization, however. What you saw was essentially what you got.

As in the 1960s, the health care executive's involvement in information system–related decisions was generally limited to working to secure the funds needed to acquire new information systems, although now executives were working with individual clinical as well as administrative departments on this issue. Most systems were still stand-alone and did not interface well with other administrative or clinical information systems in the organization.

1980s: Computers for the Masses; Age of the Cheap Machine; Arrival of the Computer Utility

Although the use of health care information systems in the 1970s could be considered an extension of the applications used in the 1960s with a slight increase in the use of clinical applications, the 1980s saw an entirely different story. Sweeping changes in how Medicare reimbursed hospitals and others for services, coupled with the advent of the microcomputer, radically changed how health care information systems were viewed and used. In 1982, Medicare shifted from a cost-based reimbursement system for hospitals to a prospective payment system based on *diagnosis related groups* (DRGs). This new payment system had a profound effect on hospital billing practices. Reimbursement amounts were now dependent on the patient's diagnosis, and the accuracy of the ICD-9-CM codes used for each patient and his or her subsequent DRG assignment became critical. Hospitals received a predetermined amount based on the patient's DRG, regardless of the cost to treat that patient. The building and revenue enhancement mode of the 1960s and 1970s was no longer always the best strategy for a hospital financially. The incentives were now directed at ordering fewer diagnostic tests, performing fewer therapeutic procedures, and planning for the patient's discharge at the time of admission. Health care executives knew they needed to reduce expenses and maximize reimbursement. Services that had once been available only in hospitals now became more widespread in less resource-intensive outpatient settings and ambulatory surgery centers. As Medicare and many state Medicaid programs began to reimburse hospitals under the DRG-based system, many private insurance plans quickly followed suit.

Hospitals were not the only ones singled out to contain health care costs. Overall health care costs in the 1980s rose by double the rate of inflation. Health insurance companies argued that the traditional *fee-for-service* method of payment to physicians failed to promote cost containment. Managed care plans began to emerge in parts of the nation, and they reimbursed physicians based on *capitated* or fixed rates.

At the same time, as changes were made in reimbursement practices, large corporations began to integrate the organizations making up the hospital system (previously a decentralized industry), enter many other health care–related businesses, and consolidate control. Overall there was a shift toward privatization and corporatization of health care. The integrated delivery system began to emerge, whereby health care organizations offered a spectrum of health care services, from ambulatory care to acute hospital care to long-term care and rehabilitation.

With these environmental changes happening in health care, the development of the *microcomputer* in the mid-1980s could not have been more timely. The microcomputer, or personal computer (PC), was smaller, often as or more powerful, and far more affordable than a mainframe computer. Health care information system vendors were developing administrative and clinical applications for a variety of health care settings and touting the possibilities available in bringing "real computing power" to the user at his or her workstation. Health care executives viewed this as an enormous opportunity for health care organizations, particularly hospitals, to acquire and implement needed clinical information systems. Again, the major focus was on revenue-generating departments.

Although most organizations had patient demographic and insurance information available in their administrative applications, rarely were they able to integrate the clinical and the financial information needed to evaluate care and the cost of delivering that care in this new environment. Most of the clinical information systems or applications were being acquired piecemeal. For example, it was not uncommon for the director of laboratory services to go out and purchase from the vendor community the "best" laboratory information system, the pharmacy director to select the "best" pharmacy system, and so forth. This concept of selecting the "best of breed" among vendors and systems became prevalent in the 1980s and still exists to some extent today. Organizations that adopted the best-of-breed approach then faced a challenge when they tried to build interfaces or integrate data so that the different systems could interoperate, or communicate with each other. Even today, system integration remains a challenge for many health care organizations despite progress in the use of interoperability standards.

The use of microcomputers was not confined to large hospitals. During this era a computer market opened among home health organizations, small hospital departments, and physician practices. These health care settings had historically lacked the financial and personnel resources to support information systems. The advent of the microcomputer brought computing capabilities to a host of these smaller organizations. It also led to users' being more demanding of information systems, asking the information system function to be more responsive.

Sharing information among microcomputers also became possible with the development of *local area networks*. A local area network (LAN) is a group of computers and associated devices that are controlled by a single organization. Usually, one or more *servers* houses applications and data storage that are then shared by multiple PC users. A LAN may serve as few as two or three users (for example, in a home network) or as many as thousands of users (for example, in a large academic medical center). Specific LAN technologies will be discussed in Chapter Eight.

1990s: Health Care Reform Initiatives; Advent of the Internet

The 1990s marked another time of great change in health care. It also marked the evolution and widespread use of the Internet along with a new focus on electronic medical records. In 1992, owing partly to the success of the DRG-based reimbursement system for hospitals, Medicare introduced a new method for reimbursing physicians. Formerly paid under a customary, prevailing, and reasonable rate methodology, physicians treating Medicare patients were now reimbursed for services under the *resource-based relative value scale* (RBRVS). The RBRVS payment method factored provider time, effort, and degree of clinical decision making into relative value units. RBRVS was initially designed to redistribute funds from specialty providers to primary care providers. That is, the system would reward financially the physicians who spent time educating patients but would discourage or limit reimbursement to highly skilled specialists who tended to perform invasive procedures and order an extensive number of diagnostic and therapeutic tests.

Under the RBRVS system, primary care physicians such as family medicine, internal medicine, and pediatric physicians began to see slight increases in reimbursement for their services, and specialty physicians such as ophthalmologists, surgeons, and radiologists experienced decreases in payments. In addition to this new payment scheme for physicians, health care organizations and communities promoted preventive medicine with the goal of promoting health and well-being and preventing disease. Much of this preventive medicine and health promotion occurred in the primary care physician's practice. The emphasis on preventive medicine was the foundation on which the concept of managed care was built. The thought was that if we educate and help keep patients well, the overall cost of providing health care services will be lower in the long run. The primary care provider was viewed as the *gatekeeper* and assumed a pivotal role in the management of the patient's care. Under this managed care model, physicians were reimbursed on a capitated or fixed rate (for example, per member per month) or some type of discounted rate (for example, preferred provider).

The changes in physician reimbursement and the increased focus on prevention guidelines and disease management in the 1990s had implications for the community-based physician practice and its use of information systems. Up until this time, most of the major information systems development had occurred in hospitals. Some administrative information systems were used in physician practices for billing purposes, but as physician payment relied increasingly on documentation substantiated in the patient's record and as computers became more affordable, physicians began to recognize the need for timely, accurate, and complete financial *and* clinical information. Early adopters of clinical information systems also found electronic prompts and preventive health reminders helpful in managing patient care more effectively and efficiently. Likewise, more vendor products designed specifically with the physician practice setting in mind were becoming available.

Health plans, particularly those with a managed care focus, began encouraging health care providers to manage the care of patients differently, particularly patients with chronic diseases. Practice guidelines and standards of care were developed and made available to physicians to use in caring for these patients. Subsequently, several vendors developed electronic *disease management programs* that facilitated the management of chronic diseases and were incorporated into clinical applications. Patients could assume a more active role in monitoring their own care. For example, clinicians at a Partners Community Hospital introduced a disease management program called Matrix that enables providers to plan, deliver, monitor, and improve the quality and outcomes of the treatment and care delivered to patients with diabetes. This program gives clinicians the tools to automate the planning and delivery of patient care as well as monitor and analyze clinical results on an ongoing basis. Disease management programs have also been shown to be effective in helping providers and patients manage mental health issues and conditions such as hypertension, asthma, and unstable angina (Raymond & Dold, 2002).

In 1991, the Institute of Medicine (IOM) published its landmark report *The Computer-Based Patient Record: An Essential Technology for Health Care.* This report brought international attention to the numerous problems inherent in paper-based medical records and called for the adoption of the computer-based patient record (CPR) as the standard by the year 2001. The IOM defined the CPR as "an electronic patient record that resides in a system specifically designed to support users by providing accessibility to complete and accurate data, alerts, reminders, clinical decision support systems, links to medical knowledge, and other aids" (IOM, 1991, p. 11). This vision of a patient's record offered far more than an electronic version of existing paper records—the IOM report viewed the CPR as a tool to assist the clinician in caring for the patient by providing him or her with reminders, alerts, clinical decision-support capabilities, and access to the latest research findings on a particular diagnosis or treatment modality. We will discuss the status of CPR systems and related concepts (for example, the electronic medical record and the electronic health record) in the next chapter. At this point in the history and evolution of health care information systems, it is important to understand the IOM report's impact on the vendor community and health care organizations. Leading vendors and health care organizations saw this report as an impetus toward radically changing the ways in which patient information is managed and patient care is delivered. During the 1990s, a number of vendors developed CPR systems. Yet only 10 percent of hospitals and less than 15 percent of physician practices had implemented them by the end of the decade (Goldsmith, 2003). These percentages are particularly low when one considers the fact that by the late 1990s, CPR systems had reached the stage of reliability and technical maturity needed for widespread adoption in health care.

Five years after the IOM report advocating computer-based patient records was published, President Clinton signed into law the Health Insurance Portability and Accountability Act (HIPAA) of 1996. HIPAA was designed to make health insurance more affordable and accessible, but it also included important provisions to simplify administrative processes and to protect the confidentiality of personal health information. All of these initiatives were part of a larger health care reform effort and a federal interest in health care IT for purposes beyond reimbursement. Before HIPAA, it was not uncommon for health care organizations and health plans to use an array of systems to process and track patient bills and other information. Health care organizations provided services to patients with many different types of health insurance and had to spend considerable time and resources to make sure each claim contained the proper format, codes, and other details required by the insurer. Likewise, health plans spent time and resources to ensure their systems could handle transactions from a host of different health care organizations, providers, and clearinghouses. The adoption of electronic transaction and code set standards and the greater use of standardized electronic transactions is expected to produce significant savings to the health care sector. In addition, the administrative simplification provisions led to the establishment of health privacy and security standards which went into effect in 2001 and 2003, respectively. It may be years before the full impact of HIPAA legislation on the health care sector is realized.

HIPAA also brought national attention to the issues surrounding the use of personal health information in electronic form. During the first half of the 1990s, microcomputers had become smaller and less expensive and were to be found not only in the workplace but in the homes of middle-class America. The Internet, historically used primarily by the U.S. Department of Defense and academic researchers, was now widely available, through the World Wide Web, to consumers, businesses, and virtually anyone with a microcomputer and a modem. Health care organizations, providers, and patients could connect to the Internet and have access to a worldwide library of resources—and at times to patient-specific health information. In the early years of its use in health care, many health care organizations and vendors used the Internet to market their services, provide health information resources to consumers, and give clinicians access to the latest research and treatment findings. Other health care organizations saw Internet use as a strategy for changing how, where, and when they delivered health care services. The overall effects of Internet resources and capabilities on health care may not be fully realized for decades to come. We do know, however, that the Internet has provided affordable and nearly universal connectivity, enabling health care organizations, providers, and patients to connect to each other and the rest of the health care system. Along with the microcomputer, the Internet is perhaps the single greatest technological advancement in this era. It revolutionized the way that consumers, providers, and health care organizations access health information, communicate with each other, and conduct business. Health futurist Jeff Goldsmith (2003) describes the Internet as "a technology enabler or, in military jargon, a force multiplier, that helps lower communications and transaction cost, time and complexity. It is also a lubricant of information flow and a solvent of organizational boundaries. It may take at least another decade before the health system realizes the full extent of its transformative potential" (pp. 30–31).

With the advent of the Internet and the availability of microcomputers, came *electronic mail* (e-mail). Consumers began to use e-mail to communicate with colleagues, businesses, family, and friends. It substantially reduced or eliminated needs for telephone calls and regular mail. E-mail is fast, easy to use, and fairly widespread. Consumers soon discovered that they could not only search the Internet for the latest information on a particular condition but could then also e-mail that information or questions to their physicians. In a 2000 survey of e-mail users, although only 6 percent of participants reported sending an e-mail message to their physician, more than half wished to do so (Baker, Wagner, Singer, & Bundorf, 2003). MacDonald (2003) and others (Moyer, Stern, Dobias, Cox, & Katz, 2002) have found that many patients are beginning to use e-mail and other online communications and are dragging their physicians along.

The use of *telemedicine* and *telehealth* has also become more prevalent during the past few decades, particularly during the 1990s with its major advancements in telecommunications. Telemedicine is the use of telecommunications for the clinical care of patients and may involve various types of electronic delivery mechanisms. It is a tool that enables providers to deliver health care services to patients at distant locations. Most telemedicine programs have been pilot programs or demonstration projects that have not endured beyond the life of specific research and development funding initiatives. Reimbursement policies for these services vary, and that has been a significant limiting factor. In 2003, federal legislation allowed health care organizations to be reimbursed for professional consultations via telecommunication systems with specific clinicians when patients are seen at qualifying sites. State reimbursement policies for telemedicine for Medicaid patients vary from state to state. And local third-party payers have individual practices for reimbursing for telemedicine services (American Telemedicine Association, 2003). Until reimbursement issues are addressed at the federal, state, and local levels, the future of telemedicine and telehealth is uncertain.

2000 to Today: Health Care IT Arrives; Patients Take Center Stage

Health care quality and patient safety emerge as top priorities at the start of the millennium. In 2000, the IOM published the report *To Err Is Human: Building a Safer Health Care System*, which brought national attention to research estimating that 98,000 patients die each year due to medical errors. A subsequent report by the Institute of Medicine Committee on Data Standards for Patient Safety, *Patient Safety: Achieving a New Standard for Care* (2004), called for health care organizations to adopt information technology capable of collecting and sharing essential health information on patients and their care. This IOM committee examined the status of standards, including standards for health data interchange, terminologies, and medical knowledge representation. Here is an example of the committee's conclusions.

As concerns about patient safety have grown, the health care sector has looked to other industries that have confronted similar challenges, in particular, to the airline industry. This industry learned long ago that information and clear communications are critical to the safe navigation of an airplane. To perform their jobs well and guide their plane safely to its destination, pilots must communicate with the airport controller concerning their destination and current circumstances (e.g., mechanical or other problems), their flight plan, and environmental factors (e.g., weather conditions) that could necessitate a change in course. Information must also pass seamlessly from one controller to another to ensure a safe and smooth journey for planes flying long distances; provide notification of airport delays or closures due to weather conditions; and enable rapid alert and response to extenuating circumstance, such as a terrorist attack.

Information is as critical to the provision of safe health care—care that is free of errors of both commission and omission—as it is to the safe operation of aircraft. To develop a treatment plan, a doctor must have access to complete patient information (e.g., diagnoses, medications, current test results, and available social supports) and to the most current science base [IOM Committee on Data Standards for Patient Safety, 2004].

Whereas *To Err Is Human* focused primarily on errors that occur in hospitals; the 2004 report examined the incidence of serious safety issues in other settings as well, including ambulatory care facilities and nursing homes. Its authors point out that earlier research on patient safety focused on errors of commission, such as prescribing a medication that has a potentially fatal interaction with another medication the patient is taking, and they argue that errors of omission are equally important. An example of an error of omission is failing to prescribe a medication from which the patient would likely have benefited (IOM, Committee on Data Standards for Patient Safety, 2003b). A significant contributing factor to the unacceptably high rate of medical errors reported in these two reports and many others is poor information management practices. Illegible prescriptions, unconfirmed verbal orders, unanswered telephone calls, and lost medical records can all place patients at risk.

Since the time the first IOM report was published, major purchasers of health care have taken a stand on improving the quality of care delivered in health care organizations across the nation by promoting the use of health care IT. The Leapfrog Group, for example, an initiative of public and private organizations that provide health care benefits to their employees, works to improve patient safety by identifying problems and proposing solutions for hospital systems. It has developed a list of criteria by which health care organizations should be judged in the future. One of the Leapfrog Group's many recommendations to improve patient safety is the widespread adoption of computerized provider order entry (CPOE) systems among health care organizations. CPOE systems will be discussed more fully in the next chapter, but in the context of today's health care information systems, they are a significant tool for decreasing errors made in the ordering and administration of medications and diagnostic and therapeutic tests.

The federal government has also responded to quality concerns by promoting health care transparency (for example, making quality and price information available to consumers) and furthering the adoption of health care IT. In 2003, the Medicare Modernization Act was passed, which expanded the program to include prescription drugs and mandated the use of electronic prescribing (*e-prescribing*) among health plans providing prescription drug coverage to Medicare beneficiaries. A year later (2004), President Bush called for the widespread adoption of electronic health record systems within the decade to improve efficiency, reduce medical errors, and improve quality of care. By 2006 he had issued an executive order directing federal agencies that administer or sponsor health insurance programs to make information about prices paid to health care providers for procedures and information on the quality of services provided by physicians, hospitals, and other health care providers publicly available. This executive order also encouraged adoption of health information technology (HIT) standards to facilitate the rapid exchange of health information (The White House, 2006). At the time of this writing, numerous other bills have been introduced into Congress, with bipartisan support, in an effort to improve the efficiency and safety of health care by promoting the rapid exchange of health information.

During this period significant changes in reimbursement practices also materialized in an effort to address patient safety and health care quality and cost concerns. Historically, health care providers and organizations have been paid for services rendered regardless of patient quality or outcome. A new method, known as *pay for performance* (P4P) or *value-based purchasing*, reimburses providers based on meeting predefined quality measures and thus is intended to promote and reward quality. The Centers for Medicare and Medicaid Services (CMS) have already notified hospitals and physicians that future increases in payment will be linked to improvements in clinical performance. Medicare has also announced it will not pay hospitals for the costs of treating certain conditions that could reasonably have been prevented—such as bedsores, injuries caused by falls, and infections resulting from the prolonged use of catheters in blood vessels or the bladder—or for treating "serious preventable" events—such as leaving a sponge or other object in a patient during surgery or providing the patient with incompatible blood or blood products. Some private health plans have followed Medicare's lead and are also denying payment for such mishaps.

Paying for quality or denying payment for serious preventable events is gaining traction. At the time of this writing over 200 P4P initiatives are underway in both the public and private sectors. And, even though P4P plans raise a number of concerns, such as which quality indicators will be used, health care organizations and providers are already required to report on a host of quality indicators, and they understand the importance of having accurate, reliable data for public reporting purposes. Many health care executives have come to realize that information technology is a necessary tool not only for enabling their providers to provide high-quality, safe, effective care in a cost-conscious environment but also for being able to report performance on key quality indicators to Medicare and other third-party payers. Once again, the bottom line depends on an organization's having ready access to high-quality data, including quality and clinical indicators.

In addition to the considerable activity that has occurred at the national level in promoting adoption of health care IT and making price and quality information publicly available, significant technological advances have occurred in information technology. Electronic devices have become smaller, more portable, less expensive, and multipurpose. Broadband access to the Internet is widely available, even in remote, rural communities; wireless technology and portable devices (personal digital assistants, multipurpose cell phones, and so forth) are ubiquitous; significant progress has been made in the area of standards (which will be discussed in Chapter Eight); podcasts, wikis, and Web 2.0 technologies have emerged; and radio-frequency identification devices (RFIDs), used more widely in other industries, have found their way into the health care marketplace (Figure 4.2). Consumers have also assumed a much more active role in managing their health and health information during the past decade by maintaining their own personal health records (PHRs). Unlike an EHR, which contains data collected and managed by a health care provider or organization, a PHR is consumer controlled. It is envisioned as a lifelong and comprehensive health record that is accessible from any place at any time (Tang, Ash, Bates, Overhage, & Sands, 2006). Health plans, insurance companies, and companies such as Google and Microsoft are making PHRs available to consumers, via secure Web sites, to store their personal health information. PHRs are described more fully in the next chapter, but they are introduced here as an important development in the evolution of health care information systems.

FIGURE 4.2. *Physician Using a PDA*

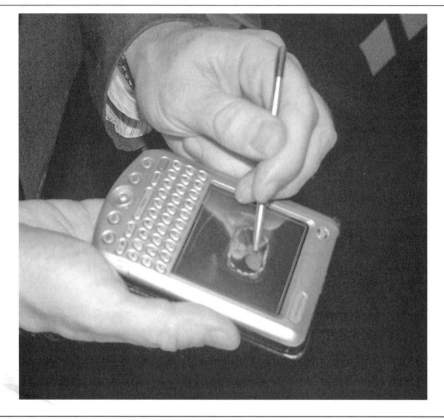

As progress is being made on a number of fronts nationally, a substantial amount of activity is also occurring at regional and local levels. Regional health information organizations (RHIOs) and health information exchange (HIE) initiatives have emerged that bring multiple stakeholders such as provider organizations (for example, hospitals, physicians, community health clinics, local public health departments, and emergency departments), health plans, payers, and consumer groups into formal partnerships to exchange health data electronically. The purpose of the exchange is to improve quality and patient safety and to address inefficiencies and rising costs in the health care system. A recent national survey reported that 120 RHIOs and HIE initiatives in various stages of development exist (eHealth Initiative, 2007). Of these organizations, 32 reported that they were fully operational and exchanging data across multiple stakeholders in their state, region, or community. Some RHIOs have not been able to sustain operations financially (Adler-Milstein, McAfee, Bates and Jha, 2007). For the most part, RHIO and HIE initiatives have migrated to a model whereby multiple, diverse stakeholders participate in the effort and share costs and governance.

At the institution level, hospitals and health system organizations continue to move forward with the adoption and implementation of clinical information systems that promote patient safety, including clinical documentation systems and bar-coding medication administration, CPOE, and electronic medical record systems. Physicians have also begun to invest in health care information systems, including EMRs, but most are in large practices of fifty or more providers. The great majority of solo and small physician practices continue to use paper-based medical record systems. Studies have shown that the relatively low adoption rates among solo and small physician practices is due to the cost of health care IT and the misalignment of incentives (DesRoches, Campbell, Rao, Donelan, Ferris, et al., 2008; Burt, Hing, and Woodwell, 2005). Patients, payers, and purchasers have the most to gain from physician use of EMR systems, yet it is the physician who generally bears the total cost. Until the incentives are appropriately aligned or the costs are shared among all stakeholders, widespread adoption of electronic medical records will likely remain low in small physician practices.

WHY HEALTH CARE LAGS IN IT

One might wonder why, with all the advances in information technology, the health care sector has been slow to adopt health care information systems, particularly clinical information systems. Other industries have automated their business processes and have used IT for years. The reasons for the slow adoption rate are varied and may not be readily apparent. First, health care information is complex, unlike simple bank transactions, for example, and it can be difficult to structure. Health care information may include text, images, pictures, and other graphics. There is no simple standard operating procedure the provider can turn to for diagnosing, treating, and managing an individual patient's care. Although there are standards of care and practice guidelines, the individual provider still plays a pivotal role in conducting the physical examination, assessment, and history of the patient. The provider relies on prior knowledge and experience and may order a battery of tests and consult with colleagues before arriving at a diagnosis or an individualized treatment plan. Terminologies used to describe health information are also complex and are not used consistently among clinicians. Second, health information is highly sensitive and personal. What could be more sensitive than a patient's personal health habits, family history, mental health, and sexual orientation? Yet such information may be relevant to the accurate diagnosis and treatment of the patient. Every patient must feel comfortable sharing such sensitive information with health care providers and confident that the information will be kept confidential and secure. Until HIPAA there were no federal laws that protected the confidentiality of all patient health information, and the state laws varied considerably. Today's younger generation, however, is very technologically savvy and far more comfortable with using the Internet for managing money, purchasing goods, seeking health information or second opinions, joining electronic support groups, and the like, so among these younger patients the concept of managing their own PHR may take off if the confidentiality and security of their health information can be assured. Third, health care IT is expensive, and currently it is the health care provider or provider organization that bears the brunt of the cost for acquiring, maintaining, and supporting these systems. It has been very difficult to make a business case for the adoption of electronic medical records in small physician practices, where the bulk of health care is delivered.

Finally, the U.S. health care system is not a single system of care but rather a conglomeration of systems, including organizations in both the public and private sectors. Even within an individual health care organization there may be a number of fragmented systems and processes for managing information. Thus another major challenge facing health care is the integration of heterogeneous systems. Some connectivity problems stem from the fact that when microcomputers became available and affordable in the last half of the 1980s, many health care organizations acquired a variety of departmental clinical systems, with little regard for how they fit together in the larger context of the organization or enterprise. There was little emphasis initially on enterprise-wide systems or on answering such questions as, Will the departmental systems communicate with each other? With the patient registration system? With the patient accounting system? To what degree will these systems support the strategic goals of the organization? As health care organizations merged or were purchased from larger organizations, the problems with integrating systems multiplied.

Integration issues may be less of an issue when a health care organization acquires an enterprise-wide system from a single vendor or when the organization itself is a self-contained system. For example, Hospital Corporation of America (HCA), a for-profit health care system comprising hundreds of hospitals throughout the nation, has adopted an enterprise-wide system from a single vendor that is used across all HCA facilities. However, rarely does a single vendor offer all the applications and functionality needed by a health care organization. Significant progress has been made in terms of interoperability standards, yet much work remains.

SUMMARY

Health care information system is a broad term that includes both administrative and clinical information systems. An information system is an arrangement of information (derived from data), processes, people, and information technology that interact to collect, process, store, and provide as output the information needed to support the health care organization. Administrative information systems contain primarily administrative or financial data and are used to support the management functions and general operations of the health care organization. Clinical information systems contain clinical, or health-related, data and are typically used by clinicians in diagnosing, treating, and managing the patient's care.

This chapter provided an overview of the history and evolution of health care information systems, including administrative and clinical applications, since the early 1960s. The information was presented in the context of the major events and issues that have been pertinent to health care, changes in reimbursement practices, advances in information technology, and the federal government's growing interest in IT.

Although it is still too early to tell what the twenty-first century holds for health care information systems, if the past is any indication health care executives should keep abreast of major health issues and concerns, proposed changes to reimbursement practices, federal IT initiatives, and advances in IT. The challenge health care organizations face is to overcome the barriers to the widespread adoption of information technology. To that end the following chapter describes a variety of clinical information systems, the major barriers to their widespread use, and the strategies health care organizations have employed to overcome these barriers.

KEY TERMS

Administrative applications (or administrative information systems)

Capitation

Clinical applications (or clinical information systems)

Computerized provider order entry (CPOE)

Diagnosis related groups (DRGs)

Dumb terminals

Electronic health record (EHR)

Electronic mail (e-mail)

Electronic medical record (EMR)

E-prescribing

Fee for service

Health care information systems

Health information exchange (HIE)

Information systems

Information technology

Local area network (LAN)

Mainframe computer

Microcomputer

Minicomputer

Pay-for-performance (P4P)

Personal health record (PHR)

Regional health information organization (RHIO)

Resource-based relative value system (RBRVS)

Shared systems

Telehealth

Telemedicine

Turnkey system

LEARNING ACTIVITIES

1. Visit at least two different types of health care organizations, and compare and contrast the history and evolution of the information systems they use. What administrative information systems does each organization use? What clinical information systems? What factors led to the adoption or implementation of these systems? What role, if any, do health care executives appear to have in decisions about today's information systems (for example, the planning, selection, implementation, or evaluation of these systems)? Has this role changed over time? Explain.

2. Explore the history and evolution of at least one of the following information technologies. Create a timeline that includes the technology's date of inception, major milestones, and use inside and outside the field of health care.

   a. Bar coding

   b. Voice recognition

   c. Wireless networks

   d. Portable devices (for example, PDAs, multipurpose cell phones)

   e. Digital imaging

    f.   Artificial intelligence

    g.   The Internet

    h.   Electronic mail (e-mail)

    i.   Wikis, blogs

    j.   Web 2.0 technologies

3.   Choose a major federal policy initiative or piece of legislation that affects health care IT, and describe the impact that it has had or will likely have in the future.

4.   If the United States went to a single-payer model for health care, how would that affect providers' spending on health care IT? If the United States went to a payment mechanism in which reimbursement was based on the quality of care, how would that affect providers' spending on health care IT?

5.   Examine the deployment of health care IT in the United Kingdom, Canada, or a European Union country. Why has health care IT evolved there in a way that is different from its evolution in the United States?

6.   Investigate the extent to which RHIOs or HIEs exist in your state or community. Select one of these initiatives, and answer these questions about it: How far along is the RHIO or HIE in its development? In its sustainability? Describe its governance structure and financing model. What factors have contributed to its current status?

7.   What impact, if any, have pay-for-performance initiatives had on the adoption of health care information systems?

CHAPTER

CURRENT AND EMERGING USE OF CLINICAL INFORMATION SYSTEMS

LEARNING OBJECTIVES

- To be able to describe the purpose, use, key attributes, and functions of some of the major types of clinical information systems used in health care, including

  Electronic medical record and electronic health record
  Computerized provider order entry
  Medication administration
  Telemedicine
  Telehealth
  E-prescribing
  Personal health record

- To be able to define the key components of an EHR system and the current status of these systems.

- To be able to discuss the major barriers to EMR and EHR adoption and the strategies being employed to overcome them.

- To be able to give examples of how clinical information systems might affect patient care safety, quality, efficiency, and outcomes.

- To be able to define health information exchange, regional health information organization, and Nationwide Health Information Network, and identify the challenges associated with sharing health information across organizational settings.

What will it take to give U.S. health care organizations and providers access to comprehensive clinical information systems that are well integrated with administrative applications—not just in large academic medical centers but also in small physician practices, nursing homes, and rural health clinics and among other health care organizations in a community? Many health care organizations have already invested considerably in implementing administrative information systems and a handful of clinical applications. They are now wrestling with how to successfully expand their clinical information system capabilities in an effort to improve patient safety, increase health care quality, and decrease costs. Examples of clinical information system expansion include everything from computerized provider order entry (CPOE) systems to medication administration systems to fully electronic medical record (EMR) systems.

To appreciate the broad spectrum of clinical information system capabilities, this chapter begins by providing the reader with a conceptual framework for understanding the major components and functions of an electronic medical record system. We view the EMR as the hub of the organization's clinical information and as a tool in improving patient care quality, safety, and efficiency. Our discussion centers on the value of EMR systems to the patient, the provider, the health care organization, and the health care community at large. We focus on two key functions that are particularly important to patient safety, CPOE and medication administration using bar-coding technology. We also explore the applications used to deliver patient care services and to interact with patients at a distance (telemedicine and telehealth), and introduce the concept and use of the personal health record (PHR) and its potential future use in health care. This section of the chapter concludes by examining how health data might be shared among different organizations within a community or region through a health information exchange (HIE) or regional health information organization (RHIO).

Implementing an EMR or any other health care information system (HCIS) in an organization does not happen overnight. It is a process that occurs over a number of years. Health care organizations today are at many different stages of information system (IS) adoption and implementation. We conclude this chapter by discussing barriers to the adoption of health care information systems (financial, cultural, and technical), along with the strategies being employed to overcome them.

THE ELECTRONIC MEDICAL RECORD

As we have discussed, patient medical records are used by health care organizations for documenting patient care, as a communication tool for those involved in the patient's care, and to support reimbursement and research. Most patient records have been kept, and are still kept, in paper form. Numerous studies have revealed the problems with paper-based medical records (Burnum, 1989; Hershey, McAloon, & Bertram, 1989; Institute of Medicine, 1991). These records are often illegible, incomplete, or unavailable when and where they are needed. They lack any type of *active* decision-support capability and make data collection and analysis very cumbersome. This passive role for the medical record is no longer sufficient in today's health care environment. Health care providers need access to active tools that afford them clinical decision-support capabilities and access to the latest relevant research findings, reminders, alerts, and other knowledge aids. The medical record of the future will likely become as critical to the accurate diagnosis and treatment of patients as the physician's stethoscope has been to detecting heart murmurs and respiratory problems.

EMR Definition and Functions

What are electronic medical records, and how do they differ from merely automating the paper record? In Chapter Four we introduced the concept of the EMR when we described the Institute of Medicine's definition of the computer-based patient record (CPR) in its 1991 report titled *The Computer-Based Patient Record: An Essential Technology for Health Care*. Since this Institute of Medicine (IOM) report was first published, a variety of terms have been used in the literature to describe EMR-related systems. By the late 1990s, the term CPR had been generally replaced with the terms *electronic medical record* (EMR) or *electronic health record* (EHR). In 2008, after having sought widespread input and consensus, the National Alliance for Health Information Technology proposed standard definitions for the electronic medical record, the electronic health record, and the personal health record (discussed later in this chapter). Table 5.1 displays these definitions. The IOM defines the EHR as a system that can perform eight electronic functions (Table 5.2); the first four functions are considered the core of an EHR.

For simplicity, we use the terms *EMR* to refer to organizational systems that include at least the four core functions and *EHR* to refer to systems that share information *across* different organizations, perhaps through a regional health information organization. An EMR (and an EHR) is able to electronically collect and store patient data, supply that information to providers on request, permit clinicians to enter orders directly into a computerized provider order entry system, and advise health care practitioners by providing decision-support tools such as reminders, alerts, and access to the latest research findings or appropriate evidence-based guidelines. These decision-support capabilities make the EMR far more robust than a digital version of the paper medical record.

TABLE 5.1. Health Information Technology Definitions

Electronic Medical Record	Electronic Health Record	Personal Health Record
An electronic record of health-related information on an individual that can be created, gathered, managed, and consulted by authorized clinicians and staff in *one* health care organization.	An electronic record of health-related information on an individual that conforms to nationally recognized interoperability standards and that can be created, managed, and consulted by authorized clinicians and staff across *more than one* health care organization.	An electronic record of health-related information on an individual that conforms to nationally recognized interoperability standards and that can be drawn from multiple sources while being managed, shared, and controlled by the individual.

Source: National Alliance for Health Information Technology, 2008.

TABLE 5.2. **Functions of an EHR System as Defined by the IOM**

Core Functions	Other Functions
Health information and data: includes medical and nursing diagnoses, a medication list, allergies, demographics, clinical narratives, and laboratory test results.	*Electronic communication and connectivity:* enables those involved in patient care to communicate effectively with each other and with the patient; technologies to facilitate communication and connectivity may include e-mail, Web messaging, and telemedicine.
Results management: manages all types of results (for example, laboratory test results, radiology procedure results) electronically.	*Patient support:* includes everything from patient education materials to home monitoring to telehealth.
Order entry and support: incorporates use of computerized provider order entry, particularly in ordering medications.	*Administrative processes:* facilitates and simplifies such processes as scheduling, prior authorizations, insurance verification; may also employ decision-support tools to identify eligible patients for clinical trials or chronic disease management programs.
Decision support: employs computerized clinical decision-support capabilities such as reminders, alerts, and computer-assisted diagnosing.	*Reporting and population health management:* establishes standardized terminology and data formats for public and private sector reporting requirements.

Source: Adapted from IOM, IOM, 2003a.

Figure 5.1 illustrates an EMR alert reminding the clinician that the patient is allergic to certain medication or that two medications should not be taken in combination with each other. Reminders might also show that the patient is due for a health maintenance test such as a mammography or a cholesterol test or for influenza vaccine (Figure 5.2).

EMR Current Adoption and Use

How widely are EMR systems used in hospitals, physician practices, and other health care organizations? What might appear on the surface to be an easy question does not have a simple answer. A number of professional organizations and researchers have attempted to estimate EMR adoption rates in recent years, yet accurately measuring adoption is difficult for several reasons. First, no one definition for the EMR (or CPR or EHR) has been used consistently among researchers. Second, organizations may be in different stages of adoption. EMR adoption does not occur at a single moment in time but rather evolves in stages over time. Further, the degree of usage and functionality can

FIGURE 5.1.   *Sample Drug Alert Screen*

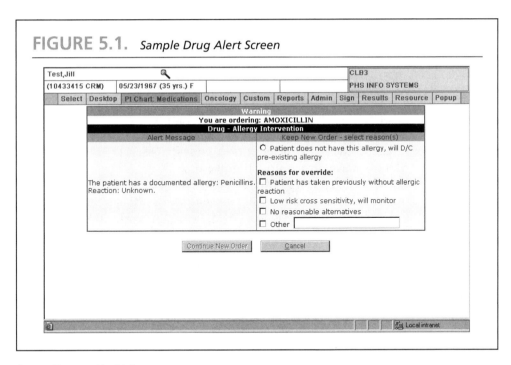

Source: Partners HealthCare

FIGURE 5.2.   *Sample EMR Screen*

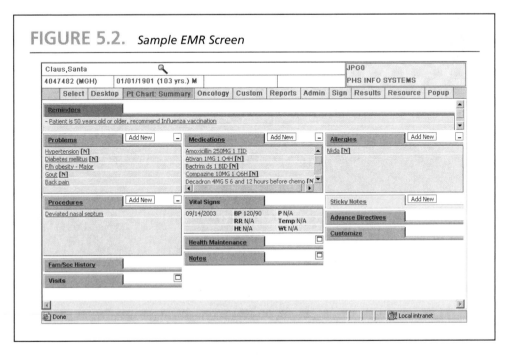

Source: Partners HealthCare

differ greatly from one organization to the next or even among divisions or departments in a single organization. It may not be clear whether health care providers use specific EMR functions such as decision support, even if they report having an EMR fully deployed. A recent statewide survey of physicians in Massachusetts illustrates this point (Simon, 2007). This research found that although nearly 29 percent of physicians reported that their practice had adopted an EMR system, less than half reported being able to transmit prescriptions to a pharmacy electronically or order laboratory tests electronically. Additionally, less than half of the physicians who had systems with clinical decision support, transmittal of electronic prescriptions, and radiology order entry actually *used* these functions most or all of the time.

Despite limitations in interpreting EMR adoption estimates, it is probably safe to say that 10 to 15 percent of hospitals have fully implemented EMR systems (American Hospital Association, 2007; Fonkych & Taylor, 2005; Poon, Jha, et al., 2006), and 20 to 25 percent of physicians in ambulatory care practice use *some* form of EMR application (Jha et al., 2006; Poon, Jha, et al., 2006). Rates of EMR adoption tend to be higher in larger facilities than in smaller ones. A 2007 report by the American Hospital Associated indicated that 11 percent of hospitals had fully implemented EMR systems, but another 57 percent had partially implemented such systems. Figure 5.3 shows the distribution by bed size of hospitals reporting fully or partially implemented EMR systems. Large, urban hospitals and teaching hospitals are much more likely to use EMRs than are rural or small community hospitals or hospitals that do not belong to a health system.

As with hospitals, the larger the physician practice, the more likely the practice is to use an EMR system (Figure 5.4). The latest results from the National Ambulatory Medical Care Survey (NAMCS) indicate that approximately 25 percent of office-based

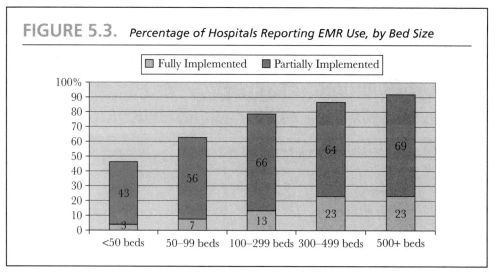

FIGURE 5.3. *Percentage of Hospitals Reporting EMR Use, by Bed Size*

Source: Adapted from American Hospital Association, 2007.

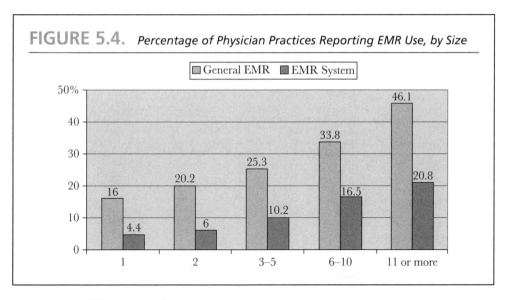

FIGURE 5.4.   *Percentage of Physician Practices Reporting EMR Use, by Size*

Source: Adapted from Burt et al., 2005.

physicians report using a fully or partially implemented EMR system in 2005, a 31 percent increase from the 18.2 percent reported in an earlier 2001 study (Burt, Hing, & Woodwell, 2005). To better understand physicians' use of EMRs, the 2005 NAMCS included questions about EMR system features that health information technology (HIT) experts consider to be the minimal requirements for a complete EMR, such as computerized orders for prescriptions, orders for tests, reporting of test results, and physician notes. When these requirements are factored in, only one in ten of the physician practices surveyed is considered to be using an EMR system. These EMR adoption percentages are low compared with those in other countries. The majority of primary care providers in Australia, Finland, the Netherlands, New Zealand, and the United Kingdom use EMR systems (Brailer & Terasawa, 2003; Schoen et al., 2007). It is worth noting however that in these countries a single-payer system exists or EMR use is government mandated.

Less is known about EMR adoption rates in settings other than hospitals and physician practices. The first and only study found of home health and hospice agencies reported that approximately 32 percent of home health agencies and 18 percent of hospice agencies are estimated to use computerized medical record systems, although it is not clear if these systems offer the level of functionality defined by the IOM (Pearson & Bercovitz, 2006). Data used in estimating these adoption rates come from the 2000 National Home and Hospice Care Survey, conducted before the latest IOM definition existed. Some states, such as California, have attempted to assess health information technology use in long-term care facilities (Hudak & Sharkey, 2007), but again, EMR functions can differ in these settings, and national estimates are nearly nonexistent.

Factors Influencing EMR Adoption

Despite the relatively low rates of EMR use in the United States, a number of factors are driving an increased interest in adopting such systems. The desires to improve patient safety, reduce medical errors, reduce duplicate services, improve organizational efficiency, optimize reimbursement, and compete locally and regionally are just a few of the many factors encouraging health care organizations and providers to take steps toward implementing an EMR system. Health care leaders are becoming increasingly aware of the potential value of EMR systems to the patient, the provider, the organization, and the health care community at large in improving quality, addressing patient safety concerns, and decreasing administrative costs. The recent focus on health information technology at the federal level is unprecedented.

Value of EMR Systems

A number of studies over the past thirty years have demonstrated the value of using EMR systems and other types of clinical information systems. The benefits fall into three major categories: (1) improved quality, outcomes, and safety; (2) improved efficiency, productivity, and cost reduction; and (3) improved service and satisfaction. Following is a discussion of each of these major categories, along with several examples illustrating the value of EMR systems to the health care process.

Improved Quality, Outcomes, and Safety Clinical information systems, including EMRs, can have a significant impact on patient quality, outcomes, and safety. Three major effects on quality are increased adherence to guideline-based care, enhanced surveillance and monitoring, and decreased medication errors. For example, several studies have shown that physicians who had access to clinical practice guidelines and features such as computerized reminders and alerts were far more likely to provide preventive care than were physicians who did not (Balas et al., 2000; Bates et al., 1999; Kuperman, Teich, Gandhi, & Bates, 2001; Teich et al., 2000; Ornstein, Garr, Jenkins, Rust, & Arnon, 1991). Other studies have found that computerized reminders used in an outpatient setting can have a significant effect on cancer prevention activities such as the performance of stool occult-blood tests, rectal examinations, breast examinations, smoking cessation counseling, and dietary counseling (Landis, Hulkower, & Pierson, 1992; McPhee, Bird, Jenkins, & Fordham, 1989; McPhee, Bird, Fordham, Rodnick, & Osborn, 1991; Yarnall et al., 1998). EMR-related systems have also been shown to improve drug prescribing and administration by providing clinicians with information on the appropriate use of antibiotics at the point of care (Berman, Zaran, & Rybak, 1992), to reduce adverse drug reactions (Bates & Gawande, 2003; Burke & Pestotnik, 1999; Evans, Pestotnik, Classen, & Burke, 1993), to improve the accuracy of drug dosing (Duxbury, 1982), and to reduce errors of omission such as failing to act on results or to carry out indicated tests (Bates & Gawande, 2003; Litzelman, Dittus, Miller, & Tierney, 1993; McDonald et al., 1984; Overhage, Tierney, Zhou, & McDonald, 1997). Bates and Gawande (2003) suggest that information technology can reduce the rate of medical errors by (1) preventing errors and adverse effects, (2) facilitating a more rapid response after an adverse event has occurred, and (3) tracking and providing feedback about adverse effects. Likewise, EMR systems can improve communication, make knowledge more readily available, require key pieces of information (such as the dose of the drug), assist with calculations, perform checks in real time, assist with monitoring, and provide decision support. If effectively incorporated into the care process, all of these features have the potential to improve quality, outcomes, and patient safety.

Improved Efficiency, Productivity, and Cost Reduction   In addition to improving the quality of care the patient receives, studies have shown that the EMR can improve efficiency, increase productivity, and lead to cost reductions (Grieger, Cohen, & Krusch, 2007; Barlow, Johnson, & Steck, 2004; Tate, Gardner, & Weaver, 1990; Tierney, Miller, Overhage, & McDonald, 1993). It is not uncommon for clinicians who do not have EMR access to order a second set of tests because the results from the first set are unavailable, so one way EMR systems improve efficiency is by making test results readily available to clinicians (Bates et al., 1999; W. Tierney, McDonald, Hui, & Martin, 1988; Tierney, Miller, & McDonald, 1990). In addition, EMR features such as computerized reminders and alerts can reduce pharmaceutical costs by prompting physicians to use generic and formulary drugs (Bates & Gawande, 2003; Donald, 1989; Garrett, Hammond, & Stead, 1986; Levit et al., 2000; Karson et al., 1999). EMRs can also provide the infrastructure necessary to measure care processes and aid in continuous quality improvement efforts (Edwards, Huang, Metcalfe, & Sainfort, 2008).

Several studies have shown that the use of EMR systems can reduce costs related to the retrieval and storage of medical records. For instance, the Memorial Sloan-Kettering Cancer Center estimated that it realized space savings of 2,000 square feet after implementing an EMR, equating to a savings of approximately $100,000 a year (Evans & Hayashi, 1994). Twenty-eight ambulatory care providers affiliated with the University of Rochester Medical Center found initial EMR costs were recaptured within sixteen months of implementation, with ongoing annual savings of $9,983 per provider (Grieger et al., 2007). Much of their savings was due to reductions in storage and retrieval costs. Savings have also been realized through the decreased use or elimination of transcription services (Renner, 1996). Others have reported that an EMR system has led to higher quality documentation, resulting in improved coding practices and subsequently higher reimbursement (Barlow et al., 2004; Bleich, Safran, & Slack, 1989; Wager, Lee, White, Ward, & Ornstein, 2000) and also in savings from lower drug expenditures, improved utilization of radiology tests, and decreased billing errors (Wang et al., 2003). As to the impact of EMRs on clinician time, results are mixed. Nurses are more likely to realize time savings in using computer systems to documentation patient information than their physician counterparts are (Poissant, Pereira, Tamblyn, & Kawasumi, 2005). This may be due in part to the fact that nurses often document using standardized forms or care plans, whereas physicians rarely use standardized templates to document their notes.

Improved Service and Satisfaction   The third category of benefits to be realized as a result of using EMR systems is improved service and satisfaction, from both the patient's and the user's perspectives. Patients whose physicians use EMR systems like the fact that their health information (health history, allergies, medications, and test results) is readily available when and where it is needed. Several qualitative studies have shown that patients' response to physicians' using an EMR in the examination room is quite positive (Ornstein & Bearden, 1994; Ridsdale & Hudd, 1994). Patients in practices that use an EMR system view their physicians as being innovative and progressive. And even though some physicians initially expressed concern that using the EMR in the examination room might distance them from patients or impede the physician-patient relationship, the majority by far of the studies in this area have shown that EMR use has had no negative impact on the physician-patient relationship (Wager et al., 2005; Gadd & Penrod, 2000; Legler & Oates, 1993; Solomon & Dechter, 1995) and can in fact enhance it by involving patients more fully in their own care (Marshall & Chin, 1998).

EMR systems can also positively affect provider and support staff satisfaction. Physicians who have successfully implemented an EMR system in their practice have reported that it has improved the quality of documentation, improved efficiency, and had a positive impact on their job satisfaction and stress levels (Wager et al., 2000, 2005, 2008). They are proud of the quality of their records and believe that their documentation is now more complete, accurate, and available and more useful in substantiating the diagnostic and procedural codes assigned for billing purposes. EMR users such as nurses and support staff have reported that the EMR has enhanced their ability to respond to patient questions promptly. Support staff who have historically been responsible for filing paper reports, pulling paper records, and processing bills, tout the many benefits of having easy access to patient information through the use of an EMR system (Wager et al., 2000).

Limitations and Need for Future Research Despite the promising work that has been done to date in evaluating EMRs, much more work is needed, particularly in studying the impact of such systems on organizations or communities that share patient data *across* organizational boundaries (creating an EHR system). Results from a recent review of the impact of health information technology on quality and safety found that the majority of research on EMRs has been limited to four academic institutions that implemented internally developed systems over many years (Chaudhry et al., 2006). In addition, studies that have examined the impact of EMR systems on efficiency have tended to focus on the user level instead of the organizational level or, ultimately, the health system level (Poissant et al., 2005). Thus an EMR might not save an individual physician time in documenting patient information, yet that information may be more complete and therefore may reduce unnecessary tests or improve the coordination of care, and thus the process may save time or money in the long run.

Noteworthy EMR Implementations

There are many examples of health care organizations that have successfully implemented EMR systems and have realized the value that comes from using them. The following examples profile the two 2007 Nicholas E. Davies Award recipients in the ambulatory care category and the 2007 recipient in the organizational category. The Nicholas E. Davies Award was established in 1994 by the Computer-Based Patient Record Institute (CPRI) to recognize organizations that have carried out exemplary implementations of EMR systems. (The Healthcare Information and Management

Systems Society [HIMSS] has administered the Davies Award since 2002, the year that CPRI merged with HIMSS.)

PERSPECTIVE

2007 DAVIES AWARD RECIPIENTS: AMBULATORY CARE CATEGORY

Valdez Family Clinic, PC   The Valdez Family Clinic is a solo family practice serving an economically disadvantaged and medically underserved community in San Antonio, Texas. Founded in 2006, it serves a largely Hispanic population, with the majority of the patients being covered by Medicare and Medicaid. Dr. Alicia Valdez, who owns the practice, recognized the need to improve clinical workflow, improve documentation, and increase the accuracy of coding.

To ensure support and buy in, Dr. Valdez included the entire staff in the EHR selection process. The staff attended a vendor trade show in March 2006. Afterward, using staff members' evaluations of what they had seen, the clinic developed an "ideal" EHR profile. Next, staff members ranked their top three product choices. The top three vendors were then invited to demonstrate their EHR systems at the clinic. MedcomSoft Record was the unanimous choice.

MedcomSoft Record is a feature-rich medical office software suite built around an EHR. Unlike interfaced systems, its full functionality is driven by a single database, using codified data captured at the point of care. The system uses the Medcin nomenclature, which enables true integration. The system also offers functions including CPOE, EKG integration, document and image management, referrals and authorizations management, billing functions, scheduling capabilities, and clinical decision support. The objective of paperless operations was set for 90 days after *go-live*, and today the clinic is completely paperless. Due to this successful implementation, the practice has realized increased efficiency, decreased labor costs, and improved billing practices.

Family Medical Specialists of Texas   Family Medical Specialists of Texas (FMS) is a three-physician practice in Plano, Texas. Founded in 2001, it is a traditional family practice in a suburban community. After being in practice for two years, FMS physicians knew they needed better tools to achieve their mission of providing unsurpassed customer service and clinical quality, and thus in 2003 they made the decision to move to an EMR system.

FMS does a lot of preventative care and chronic disease management, thus the staff were interested in an EMR that would track preventive care and provide reminders and clinical decision alerts and support. They also wanted a system that would improve physician and staff job satisfaction through improved efficiency and productivity. FMS chose GE's Centricity PM/EHR, now called Centricity Physician

(Continued)

PERSPECTIVE (*Continued*)

Office. The system offers lab, EKG, vital signs machine, secure messaging, and electronic faxing interfaces, and also interfaces with a patient portal.

The EMR was implemented over a six-week period. Everyone in the practice was involved in the process; consensus was always the goal. The practice decided to use *thick clients* (full-featured computers connected to a network) in the exam rooms, with flat panel monitors. While patients wait in an exam room for the physician to arrive, videos are available to educate or entertain patients and to market new products or services. Every new patient watches a video about FMS's Web site and how to sign up for patient portal access.

The value of the EMR to the practice has far exceeded staff expectations. Examples of some of the benefits realized include the ability to do prescription refills within an hour, a reduction in patient calls for refills, better adherence to clinical guidelines, use of an automated recall list to remind patients of appointments (which has led to a lower no-show rate), better coding, improved patient satisfaction, and improved physician lifestyle (through, for example, having remote access to patient information).

Source: Adapted from HIMSS, 2008.

2007 DAVIES AWARD RECIPIENT: ORGANIZATIONAL CATEGORY

Allina Hospitals & Clinics Allina Hospitals and Clinics of Minnesota is a nonprofit health care system including eleven hospitals and sixty-five clinics. In 2003, a new CEO and leadership team developed a systemwide strategic plan, with a major goal of implementing an EMR system. Allina's EMR system, known as Excellian, allows physicians and other caregivers immediate access to comprehensive medical record information on patients regardless of where within the Allina system they have been seen in the past. The result is care that is based on knowledge of the patient's preexisting conditions, medications being taken, and past tests and evaluations. This allows caregivers to make more informed treatment decision, avoid unnecessary tests, and provide safer, more effective care.

Allina is also using the EMR to monitor treatment regimens for patients with chronic diseases, as well as to identify patients who may be at risk for other diseases. The Allina EMR includes a patient portal that enables patients to securely access portions of their medical record, view lab results, and schedule follow-up appointments. Allina is also a founding member in the Minnesota Health Information Exchange, a public-private partnership established to link health records stored in organizations throughout Minnesota.

Source: Adapted from HIMSS, 2008.

OTHER MAJOR HCIS TYPES

In addition to EMR systems, several other clinical information systems or applications warrant discussion. The five we have selected to discuss are computerized provider order entry (CPOE), medication administration, telemedicine, telehealth, and the personal health record (PHR). We selected these systems because they have an enormous potential to improve quality, decrease costs, and improve patient safety or because they are being widely debated and are likely to be hot topics for the next few years—or because they possess both these qualities.

The first two, computerized provider order entry and medication administration systems, are applications used primarily in health care settings where tests and medications are ordered, performed, or administered. Telemedicine and telehealth are means of delivering services or communicating with patients at a distance. A personal health record is a record the patient creates, maintains, and controls. Its intent is to bring together the data and information that patients need to manage their health. The record can be maintained in paper or electronic form. Each of these information systems is described in the sections that follow, along with their current use and value to the patient care delivery process.

Computerized Provider Order Entry

One of the biggest concerns facing health care organizations today is how to keep patients safe. Several Institute of Medicine studies have brought to the forefront of people's attention the fact that an estimated 98,000 patients die each year in U.S. hospitals due to medical errors (IOM, 2000, 2001). Medication errors and adverse drug events (ADEs) top the list and are common, costly, and clinically important issues to address. A *medication error* is an error in the process of ordering, dispensing, or administering a medication, whether or not an injury occurs and whether or not the potential for injury is present. An *adverse drug event* is an injury resulting from the use of a drug, a use that may or may not have involved a medication error. Thus a medication error may lead to an adverse drug event but does not necessarily do so (Bates et al., 1999). Studies have shown that computerized provider order entry (CPOE) has the potential to reduce medication errors and adverse drug events (Bates et al., 1998; Bates & Gawande, 2003). In fact the Leapfrog Group has identified CPOE as one of three changes that it believes would most improve patient safety.

Many health care executives have taken steps to implement CPOE or are planning to do so in the near future. What is CPOE? How might it improve patient safety? How widely used are CPOE systems? We begin by defining CPOE and its major functions and then move on to discuss its current use and its potential value in improving patient safety and preventing medical errors.

Definition and Primary Functions of CPOE Systems   During a patient encounter the physician generally orders a number of diagnostic tests and therapeutic plans for the patient. In fact virtually every intervention in patient care—performing diagnostic tests, administering medications, drawing blood—is initiated by a physician's order.

Historically, physicians have handwritten these orders or called them in as verbal orders for a nurse or other health care professional to document. The ordering process itself is a critical step in the patient care process and represents a point where intervention can often prevent medication errors and improve adherence to clinical practice guidelines.

CPOE, at its most basic level, is a computer application that accepts physician orders electronically, replacing handwritten or verbal orders and prescriptions. Most CPOE systems provide physicians with decision-support capabilities at the point of ordering. For example, an order for a laboratory test might trigger an alert to the physician that the test has already been ordered and the results are pending. An order for a drug to which the patient is allergic might trigger an alert warning the physician of the patient's allergy and possibly recommending an alternative drug. If a physician orders an expensive test or medication, the CPOE system might show the cost and offer alternative tests or drugs. CPOE systems can also provide other types of clinical decision support to the physician. For instance, if the physician is ordering a series of tests and medications for a common diagnosis, the computer can offer the use of a preprogrammed, institutionally approved set of orders to facilitate the process and can recommend drug therapy to aid the physician in following accepted protocols for that diagnosis (Metzger & Turisco, 2001) (Figure 5.5). The scope of CPOE functions

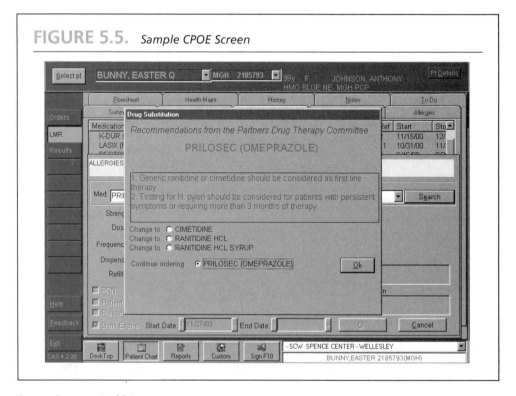

FIGURE 5.5. *Sample CPOE Screen*

Source: Partners HealthCare

and capabilities can vary considerably. The most advanced systems have sophisticated decision-support capabilities and can aid the provider in diagnosing and treating the patient by supplying information derived from knowledge-based rules and the latest research.

Current Use of CPOE   Estimating the current use of CPOE systems is almost as difficult as assessing the use of EMR systems. A CPOE system is typically an integral part of a comprehensive clinical information system or EMR system and not a stand-alone application. Most of the recent estimates of the proportion of hospitals using CPOE put it at approximately 5 to 15 percent (Blumenthal & Glaser, 2007; Cutler, Feldman, & Horwitz, 2005; Jha et al., 2006).

A study by Cutler, Feldman, and Horwitz (2005) found that CPOE adoption is related to hospital ownership and teaching status; governmental and teaching hospitals are much more likely than other hospital types are to invest in CPOE. Why the relatively low usage rate? Part of it may be due to the fact that historically, health care executives and vendors did not believe that physicians would be interested in computerized order entry, and consequently CPOE development lagged behind the development of other clinical information system components. Even among hospitals that have implemented a full or partial CPOE system, relatively few require physicians to use the system.

Value of CPOE   Despite the relatively low usage rates, CPOE systems can provide patient care, financial, and organizational benefits. Clearly, one of the fundamental reasons that CPOE has received so much attention in recent years is its potential to improve patient safety and, more specifically, reduce medication errors (Holdsworth et al., 2007; Walsh et al., 2008). A recent review of CPOE studies found that 80 percent of studies report significant reductions in total prescribing errors, 43 percent in dosing errors, and 37.5 percent in adverse drug events when CPOE rather than handwritten orders is used (Shamliyan, Duval, Jing, & Kane, 2008). The use of CPOE is also associated with a 66 percent reduction in total prescribing errors for adults and a positive tendency in children.

The benefits of using CPOE systems in outpatient settings show promise as well, yet not as much research has been done in this area. Authors of two studies have found that CPOE can lead to better adherence to clinical protocols and improvements in the stages of clinical decision making—that is, initiation, diagnosing, monitoring and tracking, and acting (Johnston, Pan, Walker, Bates, & Middleton, 2003, 2004). They also found that CPOE can lead to improved patient outcomes by reducing medical errors, decreasing morbidity and mortality, and expediting recovery times. A report from the Agency for Healthcare Research and Quality (2001) substantiates the notion that CPOE systems can significantly reduce medication errors in outpatient settings and estimates that such systems may prevent 28 to 95 percent of adverse drug events.

Besides clinical benefits, CPOE systems can also provide financial benefits to a health care organization. For example, organizations that use CPOE systems may require fewer administrative clinical staff, improve the accuracy and timeliness of billing, and increase transaction processing rates (Johnston et al., 2004). Studies have also showed reductions in medication turnaround times, elimination of transcription errors, and improvements in countersigning orders (Ahmad et al., 2002; Jensen, 2006).

Despite growing evidence that CPOE systems have positive effects on patient safety, there have been studies that raised concerns. In 2005, researchers from an academic children's hospital observed an unexpected increase in mortality after implementation of a vendor-acquired CPOE system (Han et al., 2005). Although some have challenged the methods used in this particular study, most would agree that CPOE technology is still evolving and requires ongoing assessment of systems integration and the effectiveness of the human-computer interface (Ash et al., 2007; Kilbridge, Classen, Bates, & Denham, 2006). A CPOE system does not operate in isolation. To function properly it requires seamless integration within a strong and dynamic health information architecture (Han et al., 2005). Issues such as alert fatigue and the need for ongoing system enhancements are real, and without proper management, unintended consequences can occur.

In the late 1980s, the University of Virginia experienced a great deal of resistance to its CPOE initiative. Organizational leaders underestimated the impact of CPOE on clinical workflow as well as on physicians' and nurses' time and, in retrospect, did not invest sufficient resources in the effort. Many physicians, including residents, perceived the CPOE as an Information Systems Department initiative rather than as a clinician-led effort and felt it was forced upon them and offered little flexibility. Physicians complained administration was trying to "turn them into clerks to save money." Cumbersome interfaces and time-consuming ordering processes, along with the fact that the clinical care processes were never fully redesigned, contributed to the problems encountered (Massaro, 1993a, 1993b). In 2003, Cedars-Sinai Medical Center in Los Angeles experienced some of the same problems with its CPOE system implementation and ended up "pulling the plug" on the system, as the following case study describes. As of the time of this writing, Cedars-Sinai has yet to implement CPOE.

PERSPECTIVE

CPOE IMPLEMENTATION

Cedars-Sinai Medical Center developed and implemented a computer system known as Patient Care Expert (PCX) several years ago as part of a larger project to modernize the medical center's computing infrastructure. The PCX system included a CPOE component and used browser-based technology, making the system accessible through any browser-enabled computer anytime, anywhere. Other performance criteria specified that

- "The system needed to be highly flexible, allowing for rapid modifications of content and functionality."

- "The system needed to be fully integrated with all ancillary services, patient registration, and patient accounting."

■ "The system needed to be user-friendly for large groups of users with a diverse range of familiarity and experience with computers" (Langberg, 2004).

After conducting an extensive review of existing products and obtaining broad input from administration, clinicians, and information technology experts, the Cedars-Sinai board of directors decided the organization should develop an in-house product in collaboration with Perot Systems. In August 2002, after nearly three years of development and testing, Cedars-Sinai launched a pilot program of the PCX system. This pilot involved obstetrical patients over a two-week period, during which approximately 400 patients were entered into the system. As part of the pilot, more than 140 physicians and 200 department staff members used the system to care for all obstetrical patients. Clinical staff tested the system with more than 20,000 orders. By October, more than 2,000 physicians had been trained and certified to use PCX. The pilot was felt to have been very successful, and minor changes were made to the PCX before rolling it out to other areas of the medical center. By January 2003, 700,000 orders had been placed for more than 7,000 patients—more than 10,000 orders per day. The system was operational for more than two-thirds of the medical center's inpatients. However, in late January 2003, the system was suspended after hundreds of physicians complained that the system slowed down the ordering process and said they feared that orders were getting lost in the system. The medical center had worked with a forty-physician medical executive committee throughout the development and implementation process, and the administration believed that physicians were sufficiently involved throughout the project. However, rank-and-file physicians argued that the committee did not represent their views (Chin, 2003). One physician, for example, argued that the CPOE was very cumbersome and didn't follow physician workflow. This same physician complained that to order an antibiotic, doctors had to go through three or four computer screens and wait six to eight seconds between screens (Chin, 2003). After receiving such complaints, the administration made the decision to take down the CPOE system. Those involved in the implementation reported that they found themselves managing two complex processes:

1. "*Physician change management:* Four months into 'go-live' physicians remained deeply concerned about the added time they reported in entering orders and their negative perception of the system's ease of use. Further, [it was] believed that too many physicians . . . did not have an optimal working knowledge of the system's functionality."

2. "*Workflow change management:* The procedures involved in hospital-based patient care are complex in any environment and need to be carefully and thoroughly understood in advance of automation. Additionally, CPOE will

(*Continued*)

PERSPECTIVE (*Continued*)

affect the workflow of all caregivers. [It was found that] far more operational workflow analysis and adjustment needed [to occur] after the 'go-live' than was initially anticipated" (Langberg, 2004).

Besides managing these two processes, the management team has instituted a number of system enhancements and has aggregated input from all users to enhance PCX and improve the implementation and workflow procedures. By intensifying training and support resources, and accelerating the system response time, management expects to improve physicians' experiences.

Source: Adapted from Langberg, 2004.

We will discuss a host of issues related to the implementation of CPOE and other applications more fully in Chapter Seven. At this point, however, it is important to understand that CPOE systems can have a dramatic impact on physicians—how they spend their time, their work patterns, and the functions they perform. CPOE is an expensive and complex project that touches almost all aspects of the health care operation. It is not simply a niche computer system to replace handwritten orders. Rather CPOE is a tool to aid the provider in order management. It can directly affect not only physician ordering but also physician decision making (through the decision-support features) and care planning, pharmacist decision making and workflow, nursing workflow and documentation, and communication with ancillary services. Just as automating the paper medical record is not the same as implementing an EMR system, neither is automating the ordering process the same as implementing a CPOE system. Like an EMR system, a CPOE system provides decision support and can be a useful tool to the provider in managing the patient's care more effectively.

Medication Administration Systems

Another clinical application that is being widely discussed in terms of its potential to improve patient safety is medication administration that uses a *bar-code-enabled point of care* (BPOC) approach. Like EMR and CPOE systems, medication administration systems with BPOC have the potential to address many patient safety issues, particularly those relating to correctly identifying patients and medications. Patient safety is such a complex issue that it is unlikely that it can be fixed by a single solution. The HIMSS Bar Coding Task Force argues that "unprecedented cooperation through the medical supply chain, across software vendors and within provider organizations, is required" (HIMSS, 2003, p. vii) for real change to occur.

Bar-coding technology is nothing new. It has infiltrated our lives, and we find it in grocery stores, hospitals, department stores, airports, and even in our own homes. In health care, bar-coding technology has been employed in areas such as materials management, supply inventory, and document management. However, medication administration using BPOC, which has the potential to enhance productivity, improve patient safety, and ultimately, improve quality of care, is a new area of emphasis for this technology. To be effective, medication administration BPOC systems must be combined with decision-support capabilities and enable alerts and warnings designed to prevent errors. The goal is to ensure that the five "rights" of drug administration are met, meaning getting the right drug to the right patient through the right route at the right dose at the right time (Sakowski et al., 2005).

Most medication administration BPOC systems operate in essentially the same way. At the time of admission the patient receives an identification wristband with a bar code. This wristband correctly identifies the patient by name, date of birth, medical record number, and any other important identifying information. Correctly identifying the patient is the first step in seeing that the right patient gets the right medication. Next the provider scans his or her own bar-coded identification band in order to log into the medication administration system. Bar-coding the provider or employee gives positive identification of the caregiver and ensures secure access to various information systems, according to the individual user's privileges. It also produces an audit trail showing who has accessed what systems at what time and for what information. When the provider scans the patient's bar-coded wristband, he or she has access to the physician's orders and can view what currently needs to be done for the patient. When the caregiver scans a bar-coded item or medication, that code is compared with the order profile. If it does not match, the caregiver is alerted to the discrepancy, and a potential error is averted. The scanning process might also trigger real-time documentation and billing.

Studies have shown that about half of medication errors occur during the ordering process (Hatoum, Catizone, Hutchinson, & Purohit, 1986), but errors also occur in dispensing, administering, and monitoring medications (Poon, Cina, et al., 2006; Kaushal & Bates, 2002). Medication administration systems that use BPOC can be highly effective in reducing all types of medication errors, wherever in the treatment cycle they occur (Paoletti et al., 2007; Poon, Cina, et al., 2006; Sakowski et al., 2005).

A number of resources exist to aid health care organizations in implementing BPOC. HIMSS (2003b) developed a resource guide that outlines how bar coding works, describes clinical and administrative applications that can employ bar-coding technology, and offers strategies and tips for successfully implementing bar coding in health organizations. The University HealthSystem Consortium (UHC) Bar-Coding Task Group has published recommendations for hospitals, ranging from general recommendations to technology recommendations and implementation strategies (Cummings, Bush, Smith, & Matuszewski, 2005). Additionally, the Department of Veterans Affairs (VA) has implemented BPOC in conjunction with its electronic medical record system used throughout its 163 medical centers. The VA has found that although bar-coding systems can lower medication administration errors, introducing BPOC also presents new challenges (Mills, Neily, Mims, Burkhardt, & Bagian, 2006). To address these challenges, it has employed a series of quality improvement strategies, using multidisciplinary teams to improve the safety and efficiency of the BPOC system.

Telemedicine

"Telemedicine is the use of medical information exchanged from one site to another via electronic communications to improve patients' health status" (American Telemedicine Association [ATA], 2007). It is a tool that enables providers to deliver health care services to patients at distant locations, and it is often promoted as a means of addressing the imbalances in the distribution of health care resources. Telemedicine systems have evolved over the past few decades, becoming most prevalent during the 1990s owing to major advancements in telecommunications technology and decreases in equipment and transmission costs. Telemedicine may be as simple as two health care providers discussing a case over the telephone or as sophisticated as using satellite technology and videoconferencing equipment to broadcast a consultation between providers at facilities in two countries. The first method is used daily by most health professionals, and the second is used by the military and some large medical centers.

Health care literature often uses the terms *telemedicine* and *telehealth* interchangeably. We use *telehealth* to refer to a broader view of remote health care, one that does not always involve the provision of clinical services, which is the province of telemedicine. Telehealth includes the use of technology to access remote health information, diagnostic images, and education.

Current Status and Primary Delivery Methods Most recent estimates suggest that there are over 200 telemedicine programs throughout the nation, involving close to 2,000 medical institutions (ATA, 2007). The types of telemedicine services may include everything from specialist referral services to patient consultations to remote patient monitoring. Two delivery methods can be used to connect providers to providers or providers to patients. The first is called *store and forward*. This technology is used primarily for transferring digital images from one location to another. For example, a digital image might be taken with a digital camera, stored on a server, and then sent (or forwarded) to a health care provider at another location upon request (Brown, 2003). *Teleradiology* and *teledermatology* are two telemedicine services that use store-and-forward technology. In the case of teleradiology one provider might send radiological images such as X-rays, CT scans, or magnetic resonance imaging (MRI) results to another provider to review. In the case of teledermatology a digital image of the patient's skin might be sent to a dermatologist for diagnosis or consultation. Store-and-forward technology is generally used in nonemergency situations. These images can be sent using private point-to-point networks.

The second major delivery method is known as *two-way interactive videoconferencing* and is used when a face-to-face consultation is necessary. For example, a specialty physician in an urban tertiary care hospital might consult with a primary care physician in a rural community, using high-speed or dedicated Internet lines and real-time videoconferencing capabilities. This gives patients and providers in rural communities access to providers, particularly specialists, in urban areas without having to travel. In addition, a number of peripheral devices can be linked to computers to aid in interactive examination. For example, a stethoscope can be linked to a computer, allowing the consulting physician to hear the patient's heartbeat from a distance. Remote monitoring of patients is also possible through closed-circuit television systems, and electronic monitoring of physiological vital signs can be done through existing intensive care unit (ICU) patient monitoring systems (Roberts & Sebastian, 2006).

The military and some university research centers are also developing robotic equipment for *telesurgery* applications. Telesurgery might enable a surgeon in one location to remotely control a robotic arm to perform surgery in another location. The military are developing this technology particularly for battlefield use, although some academic medical centers are also piloting telesurgery technology.

Value of Telemedicine   Telemedicine can make specialty care more accessible to rural and medically underserved communities. Through videoconferencing a patient or provider living in a rural community can consult with specialists living at a distance, and this can reduce or eliminate travel and other costs associated with delivering health care services. Kaiser Permanente conducted a study examining the impact of remote video technology on quality, use, patient satisfaction, and cost savings in the home health care setting. It found that the technology was well received by patients, capable of maintaining quality of care, and had the potential for cost savings if used as a substitute for some in-person caregiver visits (Johnston, Wheeler, Deuser, & Sousa, 2000).

Telemedicine has also shown promising results in improving access to care, quality, and outcomes for patients with chronic diseases (Barlow, Singh, Bayer, & Curry, 2007; Gambetta, Dunn, Nelson, Herron, & Arena, 2007). Researchers have found that videoconferencing can enhance the availability and use of psychiatric services for patients living in rural or remote communities (Modai et al., 2006). Remote surgery also has value. It could bring to local communities access to the top specialists in the world.

These are a few examples of the value of telemedicine. The possibilities for using telemedicine are endless. However, several major barriers must be addressed if telemedicine is to be more widely used and available. Concerns about provider acceptance, interstate licensure, overall confidentiality and liability, data standards, and lack of universal reimbursement for telemedicine services from private payers are barriers to the widespread use of telemedicine. Furthermore, its cost effectiveness has yet to be fully demonstrated.

Telehealth

In recent years patients have increasingly turned to the Internet to obtain health care information and seek health care services, and a growing number of them are interested in communicating with their physicians directly on line regarding specific health needs. Physicians, in contrast, have not adopted these tools as readily as patients would like. They fear that communicating by e-mail with patients will create more work, result in inadequate reimbursement for the increased work, and lead to an increase in liability, security, and patient privacy concerns (MacDonald, 2003).

Several studies have examined the use and impact of online communication, and specifically the use of electronic mail, between patients and their providers. In 2003, the California HealthCare Foundation reported on a study of the various methods that can be used to facilitate online communication between patient and provider (Mac-Donald, 2003). Online patient-provider communication was defined in this report as "the electronic exchange of information between the patient and member of his or her physician practice" (p. 6). Online communication from a patient may involve anything from requesting an appointment to viewing a bill to requesting prescription refills to seeking advice or a consultation via e-mail. Our discussion focuses on the use of e-mail between patients and their providers because it tends to be the most controversial and debated issue. Telehealth is also being used to capture and monitor data from patients at home. Examples of early telehealth efforts include capturing cardiac data from congestive heart failure patients at home, monitoring patient blood sugar levels through glucometers attached to cell phones, and conducting teledermatology visits with the aid of cell phone cameras. Home monitoring devices that transmit physiological data electronically to care providers are also being used in variety of different ways.

Current Use of Physician-Patient E-Mail Approximately 30 percent of physicians use e-mail to communicate with their patients, according to a survey by Manhattan Research (Stouffer, 2008). At the same time, approximately 90 percent of American adults with Internet access would like to communicate with their physicians via e-mail. Among physicians who correspond with their patients via e-mail, only one in ten does so in a consultative role (Sciamanna, Rogers, Shenassa, & Houston, 2007).

E-mail communication between physicians and patients has been used for a variety of purposes, including follow-up patient care, clarification on advice, prescription refills, and patient education. In one of the largest studies to date on the use of e-mail between physicians and patients, researchers at the University of Michigan Health System found that physicians were most amenable to e-mail communication with patients when a triage system was in place (MacDonald, 2003). The participating physicians wanted nurses and other staff members to first sort the messages and pass on only those that warranted a physician's response. The researchers found that although the e-mail system improved communication between physicians and patients, it also increased the workload for physician practices.

Some third-party payers, including Aetna and Cigna, now reimburse physicians for e-mail or Web consultations in Florida, California, Massachusetts, and New York (Stone, 2007). Even though the providers in these states who use e-mail with patients remain a minority, most say that e-mail or Web communications between patients and providers can improve the productivity of providers, reduce the number of office visits, save money, and strengthen patient-physician relations (Stone, 2007).

Value of E-Mail Communication Systems Physicians who e-mail their patients say that it allows them to leave direct responses to a patient's questions at the physician's convenience. Many physicians complain of playing "telephone tag" with their patients and having to leave messages on patients' answering machines. Liederman, Lee, Baquero, and Seites (2005) compared the number of incoming telephone calls and e-mails from patients to a group of physicians provided with a Web-messaging system (cases) to the number of calls to a group of physicians who used only telephones for communication (control group). Among case physicians the number of messages was significantly reduced during an eleven-month period. Researchers in the Department of Pediatrics at the University of Pittsburgh School of Medicine likewise found that answering patient questions by e-mail was 57 percent faster for physicians than using the telephone (Rosen & Kwoh, 2007). Patients also reported that e-mail enhanced communication with and access to the provider. Physicians who have used secure e-mail with patients realize that the efficiency of interactions between providers and patients can be enhanced even further by linking the e-mail or messaging system to the EMR system.

When a health care organization opts to institute e-mail communication between patients and clinicians or among clinicians, it must establish policies and guidelines for appropriate system use. The American Medical Association (AMA) has published guidelines for online communication, which health care facilities about to embark on such an initiative can use as a resource (AMA, 2003). Here is an example of an e-mail communication policy developed by an integrated health care network.

PERSPECTIVE

GUIDELINES FOR CLINICAL ELECTRONIC MAIL COMMUNICATION

The following guidelines should be universally applied when using electronic mail (e-mail) to communicate patient-identifiable information. Electronic mail is vulnerable to access by many individuals. Such access includes but is not limited to messages sent to the correct person and read by the wrong person (for example, family member of patient, employer of the patient, or someone at the physician's office other than the physician who is responsible for the e-mail). Additionally, the contents of an e-mail may be altered without detection. Many companies, including Partners and its entities, reserve the right to monitor their employees' e-mail messages to assure that they are being used properly. Thus, it is possible that the patient's employer could read private messages. These guidelines are recommended for e-mail communications that contain patient-identifiable information.

E-mail Guidelines Between Clinician and Patient

1. If a clinician and a patient agree to use electronic mail, patients should be informed about privacy issues. Patients should know that

   ■ Others besides the addressee may process messages during addressee's usual business hours, during addressee's vacation or illness, and so forth.

   ■ E-mail can occasionally be sent to the wrong party.

(Continued)

PERSPECTIVE (*Continued*)

- E-mail communication will not necessarily be a part of the patient's medical record.
- E-mail can be accessed from various locations.
- Information may be sent via e-mail to other care providers.
- The Internet does not typically provide a secure media for transporting confidential information unless both parties are using encryption technologies.
- Automatic forwarding of e-mail is allowed within the harvard.edu and Partners.org community. Messages can, however, be forwarded to another recipient at the sender's discretion.

2. Clinical interactions conducted by e-mail that a clinician believes should be part of the medical record should be stored in the patient's electronic or paper medical record.

3. If the patient's health information/treatment includes particularly sensitive information, ask the patient to decide whether this information may be referenced in e-mail, or should not be shared. Such information might include references to HIV status, substance abuse, sexually transmitted diseases, sexual assault, cancer, abortion, domestic violence, or confidential details of treatment with a psychotherapist, psychologist, or social worker. Until the patient's preference is known, content of this kind in an e-mail should be avoided.

4. Patients should be asked to write the category of transaction, for example, status, appointment, in the subject line of a message so that clinicians can more easily sort and prioritize their e-mails.

5. When available, clinicians and patients should use encryption technology for transmitting patient-identifiable information. Judgment should be used in the type of medical information that is transmitted, recognizing the increased vulnerability.

6. When possible, clinicians and patients should use a Read Receipt in order to acknowledge that they have read the message that was sent.

7. Patient-identifiable information should not be forwarded to a third party (nonclinician) without the patient's prior consent.

E-Mail Guidelines Between Clinicians

1. If clinicians agree to use e-mail to communicate patient-identifiable information between one another, both parties should be knowledgeable about privacy issues:

- Others besides the addressee may process messages during addressee's usual business hours, during addressee's vacation or illness, and so forth.

- E-mail can occasionally go to the wrong party.

- E-mail communication will not necessarily be a part of the patient's medical record (see item 5 below).

- E-mail can be accessed from various locations.

- Information may be sent via e-mail to other care providers.

- The Intranet provides a reasonable level of security.

- The Internet does not typically provide a secure medium for transporting confidential information unless both parties are using encryption technologies.

2. The following statement should be added to each e-mail that leaves the Intranet:

THE INFORMATION TRANSMITTED IN THIS E-MAIL IS INTENDED ONLY FOR THE PERSON OR ENTITY TO WHICH IT IS ADDRESSED AND MAY CONTAIN CONFIDENTIAL AND/OR PRIVILEGED MATERIAL. ANY REVIEW, RETRANSMISSION, DISSEMINATION OR OTHER USE OF OR TAKING OF ANY ACTION IN RELIANCE UPON THIS INFORMATION BY PERSONS OR ENTITIES OTHER THAN THE INTENDED RECIPIENT IS PROHIBITED. IF YOU RECEIVED THIS E-MAIL IN ERROR, PLEASE CONTACT THE SENDER AND DELETE THE MATERIAL FROM ANY COMPUTER.

3. The category of transaction, for example, consult request, should be stated in the subject line of each e-mail message for clarification or filtering.

4. Changes should not be made to someone else's message and forwarded to others without making it clear where changes were made.

5. Discretion should be used when printing e-mail messages because printing all messages may defeat the purpose of e-mail (paperless medium) and may create confidentiality issues. However, clinical interactions conducted by e-mail that a clinician believes should be part of the medical record should be stored in the patient's electronic or paper medical record.

Source: Partners HealthCare

Personal Health Record

With the advent of the Internet, including e-mail, Web logs (blogs), and other Web-based technologies, patients or consumers have assumed a much more active role in managing their own health care. To empower consumers in recent years, the concept of a personal health record (PHR) has emerged. Although a PHR could be in paper or electronic format, the vision is that the electronic PHR would enable individuals to keep their own health records, and they could share information electronically with their physicians or other health care professionals and receive advice, reminders, test results, and alerts from them. Unlike the EMR (or EHR), which is managed by health care provider organizations, the PHR is managed by the consumer. It may include both health information and wellness information, such as an individual's exercise and diet. The consumer decides who has access to the information and controls the content of the record.

PHRs are at an earlier stage of development than EHRs, and they can take one of several different types. A PHR can be as simple as a form created by an individual to record important health information (for example, medications, surgeries, vaccinations, and allergies) or as complex as a Web-based system accessed and populated by individuals, health care providers, insurers, pharmacies, employers, and companies providing health-related content (Gearon, 2007). In some cases, health care organizations host *patient portals*, giving patients' access to their EMR or specific information such as laboratory test results or radiology reports. Some insurance companies also provide PHRs to their beneficiaries, giving them online access to reports derived from their claims data, including lists of health problems, medications, and reminders about pending preventive care services (Blumenthal & Glaser, 2007; Halamka, Mandl, & Tang, 2008; Ball, Smith, & Bakalar, 2007). Employers recognize that employees are taking on greater financial responsibility for their own care and therefore may benefit from having greater access to and control over their health and claims data. Even Microsoft and Google now offer PHRs to consumers.

What is the value of the PHR and how does it relate to the EMR? Tang & Lansky (2005) believe the PHR enables individuals to serve as "copilots" in their own care. Patients can receive customized content based on their needs, values, and preferences. PHRs should be lifelong and comprehensive and should support information exchange and portability. Patients are often seen by multiple health care providers in different settings and locations over the course of a lifetime. In our fragmented health care system, this means patients are often left to consolidate information from the various participants in their care. A PHR that brings together important health information across an individual's lifetime and that is safe, secure, portable, and easily accessible can reduce costs by avoiding unnecessary duplicate tests and improving health care communications.

PHRs may be particularly helpful to patients with chronic illnesses in enabling them to track their diseases in conjunction with their providers, prompting earlier intervention when they encounter a deviation or problem (Tang, Ash, Bates, Overhage, & Sands, 2006). In addition, PHRs may make it easier for caregivers to care for their loved ones by providing those caregivers with access to complete information. Research in this area is in its early stages; however, experts agree that the value of the PHR is greatest when the PHR is integrated with the provider's EMR (Tang et al., 2006).

The growing prevalence of PHRs will create many policy and technical challenges for health care organizations, payers, and employers, as well as great opportunity. Early adopters have found that a number of important considerations need to be addressed, such as what information (for example, problem lists, medications, laboratory and diagnostic test results, clinical notes) should be shared with patients, how should patients be authenticated to access their PHRs, what access should minors have, and should the PHR include secure clinician and patient messaging (Halamka et al., 2008). In the future, demand for PHR functionality will likely increase, so health care leaders will need to examine the extent to which they are equipped to meet consumer expectations.

FITTING APPLICATIONS TOGETHER

How are the clinical information systems and applications discussed in this chapter related? How can they fit together? We view the patient's electronic medical record as the hub of all the clinical information gathered by a health care organization (Figure 5.6). The data that eventually make up each patient's record originate from a variety of sources, both paper and electronic. In an electronic environment the data are typically captured by a host of different applications, including but not limited to

- *Registration systems:* patient demographic information, health insurance or payer, provider's name, date, reason for visit or encounter, and so forth

- *Accounting systems:* patient billing information such as final diagnosis and procedure codes, charges, dates of services provided, and so forth

- *Ancillary services:* laboratory, radiology, pharmacy, and so forth

- *CPOE systems:* physician's orders, date, time, status, and so forth

- *Medication administration systems:* medications ordered, dispensed, administered, and so forth

- *Other clinical and administrative systems:* nursing, physical therapy, and nutrition education documentation; scheduling information; and so forth

- *Knowledge-based reference systems:* access to Medline, the latest research findings, practice guidelines, and so forth

- *Telemedicine and telehealth systems:* documentation of provision of health care services, online communication with patients and providers, and so forth

Sometimes these applications are all components of a single vendor package. More commonly, however, especially in larger facilities, these applications have been acquired or developed over the past twenty to thirty years. The challenge many health care organizations now face is how to bring the patient's clinical data and administrative data together—how to make all the systems containing these data function as a single,

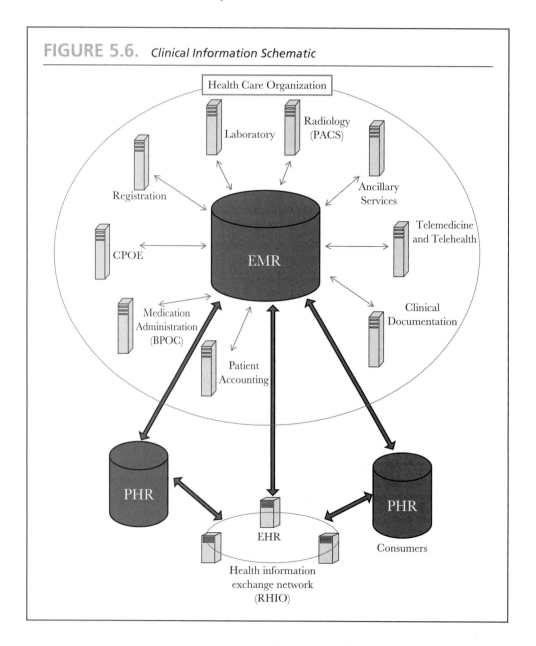

FIGURE 5.6. *Clinical Information Schematic*

seamless, integrated application. If we are to realize the goal of the electronic health record (EHR)—that is, the capturing of patient information throughout the patient's lifetime and the sharing of health information among different organizations—we must begin developing organizational EMR systems that can connect with other organizations, pharmacies, laboratories, insurers, and the like, as well as with the patient's personal health record.

INFORMATION EXCHANGE ACROSS BOUNDARIES

A central component of U.S. health care information technology strategy has been to further the adoption of interoperable EHR systems—that is, to further the exchange of health information across organizations.

A *health information exchange* (HIE) consists of the technology, standards, and governance that enable the exchange of data between the information systems of various health care stakeholders. There are diverse types of HIEs. A HIE can be dedicated to moving medication-related transactions (new prescription requests, renewals, and refills) between EHRs and pharmacies. A HIE can be used to exchange a patient's health data between two or more providers. A freestanding radiology center can use a HIE to move images and reports between its picture archiving and communication system (PACS) and provider EMR systems.

A *regional health information organization* (RHIO) is an organization that provides an HIE to health care stakeholders in a specific region, for example, a city or multicounty area. The RHIO is governed by regional stakeholders—for example, providers, health plans, and diagnostic centers. The HIE, sponsored and supported by the RHIO, enables a broad exchange of data between stakeholders. By *broad* we mean that the exchange supports the full set of patient data contained in an EHR.

The Nationwide Health Information Network (NHIN) that is in development is intended to provide the technology, standards, and governance to connect all HIEs. Hence the NHIN is expected to connect RHIOs in cities such as San Antonio, Cleveland, and Seattle and HIEs that focus on medication transactions and clinical laboratory transactions. The NHIN can be viewed as the interstate highway system that will connect the roads in individual towns and cities.

HIEs, RHIOs, and the NHIN are in their infancy. These efforts face daunting challenges of developing sustainable business models, managing patient privacy, ensuring effective governance, implementing data standards, and creating scalable technologies. Although having a goal of nationwide interoperability is correct, achieving that goal will be a multiyear and complex undertaking.

OVERCOMING BARRIERS TO ADOPTION

What do the EMR, EHR, CPOE, telemedicine, telehealth, and many other clinical applications have in common? They all affect the ways providers deliver care to or communicate with patients, and they all confront the same barriers impeding their widespread adoption and use. Most of these barriers can be categorized as (1) financial, (2) organizational or behavioral, or (3) technical. Financial barriers include lack of the capital or other financial resources needed to develop, acquire, implement, and support a health care information system. Organizational and behavioral barriers relate to provider use and acceptance of such systems. And technical barriers include everything from the work needed to build system interfaces to a lack of adequate definitions and standards for data interchange. Although all three types of barriers typically affect all clinical applications, the actual impact of any one barrier may vary considerably. For example, the lack of financial resources or of reimbursement for EMR systems has slowed their implementation but not stopped it. Conversely, the lack of financial resources or of reimbursement for telemedicine services has been devastating to telemedicine programs, and many programs have not survived these financial difficulties.

Financial Barriers

EMR and related systems can be expensive to develop, implement, and support, and currently, health care organization are receiving little or no reimbursement for the improved care that can result from using them. A health care organization might invest a significant amount of money, personnel, and other resources in an EMR system and yet not realize a positive financial return on its investment (particularly at first), even if it realizes a return in terms of quality. This situation often makes it very difficult for health care executives to justify the EMR investment, especially in times when capital is tight.

The up-front investment necessary to acquire an EMR for the small physician practice is substantial. Seventy-eight percent of physician in the United States practice in groups of eight or fewer, yet it is the small practice that is least likely to adopt an EMR system. Estimates of the cost of acquiring and installing an EMR system range from $15,000 to $50,000 (Miller, West, Brown, Sim, & Ganchoff, 2005; Baron, Fabens, Schiffman, & Wolf, 2005), with another amount equal to 15 to 20 percent of the acquisition cost needed to support the system. Physicians bear the cost of an EMR system, but the majority of the benefits are realized by patients, payers, and purchasers. Second, EMRs can negatively impact productivity, particularly during the initial months after implementation. One study found that practices experienced a 10 to 15 percent reduction in productivity for at least several months following EMR adoption (Gans, Kralewski, Hammons, & Dowd, 2005). Small physician practices tend to be highly risk averse and are fearful about the possibility of implementation failures. Thus the misalignment of incentives is a huge barrier.

The reimbursement concerns may be on the verge of decreasing, however. A number of studies are currently investigating the use of various financial incentives to encourage and reward health care organizations that use EMR systems. Here are five of the major current approaches (Mendelson, 2003[adapted]).

1. *Payment differentials:* using bonuses or add-on payments that reward providers or delivery systems, or both, for adoption and diffusion of health care information systems that improve quality of care.

2. *Cost differentials:* using patient copayments or deductibles that vary by provider, based on predetermined quality measures. The intent is to steer patients to providers that have adopted health care information systems or achieved certain quality outcomes.

3. *Innovative reimbursement:* offering reimbursement for new categories of care or service that are directly related to the use of health care information systems (for example, the virtual provider-patient visit).

4. *Shared risk:* making a portion of provider fees or rate increases contingent on technology implementation or quality improvements.

5. *Combined programs:* combining two or more of the first four approaches, often with the included benefit of public disclosure of provider progress or outcomes.

Beyond changes in reimbursement, in August 2006, the Centers for Medicare and Medicaid Services (CMS) and the U.S. Department of Health and Human Services (HHS) Office of the Inspector General expanded exceptions to the Stark and antikickback regulations, permitting hospitals to offer computerized health information systems (or access to such systems) to physician practices, potentially at a significantly greater discount than the practices could obtain if they purchased the systems individually. To meet requirements, any donated system must be "necessary and used predominately" to create, maintain, transmit, and receive electronic medical records (HHS, 2006). Although it is too early to predict the full impact of the new regulations on the adoption of EMRs, they are a positive step toward adoption of interoperable electronic health records.

Behavioral Barriers

In addition to the financial barriers, many behavioral or organizational barriers impede the adoption of EMR systems and other clinical applications. These barriers can be equally difficult to overcome as the financial barriers. They include everything from lack of physician acceptance to changes in workflow to differences in state licensing regulations.

EMR and other clinical information systems may alter the way that providers interact with patients and render patient care services. They often require that providers enter visit notes directly into the system, respond to system reminders and alerts, and give complete documentation. Studies have shown that the EMR, CPOE, and other clinical information applications can be difficult to incorporate into existing workflow processes and may require additional time (Poissant et al., 2005; Poon et al., 2004). When a system is initially implemented, it invariably adds time to the physician's day. This may seem contrary to one of the reasons for implementing EMR systems, to save time. In truth, EMR systems require that physicians respond to reminders, alerts, and other knowledge aids—all of which can lead to better patient care but may also require more time. For instance, suppose a physician is treating a patient with diabetes mellitus. The EMR might remind the physician to follow clinical practice guidelines for treating diabetes, which include conducting an eye exam and checking the patient's hemoglobin A1C levels—both of which take time. Without the EMR reminder, these tasks might have been forgotten. Unfortunately, most physicians receive no reimbursement or compensation for using EMR systems or for providing good-quality care. Until financial and reimbursement incentives are aligned with EMR use, lack of physician acceptance will likely remain a critical barrier to system adoption.

This is not to say that all health care organizations have been unable to gain physician acceptance. Strong leadership support, initial and ongoing training, sufficient time to learn the intricacies of the system, and evidence that the system is well integrated with patient care workflow are all important factors in gaining physician acceptance and use. Physicians need to realize the value that comes from using the clinical application—or they simply won't use it. This value may be improved patient services, improved quality of care, more highly satisfied patients, or happier staff, or something more personal to the physician such as improved quality of documentation, less stress, and more leisure time. Factors leading to physician acceptance of clinical information systems will be discussed further in Chapter Seven.

When it comes to telemedicine and telehealth systems, things such as differences in state laws and in standard medical practice can affect physicians' attitudes and impede adoption. Many states will not permit out-of-state physicians to practice in their state unless licensed by them. Some physicians are concerned about medical liability issues and the lack of hands-on interaction with patients. Many physicians still prefer to meet with the patient and conduct the examination in person for fear of litigation or of missing important information.

Technical Barriers

The third broad category of barriers to adopting EMR systems involves technology; health care organizations must implement the technologies necessary to support and sustain these systems. They must choose these technologies wisely—understanding how emerging technologies fit with existing technologies, and engaging in continuing development and refinement of standards and data definitions.

Getting your arms around health care information standards is not an easy task. Many of the standards issues in health care also exist for the general business community; others are specific to health care. One thing is clear—standards are what enable different computer systems from different vendors and different health care organizations to share data. We discuss standards that affect health care information systems and how these standards are developed in greater detail in Chapter Nine. In the context of the present discussion, what is important to understand is that inadequate standards combined with rapidly changing technologies can be a barrier to widespread EMR adoption and use. To aid health care executives and providers in acquiring EMR products that adhere to national standards, the Certification Commission for Healthcare Information Technology (CCHIT) was established in 2004. Since then, CCHIT has developed criteria and a process for certifying ambulatory care and inpatient EMR and EHR systems (CCHIT, 2008).

Significant work has occurred nationally in terms of standards development in recent years. The Healthcare Information Technology Standards Panel (HITSP), established in 2005, has brought together experts from across the health care community—from consumers to physicians, nurses, and hospitals; from those who develop health care IT products to those who use them; and from the governmental agencies that monitor the U.S. health care system to those organizations that actually write the standards (HITSP, 2008). Although widespread interoperability remains a goal, all the right players seem to be working together toward its achievement.

Despite these and other barriers to the widespread adoption of interoperable EHR systems, the desire to overcome them is extraordinarily strong. Our health care system is faced with rising costs, excessive variation in care, and antiquated paper-based record systems that are woefully inadequate. Public and private sector organizations and also consumers are demanding more. With collaboration, appropriate policy changes, and strong leadership, we expect that interoperable EHRs are achievable in the years to come.

SUMMARY

This chapter provided an overview of six clinical information applications: EMR, CPOE, medication administration, telemedicine, telehealth, and the PHR. We described each application and discussed its current use and its value to the patient, the provider, the health care organization, and the community at large. Special attention was given to the electronic medical record at the organizational level and the benefits it offers. These benefits include (1) improved quality, outcomes, and safety; (2) improved efficiency, productivity, and cost reduction; and (3) improved service and satisfaction. Despite the many benefits and advantages found in using EMR systems, the reality is that they are not widely used in health care today. The financial, behavioral, and technical barriers to their use were discussed here, along with some of the strategies employed to overcome these barriers.

KEY TERMS

Computerized provider order entry (CPOE)
Electronic health record (EHR)
Electronic mail (e-mail)
Electronic medical record (EMR)
E-prescribing
Health information exchange (HIE)

Medication administration systems
Nationwide Health Information Network (NHIN)
Personal health record (PHR)
Telehealth
Telemedicine

LEARNING ACTIVITIES

1. Search the Internet and find five health care information system vendors that offer EMR products. Compare and contrast the functions and features of each product. How do these systems compare with the IOM's definitions of the EHR?

2. Search the clinical management literature and find at least one article describing the adoption or use of (a) an EMR system, (b) a CPOE system, (c) a medication administration system using BPOC, (d) a telemedicine system, (e) a telehealth system, (f) a PHR, or (f) other clinical information system or application. Summarize the article for your classmates, and discuss it with them. What are the key points of the article? What lessons learned does it describe?

3. Visit a health care organization that uses one of the clinical applications described in this chapter. Find out how the application's value is measured or assessed. What do providers think about it? Health care executives? Nurses? Support staff? What impact has it had on patient care?

4.   Investigate what efforts are being made nationally and in your state (in both the public and private sectors) to further the adoption of EMR systems. How likely are these efforts to work? What concerns do you have about them? What else do you think is needed to further the adoption of EMR systems?

5.   Investigate the extent to which health information exchange initiatives or RHIOs exist in your community. How are they being used? To what extent are they achieving their objectives?

6.   Three broad categories of barriers to health information technology are discussed in this chapter. What other barriers are there beyond these? What strategies are being employed to overcome these other barriers?

CHAPTER

6

SYSTEM ACQUISITION

LEARNING OBJECTIVES

- To be able to explain the process a health care organization generally goes through in selecting a health care information system.

- To be able to describe the systems development life cycle and its four major stages.

- To be able to discuss the various options for acquiring a health care information systems (for example, purchasing, leasing, contracting with an application service provider, building a system in-house) and the pros and cons of each.

- To be able to discuss the purpose and content of a request for information and request for proposal in the system acquisition process.

- To gain insight into the problems that may occur during the system acquisition process.

- To gain an understanding of the health care IT industry and the resources available for identifying health care IT vendors and learning about their history, products, services, and reputation.

By now you should have an understanding of the various types of health care information systems and the value they can bring to health care organizations and the patients they serve. This chapter describes the typical process a health care organization goes through in acquiring or selecting a new clinical or administrative application. Acquiring an information system (IS) application can be an enormous investment for health care organizations. Besides the initial cost, there are a host of long-term costs associated with maintaining, supporting, and enhancing the system. Health care professionals need access to reliable, complete, and accurate information in order to provide effective and efficient health care services and to achieve the strategic goals of the organization. Selecting the right application, one that meets the organization's needs, is a critical step. Too often information systems are acquired without exploring all options, without evaluating costs and benefits, and without gaining sufficient input from key constituent user groups. The results can be disastrous.

This chapter describes the people who should be involved, the activities that should occur, and the questions that should be addressed in acquiring any new information system. The suggested methods are based on the authors' years of experience and on countless case studies of system acquisition successes and failures published in the health care literature.

SYSTEM ACQUISITION: A DEFINITION

In this book *system acquisition* refers to the process that occurs from the time the decision is made to select a new system (or replace an existing system) until the time a contract has been negotiated and signed. System implementation is a separate process described in the next chapter, but both are part of the systems development life cycle. The actual system selection, or acquisition, process can take anywhere from a few days to a couple of years, depending on the organization's size, structure, complexity, and needs. Factors such as whether the system is deemed a priority and whether adequate resources (time, people, and funds) are available can also directly affect the time and methods used to acquire a new system (McDowell, Wahl, & Michelson, 2003).

Prior to arriving at the decision to select a new system, the health care executive team should engage in a strategic IS planning process, in which the strategic goals of the organization are formulated and the ways in which information technology (IT) will be employed to aid the organization in achieving its strategic goals and objectives are discussed. We discuss the need for aligning the IT plans with the strategic goals of the organization and for determining IT priorities in Chapter Twelve. In this chapter, we assume that a strategic IT plan exists, IT priorities have been established, the new system has been adequately budgeted, and the organization is ready to move forward with the selection process.

SYSTEMS DEVELOPMENT LIFE CYCLE

No board of directors would recommend building a new health care facility without an architect's blueprint and a comprehensive assessment of the organization's and the community's needs and resources. The architect's blueprint helps ensure that the new facility has a strong foundation, is well designed, fosters the provision of high-quality care, and has the potential for growth and expansion. Similarly, the health care organization needs a blueprint to aid in the planning, selection, implementation, and support of a new health care information system. The decision to invest in a health care information system should be well aligned with the organization's overall strategic goals and should be made after careful thought and deliberation. Information systems are an investment in the organization's infrastructure, not a one-time purchase. Health care information systems require not only up-front costs and resources but also ongoing maintenance, support, upgrades, and eventually, replacement.

The process an organization generally goes through in planning, selecting, implementing, and evaluating a health care information system is known as the *systems development life cycle* (SDLC). Although the SDLC is most commonly described in the context of software development, the process also applies when systems are purchased from a vendor or leased through an *application service provider* (ASP). An ASP is a company that deploys, hosts, and manages one or more clinical or administrative information systems through centrally located servers (generally via the Internet), often on a fixed, per use basis or on a subscription basis. Regardless of how the system is acquired, most health care organizations follow a structured process for selecting and implementing a new computer-based system. The systems development process itself involves participation from individuals with different backgrounds and areas of expertise. The specific mix of individuals depends on the nature and scope of the new system.

Many SDLC frameworks exist, but most have four general phases, or stages—planning and analysis, design, implementation, and support and evaluation (Wager & Lee, 2006) (see Figure 6.1). Each phase has a number of tasks that need to be performed. In this chapter we focus on the first two phases; Chapter Seven focuses on the last two.

The SDLC approach assumes that this four-phase life of an IS starts with a need and ends when the benefits of the system no longer outweigh its maintenance costs, at which point the life of a new system begins (Oz, 2006). Hence, the entire project is called a *life cycle*. After the decision has been made to explore further the need for a new information system, the feasibility of the system is assessed and the scope of the project defined (in actuality it is at times difficult to tell when this decision making ends and analysis begins). The primary focus of this *planning and analysis phase* is on the business problem, or the organization's strategy, independent of any technology that can or will be used. During this phase, it is important to examine current systems and problems in order to identify opportunities for improvement. The organization should assess the feasibility of the new system—is it technologically, financially, and operationally feasible? Furthermore, sometimes it is easy to think that implementing a new IS will solve all information management problems. Rarely, if ever, is this the case. But by critically evaluating existing systems and workflow processes, the health care team might find that current problems are rooted in ineffective procedures or lack of sufficient training. Not always is a new system needed nor *the* answer to a problem.

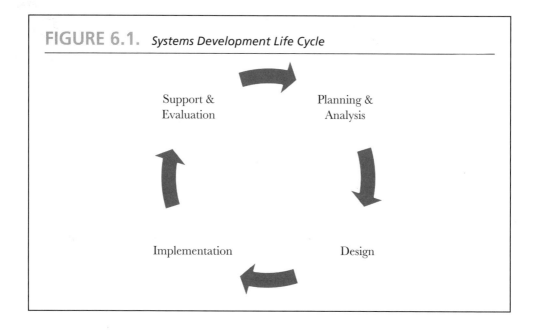

FIGURE 6.1. *Systems Development Life Cycle*

Once it is clear that a new IS is needed, the next step is to assess the information needs of users and define the functional requirements: what functions must the system have to fulfill the need? This process can be very time consuming. However, it is vital to solicit widespread participation from end-users during this early stage—to solicit and achieve buy-in. As part of the needs assessment, it is also helpful to gather, organize, and evaluate information about the environment in which the new system is to operate. Through defining system requirements the organization specifies what the system should be able to do and the means by which it will fulfill its stated goals.

Once the team knows what the organization needs, it enters the second stage, the *design phase*, where it considers all its options. Will the new system be designed in-house? Will the organization contract with an outside developer? Or will the organization purchase a system from a health information systems vendor or contract with an ASP? A large majority of health care organizations purchase a system from a vendor or at least look first at the systems available on the market. System design is the evaluation of alternative solutions to address the business problem. It is generally in this phase that all alternatives are considered, a cost-benefit analysis is done, a system is selected, and vendor negotiations are finalized.

 After the contract has been finalized or the system has been chosen, the third phase, *implementation*, begins. The implementation phase requires significant allocation of resources in completing tasks such as conducting workflow and process analyses, installing the new system, testing the system, training staff, converting data, and preparing the organization and staff for the go-live of the new system. Finally, once the system is put into operation, the *support and evaluation phase* begins. It is common to underestimate the staff and resources needed to effectively keep new and existing information systems functioning properly. No matter how much time and energy was spent on the design and build of the application, you can count on the fact that changes will need to be made, glitches fixed, and upgrades installed. Likewise, most mission-critical systems need to be functioning 99.99 percent of the time, that is, with little downtime. Sufficient resources (people, technology, infrastructure, upgrades) need to be allocated to maintain and support the new system. Although support costs can vary widely from system to system, in most industries up to 80 percent of the IS budget in spent on maintenance (Oz, 2006). The major reason for this significant proportion is that support is the longest phase in a system's life cycle.

Moreover, maintaining and supporting the new system is not enough. Health care executives and boards want to know the value of the IT investment, thus the degree to which the new system has achieved its goals and objectives should be assessed. Eventually, the system will be replaced and the SDLC process begins again.

With this general explanation of the SDLC established, we begin by focusing on the first two phases—the planning and analysis phase and the design phase. Together they constitute what we refer to as the *system acquisition process.*

SYSTEM ACQUISITION PROCESS

To gain an understanding of and appreciation for the activities that occur during the system acquisition process, we will follow a health care facility through the selection process for a new information system—specifically, an electronic medical record (EMR) system. In this case the organization, which we will call Valley Practice, is a multiphysician primary care practice.

What process should the practice use to select the EMR? Should it purchase a system from a vendor, contract with an application service provider, or seek the assistance of a system developer? Who should lead the effort? Who should be involved in the process? What EMR products are available on the market? How reputable are the vendors who develop these products? These are just a few of the many questions that should be asked in selecting a new IS.

Although the time and the resources needed to select an EMR (or any health care information system) may vary considerably from one setting to another, some fundamental issues should be addressed in any system acquisition initiative. The sections that follow the scenario describe in more detail the major activities that should occur (Exhibit 6.1), relating them to the multiphysician practice scenario. We assume that the practice wishes to purchase (rather than develop) an EMR system. However, we briefly describe other options and point out how the process may differ when the EMR acquisition process occurs in a larger health care setting, such as a hospital.

EXHIBIT 6.1. *Overview of System Acquisition Process*

- Establish project steering committee and appoint project manager.
- Define project objectives and scope of analysis.
- Screen the marketplace and review vendor profiles.
- Determine system goals.
- Determine and prioritize system requirements.
- Develop and distribute a request for proposal (RFP) or a request for information (RFI).
- Explore other options for acquiring system.

  Application service provider.

  Contract with system developer or build in-house.

- Evaluate vendor proposals.

  Develop evaluation criteria.

  Hold vendor demonstrations.

  Make site visits and check references.

  Prepare vendor analysis.

- Conduct cost-benefit analysis.
- Prepare summary report and recommendations.
- Conduct contract negotiations.

CASE STUDY

Acquiring an EMR System Valley Practice provides patient care services at three locations, all within a fifteen-mile radius, and serves nearly 100,000 patients. Valley Practice is owned and operated by seven physicians; each physician has an equal partnership. In addition to the physicians the practice employs nine nurses, fifteen support staff, a business officer manager, an accountant, and a chief executive officer (CEO).

During a two-day strategic planning session, the physicians and management team created a mission, vision, and set of strategic goals for Valley Practice. The mission of the facility is to serve as the primary care "medical home" of individuals within the community, regardless of the patients' ability to pay. Valley Practice wishes to be recognized as a "high-tech, high-touch" practice that provides high-quality, cost-effective patient care using evidence-based standards of care. Consistent with its mission, one of the practice's strategic goals is to replace its current paper-based medical record with an EMR system. Such a system should enable providers to care for patients using up-to-date, complete, accurate information, anywhere, anytime.

Dr. John Marcus, the lead physician at Valley Practice, asked Dr. Julie Brown, the newest partner in the group, to lead the EMR project initiative. Dr. Brown joined the practice two years ago after completing an internal medicine residency at an academic medical center that had a fully integrated EMR system available in both the hospital and its ambulatory care clinics. Of all the physicians at Valley Practice, Dr. Brown has had the most experience using an EMR. She has been a vocal advocate for implementing an EMR and believes it is essential to enabling the facility to achieve its strategic goals.

Dr. Brown agreed to chair the project steering committee. She invited other key individuals to serve on the committee, including Dr. Renee Ward, a senior physician in the practice; Mr. James Rowls, the CEO; Ms. Mary Matthews, RN, a nurse; and Ms. Sandy Raymond, the business officer manager. Dr. Brown suggested that the committee contract with a health care IT consultant to guide committee members through the system acquisition process. The physician partners approved this request, and the committee retained the services of Ms. Sheila Moore, a consultant with HIT Consulting Solutions, who came highly recommended by a colleague of Dr. Marcus's.

After the project steering committee was formed, Dr. Marcus met with the committee to outline its charge and deliverables. Dr. Marcus expressed his appreciation to Dr. Brown and all of the members of the committee for their willingness to participate in this important initiative. He assured them that they had his full support and the support of the entire physician team.

Dr. Marcus reviewed with the committee the mission, vision, and strategic goals of the practice as well as the committee's charge. The committee was asked to fully investigate and recommend the top three EMR products available in the vendor community. He stressed his desire that the committee members would focus on EMR vendors that have experience and a solid track record in implementing systems in physician practices similar to theirs and that have products certified by the Certification Commission for Healthcare Information Technology (CCHIT).

Dr. Marcus felt strongly that the EMR system needed to enable providers to access patient information from any of Valley Practice's three sites and from their homes. He also spoke of the need for the system to provide health maintenance reminders, drug interactions, and access to clinical practice guidelines or standards of care. One goal was to eventually rid Valley Practice of paper records and significantly decrease the amount of dictation and transcription currently being done. Dr. Ward, Mr. Rowls, and Ms. Matthews assumed leadership roles in verifying and prioritizing the requirements expressed by the various user groups.

Under the leadership of Dr. Brown the members of the project steering committee established five project goals and the methods they would use to guide their activities. Ms. Moore, the consultant, assisted them in clearly defining these goals and discussing the various options for moving forward. They agreed to consider EMR products from only those vendors that had five or more years of experience in the industry and had a solid track record of implementations (which they defined as having done twenty-five or more).

The five project goals were based on Valley Practice's strategic goals. These project goals were circulated for discussion and approved by the CEO and the physician partners. Once the goals were agreed upon, the project steering committee appointed a small task group of committee members to carry out the process of defining system functionality and requirements.

(Continued)

CASE STUDY (*Continued*)

Because staff time was limited, the task group conducted three separate focus groups during the lunch period—one with the nurses, one with the support staff, and a third with the physicians. Ms. Moore, the consultant, conducted the focus groups, using a semistructured nominal group technique.

Concurrently with the requirements definition phase of the project, Mr. Rowls and Dr. Brown, with assistance from Ms. Moore, screened the EMR vendor marketplace. They reviewed the literature, consulted with colleagues in the state medical association, and surveyed practices in the state that they knew used an EMR system. Mr. Rowls made a few phone calls to chief information officers (CIOs) in surrounding hospitals who had experience with ambulatory care EMRs to get their advice. This initial screening resulted in the identification of eight EMR vendors whose products and services seemed to meet Valley Practice's needs.

Given the fairly manageable number of vendors, Ms. Moore suggested that the project steering committee use a short-form request for proposal (RFP). This form had been developed by her consulting firm and had been used successfully by other physician practices to identify top contenders. The short-form RFPs were sent to the eight vendors; six responded. Each of these six presented an initial demonstration of its EMR system on site. Following the demonstrations, the practice staff members completed evaluation forms and ranked the various vendors. After reviewing the completed RFPs and getting feedback on the vendor presentations, the committee determined that three vendors had risen to the top of the list.

Dr. Brown and Dr. Ward visited four physician practices that used EMR systems from these three finalists. Mr. Rowls checked references and prepared the final vendor analysis. A detailed cost-benefit analysis was conducted, and the three vendors were ranked. All three vendors, in rank order, were presented in the final report given to Dr. Marcus and the other physician partners.

Dr. Marcus, Dr. Brown, and Mr. Rowls spent four weeks negotiating a contract with the top contender. It was finalized and approved after legal review and after all the partners agreed to it.

Establish a Project Steering Committee

One of the first steps in any major project such as an EMR acquisition effort is to create a *project steering committee*. This committee's primary function is to plan, organize, coordinate, and manage all aspects of the acquisition process. Appointing a project manager with strong communication skills, organizational skills, and leadership abilities is critical to the project. In our Valley Practice case the project manager was a physician partner. In larger health care organizations such as hospitals, where a CIO is employed, the CIO would likely be involved in the effort and might also be asked to lead it.

Increasingly, clinicians such as physicians and nurses with training in informatics are being called on to lead clinical system acquisition and implementation projects. Known as *chief medical informatics officers* or *nursing informatics officers*, these individuals bring to the project a clinical perspective as well as an understanding of IT and information management processes. Regardless of the discipline or background of the project manager (for example, IT, clinical, or administrative), he or she should bring to the project passion, interest, time, strong interpersonal and communication skills, and project management skills, and should be someone who is well respected by the organization's leadership team and who has the political clout to lead the effort effectively.

Pulling together a strong team of individuals to serve on the project steering committee is also important. These individuals should include representatives from key constituent groups in the practice. At Valley Practice, a physician partner, a nurse, the business officer manager, and the CEO agreed to serve on the committee. Gaining project buy-in from the various user groups should begin early. This is a key reason for inviting representatives from key constituent groups to serve on the project steering committee. They should be individuals who will use the EMR system directly or whose jobs will be affected by it.

Consideration should also be given to the size of the committee; typically, having five to six members is ideal. In a large facility, however, this may not be possible. The committee for a hospital might have fifteen to twenty members, with representatives from key clinical areas such as laboratory medicine, pharmacy, and radiology in addition to representatives from the administrative, IT, nursing, and medical staffs.

It is important to have someone knowledgeable about IT serving on the project steering committee. This may be a physician, a nurse, the CEO, or an outside consultant. In a physician group practice such as Valley Practice, having an in-house IT professional is rare. The committee chair might look internally to see if someone has the requisite IT knowledge, skills, and interests and also the time to devote to the project, but also might look externally for a health care IT professional who might serve in a consultative role and help the committee direct its activities appropriately.

Define Project Objectives and Scope of Analysis

Once the project steering committee has been established, its first order of business is to clarify the charge to the committee and to define project goals. The charge describes the scope and nature of the committee's activities. The charge usually comes from senior leadership or a lead physician in the practice. Project goals should also be established and communicated in well-defined, measurable terms. What does the committee expect to achieve? What process will be used to ensure the committee's success? How will milestones be acknowledged? How will the committee communicate progress and resolve problems? What resources (such as time, personnel, and travel expenses) will the committee need to carry out its charge? What method will be used to evaluate system options? Will the committee consider contracting with a system developer to build a system or outsourcing the system to an application service provider? Or is the committee only considering systems available for purchase from a health care information systems vendor?

Once project goals are formulated, they can guide the committee's activities and also clarify the resources needed and the likely completion date for the project. Here are some examples of typical project goals:

- Assess the practice's information management needs, and establish goals and objectives for the new system based on these needs.

- Conduct a review of the literature on EMR products and the market resources for these products.

- Investigate the top ten EMR system vendors for the health care industry.

- Visit two to four health care organizations similar to ours that have implemented an EMR system.

- Schedule vendor demonstrations for times when physicians, nurses, and others can observe and evaluate without interruptions.

As part of the goal-setting process, the committee should determine the extent to which various options will be explored. For example, the Valley Practice project steering committee decided at the onset that it was going to consider only EMR products available in the vendor community and specifically only those approved by the Certification Commission for Healthcare Information Technology (CCHIT). As discussed in Chapter Five, CCHIT, established in 2004, has developed and implemented standards-based certification of EMR and EHR products for both ambulatory and inpatient care settings (CCHIT, 2008). Users can be assured that certified products meet certain standards for content, functionality, and interoperability.

The committee felt CCHIT certification was important and further stipulated that it would consider only vendors with experience (for example, five or more years in the industry) and those with a solid track record of system installations (for example, twenty-five or more installations). The committee members felt the practice should contract with a system developer only if they were unable to find a suitable product from the vendor community—their rationale being that the practice wanted to be known as high-tech, high-touch. They also believed it was important to invest in IT personnel who could customize the application to meet practice needs and who would be able to assist the practice in achieving project and practice goals.

Screen the Marketplace and Review Vendor Profiles

Concurrently with the establishment of project goals, the project steering committee should conduct its first, cursory review of the EMR marketplace and begin investigating vendor profiles. Many resources are available to aid the committee in this effort. For example, the Valley Practice committee might obtain copies of recent market analysis reports—from research firms such as Gartner or KLAS—listing and describing the vendors that provide EMR systems for ambulatory care facilities. The committee might also attend trade shows at conferences of professional associations such as the Healthcare Information and Management Systems Society (HIMSS) and the American Medical Informatics Association (AMIA). (Appendix A provides an overview of the health care IT industry and describes a variety of resources available to health care organizations interested in learning about health care IT products, such as EMR systems, available in the vendor community.)

Determine System Goals

Besides identifying project goals, the project steering committee should define system goals. System goals can be derived by answering questions such as: What does the organization hope to accomplish by implementing an EMR system? What is it looking for in a system? If the organization intends to transform existing care processes, can the system support the new processes? Such goals often emerge during the initial strategic planning process when the decision is made to move forward with the selection of the new system. At this point, however, the committee should state its goals and needs for a new EMR system in clearly defined, specific, and measurable terms. For example, a system goal such as "select a new EMR system" is very broad and not specific. Here are some examples of specific and measurable goals for a physician practice.

Our EMR system should

- Enable the practice to provide service to patients using evidence-based standards of care.
- Aid the practice in monitoring the quality and costs of care provided to the patients served.
- Provide clinicians with access to accurate, complete, relevant patient information, on site and remotely.
- Improve staff efficiency and effectiveness.

These are just a few of the types of system goals the project steering committee might establish as it investigates a new EMR for the organization. The system goals should be aligned with the strategic goals of the organization and should serve as measures of success throughout the system acquisition process.

Determine and Prioritize System Requirements

Once the goals of the new system have been established, the project steering committee should begin to determine system requirements. These requirements may address everything from what information should be available to the provider at the point of care to how the information will be secured to what type of response time is expected. The committee may use any of a variety of ways to identify system requirements. One approach is to have a subgroup of the committee conduct focus-group sessions or small-group interviews with the various user groups (physicians, nurses, billing personnel, and support staff). A second approach is to develop and administer a written survey, customized for each user group, asking individuals to identify their information needs in light of their job role or function. A third is to assign a representative from each specific area to obtain input from users in that area. For example, the nurse on the Valley Practice project steering committee might interview the other nurses; the business office manager might interview the support staff. System requirements may also emerge as the committee examines templates provided by consultants or peer institutions, looks at vendor demonstrations and sales material, or considers new regulatory requirements the organization must meet.

The committee may also use a combination of these or other approaches. At times, however, users do not know what they want or will need. Hence it can be extremely helpful to hold product demonstrations, meet with consultants, or visit sites already using EMR systems, so that those who will use or be affected by the EMR can see and hear what is possible. Whatever methods are chosen to seek users' information system needs, the end result should be a list of requirements and specifications that can be prioritized, or ranked. This ranking should directly reflect the specific strategic goals and circumstances of the organization.

The system requirements and priorities will eventually be shared with vendors or the system developer; therefore it is important that they be clearly defined and presented in an organized, easy-to-understand format. For example, it may be helpful to organize the requirements into categories such as *software* (system functionality, software upgrades), *technical infrastructure* (hardware requirements, network specifications, backup, disaster recovery, security), and *training and support* (initial and ongoing training, technical support). These requirements will eventually become a major component of the request for proposal (RFP) submitted to vendors or other third parties (discussed further later in this chapter).

Develop and Distribute the RFP or RFI

Once the organization has defined its system requirements, the next step in the acquisition process is to package these requirements into a structure that a third party can respond to, whether that third party be a development partner or a health information systems vendor. Many health care organizations package the requirements into a *request for proposal* (RFP). The RFP provides the vendor with a comprehensive list of system requirements, features, and functions and asks the vendor to indicate whether its product or service meets each need. Vendors responding to an RFP are also generally required to submit a detailed and binding price quotation for the applications and services being sought.

RFPs tend to be highly detailed and are therefore time consuming and costly to develop and complete. However, they provide the health care organization and each vendor with a comprehensive view of the system needed. Health care IT consultants can be extremely resourceful in assisting the organization with developing and packaging the RFP. An RFP for a major health care information system acquisition generally contains the following information (sections marked with an asterisk [*] are completed by the vendor; the other sections are completed by the organization issuing the RFP):

- *Instructions for vendors:*

  Proposal deadline and contact information: where and when the RFP is due; whom to contact with questions.

  Confidentiality statement and instructions: a statement that both the RFP and the responses provided by the vendor are confidential and are proprietary information.

  Specific instructions for completing the RFP and any stipulations with which the vendor must comply in order to be considered.

- *Organizational objectives:* type of system or application being sought; information management needs and plans.

■ *Background of the organization:*

Overview of the facility: size, types of patient services, patient volume, staff composition, strategic goals of organization.

Application and technical inventory: current systems in use, hardware, software, network infrastructure.

■ *System goals and requirements:* goals for the system and functional requirements (may be categorized as mandatory or desirable and listed in priority order). Typically this section includes application, technical, and integration requirements.

■ *Vendor qualifications:* *general background of vendor, experience, number of installations, financial stability, list of current clients, standard contract, and implementation plan.

■ *Proposed solutions:* *how vendor believes its product meets the goals and needs of the health care organization. Vendor may include case studies, results from system analysis projects, and other evidence of the benefits of its proposed solution.

■ *Criteria for evaluating proposals:* how the health care organization will make its final decisions on product selection.

■ *General contractual requirements:* *such as warranties, payment schedule, penalties for failure to meet schedules specified in contract, vendor responsibilities, and so forth.

■ *Pricing and support:* *quote on cost of system, using standardized terms and forms.

RFPs are not the only means by which to solicit information from vendors. A second approach that is often used is the *request for information* (RFI). An RFI is considerably shorter than an RFP and less time consuming to develop and is designed to obtain basic information on the vendor's background, product description, and service capabilities. Some health care organizations send out an RFI before distributing the RFP, in order to screen out vendors whose products or services are not consistent with the organization's needs. Rather than seeking a specific quotation on price as the RFP does, the RFI simply asks the vendor to provide its guidelines for calculating the purchase price (DeLuca & Enmark, 2002).

How does one decide whether to use an RFP, an RFI, both, or neither during the system acquisition process? Several factors should be considered. Although time consuming to develop, the RFP is useful in forcing a health care organization to define its system goals and requirements and prioritize its needs. The RFP also creates a structure for objectively evaluating vendor responses and provides a record of documentation throughout the acquisition process. System acquisition can be a highly political process; by using an RFP the organization can introduce a higher degree of objectivity into that process. RFPs are also useful data collection tools when the technology being selected is established and fully developed, when there is little variability between vendor products and services, when the organization has the time to fully evaluate all options, and when the organization needs strong contract protection from the selected vendor (DeLuca & Enmark, 2002).

There are also drawbacks to RFPs. Besides taking considerable time to develop and review, they can become cumbersome, so detail oriented that they lose their effectiveness. For instance, it is not unusual to receive three binders full of product and service information from one vendor. If ten vendors respond to an RFP (about five is ideal), the project steering committee may be overwhelmed and find it difficult to wade through and differentiate among vendor responses. Having too much information to summarize can be as crippling to a committee in its deliberations as having too little.

Therefore a scaled-back RFP or an RFI might be a desirable alternative. An RFI might be used when the health care organization is considering only a small group of vendors or products or when it is still in the exploratory stages and has not yet established its requirements. Some facilities use an even less formal process consisting primarily of site visits and system demonstrations.

Regardless of the tool(s) used, it is important for the health care organization to provide sufficient detail about its current structure, strategic IT goals, and future plans that the vendor can respond appropriately to its needs. Additionally, the RFP or RFI (or variation of either) should result in enough specific detail that the organization gets a good sense of the vendor—its services, history, vision, stability in the marketplace, and system or product functionality. The organization should be able to easily screen out vendors whose products are undeveloped or not yet fully tested (DeLuca & Enmark, 2002).

Explore Other Acquisition Options

In our Valley Practice case the physicians and staff opted to acquire an EMR system from the vendor community. Organizations like Valley Practice often turn to the market for products that they will run on their own IT infrastructure. But there are times when they do not go to the market—they chose to leverage someone else's infrastructure (by contracting with an application service provider) or they build the application (by contracting with a system developer or using in-house staff).

Contract with an Application Service Provider   In recent years, with wider availability of high-speed or broadband Internet connections, more sophisticated vendor solutions, and a growing number of options for hosting software, the *application service provider* (ASP) approach has emerged as an alternative to buying, installing, and maintaining information systems. An ASP is an organization with whom health care providers contract on a subscription basis to deliver an application and provide the associated services to support it. It's somewhat analogous to the option of leasing rather than purchasing a car. ASPs are also similar in concept to the shared-systems option used by many hospitals in the 1960s and 1970s, when they could not afford or did not have the IT staff available in-house to run and support software applications and hardware. In essence, another organization houses and maintains the clinical or administrative application and related hardware; the health care organization or provider simply accesses the system remotely over a network connection and pays the monthly or negotiated fees. It is worth noting that some ASPs do not physically host the application but instead contract with a third-party data center to do so (Fortin & MacDonald, 2006).

Regional health information organizations (RHIOs) could serve as ASPs as they mature and expand their capabilities.

Why might a health care organization consider contracting with an ASP rather than purchasing an EMR system (or other application) from a vendor? There are several reasons. First, the facility may not have the IT staff needed to run or support the desired system. Hiring qualified personnel at the salaries they demand may be difficult, and retaining them may be equally challenging. Second, ASPs typically enable health care organizations to use clinical or administrative applications with fewer up-front costs and less capital. For a small physician practice these financial arrangements can be particularly appealing. Because ASPs offer fixed monthly fees or fees based on usage, organizations are better able to predict costs. Third, by contracting with an ASP, the health care organization can focus on its core business and not get bogged down in IT support issues, although it may still have to deal with issues of system enhancements, user needs, and the selection of new systems. Other advantages to using ASPs are rapid deployment and 24/7 technical support.

ASPs also have some disadvantages and limitations that the health care organization should consider in its deliberations. Although rapid deployment of the application can be a tremendous advantage to an organization, the downside is the fact that the application will likely be a standard, off-the-shelf product, with little if any customization. This means that the organization has to adapt or mold its operations to the application rather than tailoring the application to meet the operational needs of the organization. A second drawback deals with technical support. Although technical support is generally available from an ASP, it is unrealistic to think that the ASP's support personnel will have intimate knowledge of the organization and its operations. Frustrations can mount when one lacks in-house IT technical staff when and where they are needed. Third, health care providers have long been concerned about data ownership, security, and privacy — worries that increase when another organization hosts their clinical data and applications. How the ASP will secure data and maintain patient privacy should be clearly specified in the contract. Likewise, to minimize downtime, the ASP should have clear plans for backing up data, preventing disasters, and recovering data.

First Consulting recently prepared a report for the California HealthCare Foundation outlining the latest developments, benefits, challenges, issues, and concerns related to the ASP model for ambulatory clinical applications (Fortin & MacDonald, 2006). It suggests health care leaders ask themselves four important questions in deciding whether an ASP approach is the right choice for their organization:

■ How will the application fit into the organization's overall IT plans?

■ To what extent can the organization support locally installed software?

■ How willing is the organization to have another organization host a clinical application?

■ What financial resources does the organization have (Fortin & MacDonald, 2006, p. 15)?

As the industry matures, we will likely see different variations and greater choices among organizations serving as ASPs. The health care executive considering whether an ASP is the right choice should thoroughly research the company and its products and consider factors such as company viability, target market, functionality, integration, implementation and training, help desk support, security, pricing, and service levels. It is important to be able to trust the ASP and to choose one wisely.

Contract with a System Developer or Build In-House A second alternative to purchasing a system from a vendor is to contract with a developer to design a system for your organization. The developer may be employed in-house or by an outside firm. Working with a system developer can be a good option when the health care organization's needs are highly uncertain or unique and the products available on the market do not adequately meet these needs. Developing a new or innovative application can also give the organization a significant competitive advantage. The costs and time needed to develop the application can be significant, however. It is also important to consider the long-term costs. Should the developer leave, how difficult would it be to hire and retain someone to support and maintain the system? How will problems with the system be addressed? How will the application be upgraded? What long-term value will it bring the organization? These are a few of the many questions that should be addressed in considering this option. It is rare for a health care organization to develop its own major clinical information system.

Evaluate Vendor Proposals In the Valley Practice case the project steering committee decided to focus its efforts at first on considering only EMR products available for purchase in the vendor community. The committee came to this conclusion after its initial review of the EMR marketplace. Committee members felt there were a number of vendors whose products appeared to meet practice needs. They also felt strongly that in-house control of the EMR system was important to achieving the practice goal of becoming a high-tech, high-touch organization, because they wanted to be able to customize the application. Realizing this, the committee had budgeted for an IT director and an IT support staff member. Members felt that the long-term cost savings from implementing an EMR would justify these two new positions.

Develop Evaluation Criteria The project steering committee at Valley Practice decided to go through the RFP process. It developed criteria by which it would review and evaluate vendor proposals. Criteria were used to grade each vendor's response to the RFP. Grading scales were established so the committee could accurately compare vendors' responses. These grading scales involved assigning more weight to required items and less weight to those deemed merely desirable. Categories of "does not meet requirement," "partially meets requirement," and "meets requirement" were also used. RFP documents were compared item by item and side by side, using the grading scales established by the committee (see Table 6.1 for sample criteria). To avoid information overload, a common condition in the RFP review process, the project steering committee focused on direct responses to requirements and referred to supplemental information only as needed. Summary reports of each vendor's response to the RFP were then prepared by a small group of committee members and distributed to the committee at large.

TABLE 6.1. **Sample Criteria for Evaluation of RFP Responses**

Type of Application: *Electronic Medical Record System*
Vendor Name: *The EMR Company*

Criteria	Meets Requirement	Partially Meets Requirement	Does Not Meet Requirement
1. Alerts user to possible drug interactions	x		
2. Provides user with list of alternate drugs	x		
3. Advises user on dosage based on patient's weight	x		
4. Allows user to enter over-the-counter medications		x (on different screen)	
5. Allows easy print out of prescriptions	x		

Hold Vendor Demonstrations   During the vendor review process, it is important to host vendor system demonstrations. The purpose of these demonstrations is to give the members of the health care organization an opportunity to (1) evaluate the look and feel of the system from a user's point of view, (2) validate how much the vendor can deliver of what has been proposed, and (3) narrow the field of potential vendors (Superior Consultant Company, 2004). It is often a good idea to develop demonstration scripts and require all vendors to present their systems in accordance with these scripts. Scripts generally reflect the requirements outlined in the RFP and contain a moderate level of detail. For example, a script might require demonstrating the process of registering a patient or renewing a prescription. The use of scripts can ensure that all vendors are evaluated on the same basis or functionality. At the same time, it is important to allow vendors some creativity in presenting their product and services. When scripts are used, they need to be provided to vendors at least one month in advance of the demonstration, and both vendors and health care organization must adhere to them.

Criteria should be developed and used in evaluating vendor demonstrations, just as they are for reviewing vendor responses to the RFP.

Make Site Visits and Check References   After reviewing the vendors' RFPs and evaluating their product demonstrations, it is advisable to make site visits and check references. By visiting other facilities that use a vendor's products, the health care organization should gain additional insight into what the vendor would be like as a potential partner. It can be extremely beneficial to visit organizations similar to yours. For instance, in the Valley Practice case, representatives from key practice constituencies decided to visit other ambulatory care practices to see how a specific system was being used, the problems that had been encountered, and how these problems had been addressed.

How satisfied are the staff with the system? How responsive has the vendor been to problems? How quickly have problems been resolved? To what degree has the vendor delivered on its promises? Hearing answers to such questions firsthand from a variety of users can be extremely helpful in the vendor review process.

Other Strategies for Evaluating Vendors   A host of other strategies can be used to evaluate a vendor's reputation and product and service quality. Organizational representatives might attend vendor user-group conferences, review the latest market reports, consult with colleagues in the field, seek advice from consultants, and request an extensive list of system users.

Prepare a Vendor Analysis   Throughout the vendor review process, the project steering committee members should have evaluation tools in place to document their impressions and the views of others in the organization who participate in any or all of the review activities (review of RFPs, system demonstrations, site visits, reference checks, and so forth). The committee should then prepare vendor analysis reports that summarize the major findings from each of the review activities. How do the vendors compare in reputation? In quality of their product? In quality of service? How do the systems compare in terms of their initial and ongoing costs? To what degree is the vendor's vision for product development aligned with the organization's strategic IT goals?

Conduct a Cost-Benefit Analysis

The final analysis should include an evaluation of the cost and benefits of each proposed system. Figure 6.2 shows a comparison of six vendor products. Criteria were developed to score and rank each vendor's system. As the figure illustrates, the selection committee ranked vendor 4 the top choice.

The capital cost analysis may include software, hardware, network or infrastructure, third-party, and internal capital costs. The total cost of ownership should factor in support costs and the costs of the resources needed (including personnel) to implement and support the system. Once the initial and ongoing costs are identified, it is important to weigh them against the benefits of the systems being considered. Can the benefits be quantified? Should they be included in the final analysis?

Prepare a Summary Report and Recommendations

Assuming the capital cost analysis supports the organization in moving forward with the project, the project steering committee should compile a final report that summarizes the process and results from each major activity or event. The report may include

System goals and criteria

Process used

FIGURE 6.2. *Cost-Benefit Analysis*

Vendor	50 MDs	10 MDs	5 MDs	1 MD	Fin.	Tech.	Interop.	Dec. Support	Clin./ Oper. Rank	Clin./ Oper. Points
Vendor 1	$5,588	$6,178	$6,806	$13,449	3	4	4.4	3.8	2	68
Vendor 2	$6,413	$6,594	$7,413	$13,373	3	4	3.4	2.9	5	27
Vendor 3	$3,378	$4,360	$5,130	$8,842	3	4	1.9	4.2	4	28
Vendor 4	$6,899	$6,086	$7,678	$15,437	5	4	4.1	4.3	1	70
Vendor 5	$5,945	$8,494	$9,543	$34,308	4	3	3.5	3.9	6	25
Vendor 6	$4,468	$4,580	$5,654	$12,927	3	3	2.4	4.1	3	46

Note: Fin. = Financial; Tech. = Technical; Interop. = Interoperability; Dec. Support = Decision Support; Clin./Oper. Rank = Clinical and Operational Rank; Clin./Oper. Points = Clinical and Operational Points

Source: Partners HealthCare

Results of each activity and conclusions

Cost-benefit analysis

Final recommendation and ranking of vendors

It is generally advisable to have two or three vendors in the final ranking, in the event that problems arise with the first choice during contract negotiations, the final step in the system acquisition process.

Conduct Contract Negotiations

The final step of the system acquisition process is to negotiate a contract with the vendor. This too can be a time-consuming process, and therefore it is helpful to seek expert advice from business or legal advisers. The contract outlines expectations and performance requirements, who is responsible for what (for example, training, interfaces, support), when the product is to be delivered (and vendor financial liability for failing to deliver on time), how much customization can be performed by the organization purchasing the system, how confidentiality of patient information will be handled, and when payment is due. The devil is in the details, and although most technical terms are common between vendors, other language and nuances are not. Establish a schedule and a preimplementation plan that includes a timeline for implementation of the applications and an understanding of the resource requirements for all aspects of the implementation, including cultural change management, workflow redesign, application implementation, integration requirements, and infrastructure development and upgrades, all of which can consume substantial resources.

PROJECT MANAGEMENT TOOLS

Throughout the course of the system acquisition project, a lot of materials will be generated, many of which should be maintained in a project repository. A *project repository* serves as a record of the project steering committee's progress and activities. It includes such information and documents as minutes of meetings, correspondence with vendors, the request for proposal or request for information, evaluation forms, and summary reports. This repository can be extremely useful when there are changes in staff or in the composition of the committee and when the organization is planning for future projects. The project manager should assume a leadership role in ensuring that the project repository is established and maintained. Here is a sample of the typical contents of a project repository.

PERSPECTIVE

SAMPLE CONTENTS OF A PROJECT REPOSITORY

- Committee charge and membership (including contact information)
- Project objectives (including method that will be used to select system)
- System goals
- Timeline of committee activities (for example, Gantt chart)
- System requirements (mandatory, desirable)
- Request for proposal
- Request for information
- Evaluation forms for

    Responses to RFPs

    Vendor demonstrations

    Site visits

    Reference checks

- Summary report and recommendations
- Project budget and resources

FIGURE 6.3. *Example of a Simple Gantt Chart*

ID	EMR Selection Project	Start	End	Jan 2009		Feb 2009		Mar 2009	
				1/16 1/23 1/30	2/6 2/13 2/20	2/27 3/6	3/13 3/20 3/27 4/3
1	Define project objectives	1/17/2009	1/17/2009				
2	Conduct preliminary review of vendors	1/21/2009	2/8/2009	▓			
3	Determine system requirements	1/21/2009	3/15/2009	▓▓▓▓▓			
4	Conduct focus groups	2/1/2009	2/28/2009		▓▓		
5	Survey key user groups	2/1/2009	3/10/2009		▓▓▓		
6	Develop and administer RFP	3/15/2009	4/15/2009			▓	
7	Hold vendor demonstrations	4/15/2009	4/29/2009				
8	Conduct cost-benefit analysis	5/2/2009	5/13/2009				

Managing the various aspects of the project and coordinating activities can be a challenging task, particularly in large organizations or when a lot of people are involved and many activities are occurring simultaneously. It is important that the project manager helps those involved to establish clear roles and responsibilities for individual committee members, to set target dates, and to agree upon methods for communicating progress and problems. Many project management tools exist that can be useful here. For example, a simple Gantt chart (Figure 6.3) can document project objectives, tasks and activities, responsible parties, and target dates and milestones. A Gantt chart can also display a graphical representation of all project tasks and activities, showing which ones may occur simultaneously and which ones must be completed before another task can begin. Other tools enable one to allocate time, staff, and financial resources to each activity. (Gantt charts and other timelines can be created with software programs such as Visio, Microsoft Project, or SmartDraw. A discussion of these tools is beyond the scope of this book but can be found in most introductory project management textbooks.)

It is important to clearly communicate progress both within the project steering committee and to individuals outside the committee. Senior management should be kept apprised of project progress, budget needs, and committee activities. Regular updates should be provided to senior management as well as other user groups involved in the process. Communication can be both formal and informal—everything from periodic update reports at executive meetings to facility newsletter briefings to informal discussions at lunch.

THINGS THAT CAN GO WRONG

Managing the system acquisition process successfully requires strong and effective leadership, planning, organizational, and communication skills. Things can and do go wrong. Upholding a high level of objectivity and fairness throughout the acquisition process is important to all parties involved. Failing to do so can dampen the overall success of the project. Following is a list of some common pitfalls in the system acquisition process, along with strategies for avoiding them.

- *Failing to manage vendor access to organizational leadership.* The vendor may schedule private time with the CEO or a board member in the hope of influencing the decision and bypassing the project steering committee entirely. It is not unusual to hear that processes or decisions have been altered after the CEO has been on a golf outing or taken a trip to the Super Bowl with a vendor. The vendor may persuade the CEO or a board member to overturn or question the decisions of the project steering committee, crippling the decision process. Hence it should be clearly communicated to all parties (senior management, board, and vendor) that all vendor requests and communication should be channeled through the project steering committee.

- *Failing to keep the process objective (getting caught up in vendor razzle-dazzle).* Related to the need to manage vendor access to decision makers is the need to keep the process objective. The project steering committee should assume a leadership role in ensuring that there are clearly defined criteria and methods for selecting the vendor. These criteria and methods should be known to all the parties involved and should be adhered to. Additionally, it is important that the committee and other organizational representatives remain unbiased and not get so impressed with the vendor's razzle-dazzle (in the form, for example, of exquisite dinners or fancy gadgets) that they fail to assess the vendor or the product objectively. Consider the politics of a situation but do not allow the vendor to drive the result—take the high road to avoid the appearance of favoritism.

- *Overdoing or underdoing the RFP.* Striking a balance between too much and too little information and detail in the RFP and also determining how much weight to give to the vendors' responses to the RFP can be challenging. The project steering committee should err on the side of being *reasonable*—that is, the committee should include enough information and detail that the vendor can appropriately respond to the organization's needs and should give the vendor responses to the RFP appropriate consideration in the final decision. Organizations should also be careful that they do not assign either too much or too little weight to the RFP process.

- *Failing to involve the leadership team and users extensively during the selection process.* A sure way to disenchant the leadership team and end-users is to fail to involve them adequately in the system acquisition process. There should be ample opportunity for people at all levels of the organization who will use or be affected by the new information system to have input into its selection. Involvement can include everything from being invited and encouraged to attend vendor presentations during uninterrupted time to being asked to join a focus group where user input is sought. It is important that the project steering committee seek input and involvement throughout the acquisition process, not simply at the end when the decision is nearly final. Far too often information system projects fail because the leadership team and end-users were not actively involved in the selection of the new system.

■ *Turning negotiations into a blood sport.* You want to negotiate a fair deal with the vendor and not leave the vendor's people feeling as though they have just been "beaten" in a contest. A lopsided deal results in a disenchanted partner and can create a bad climate. Understand what is required from all parties and establish performance criteria for payments and remedies for nonperformance. It is important to form a healthy, respectful, long-term relationship with the vendor.

These are just a few of the many issues that can arise during the system acquisition process that the health care executive should be aware of. Failing to appropriately address these issues can interfere with the organization's ability to successfully select and implement a system that will be adopted and widely used.

SUMMARY

Acquiring or selecting a new clinical or administrative information system is a major undertaking for a health care organization. It is important that the process be managed effectively. Although the time and resources needed to select a new system will vary depending on the size, complexity, and needs of the organization, certain fundamental issues should be addressed in any system acquisition project.

This chapter discussed the various activities that occur in the system acquisition process. These activities were presented in the context of a multiphysician group practice that wishes to replace its current paper record with an EMR system by acquiring a system from a reputable vendor. Key activities in the system selection process are (1) establishing a project steering committee and appointing a strong project manager to lead the effort, (2) defining project objectives, (3) screening the vendor marketplace, (4) determining system goals, (5) establishing system requirements, (6) developing and administering a request for proposal or request for information, (7) evaluating vendor proposals, and (8) conducting a cost-benefit analysis on the various options. Other options such as contracting with an application service provider (ASP) or a system developer were also discussed. Finally, this chapter presented some of the issues that can arise during the system selection process and outlined the importance of documenting and communicating project activities and progress.

KEY TERMS

Acquisition process

Application service provider (ASP)

Contract negotiations

Cost-benefit analysis

Project repository

Project steering committee

Request for information (RFI)

Request for proposal (RFP)

Systems development life cycle (SDLC)

Planning and analysis phase

Design phase

Implementation phase

Support and evaluation phase

LEARNING ACTIVITIES

1. Interview a health care executive regarding the process last used by his or her organization to acquire a new information system. How did that process compare with the system acquisition process described in this chapter?

2. Assume you are part of a project steering committee in a rural nonprofit hospital. The hospital is interested in acquiring a new provider order entry system. You offer to screen the marketplace to see what types of computerized provider order entry systems are available. Prepare a fifteen-minute summary report of your findings to the committee at large.

3. Conduct a literature review (including an Internet search) to learn about application service provider (ASP) organizations that offer EMR systems to physician practices. Briefly summarize the EMR products available from at least three different ASPs. What criteria might you use to compare them? How do they differ in terms of service, support, and financing arrangements?

4. Find and critique a sample RFP for a health care organization. What did you like about it? What aspects of it did you feel could be improved? Explain.

5. This chapter described a typical physician practice that wishes to select an EMR system. Using the information in the Valley Practice scenario, draft a script for vendors to use in demonstrating their product and services to Valley Practice staff. Include a description of the process you used to arrive at the script.

6. Working with your classmates (in small groups), assume that you are a Valley Practice committee member interested in obtaining user feedback on the EMR vendor demonstrations. Develop a survey instrument that might be used to solicit and summarize participants' responses to each vendor demonstration. Swap the survey your group designed with another group's survey; critique each other's work.

CHAPTER

7

SYSTEM IMPLEMENTATION AND SUPPORT

LEARNING OBJECTIVES

■ To be able to discuss the process that a health care organization typically goes through in implementing a health care information system.

■ To be able to appreciate the organizational and behavioral factors that can affect system acceptance and use and strategies for managing change.

■ To be able to develop a sample system implementation plan for a health care information system project, including the types of individuals who should be involved.

■ To gain insight into many of the things that can go wrong during system implementations and strategies health care managers can employ to alleviate potential problems.

■ To be able to discuss the importance of training, technical support, infrastructure, and ongoing maintenance and evaluation of any health care information system project.

Once a health care organization has finalized its contract with the vendor to acquire an information system, the system implementation process begins. Selecting the right system does not ensure user acceptance and success; the system must also be incorporated effectively into the day-to-day operations of the health care organization and adequately supported or maintained. Whether the system is built in-house, designed by an outside consultant, leased from an application service provider (ASP), or purchased from a vendor, it will take a substantial amount of planning and work to get the system up and running smoothly and integrated into operations.

This chapter focuses on the two final stages of the system development life cycle, implementation and then support and evaluation. It describes the planning and activities that should occur when implementing a new system. Our discussion focuses on a vendor-acquired system; however, many of the activities described also apply to systems designed in-house or by an outside developer or acquired through an ASP.

Implementing a new system (or replacing an old system) can be a massive undertaking for a health care organization. Not only are there workstations to install, databases to build, and networks to test but there are also processes to redesign, users to train, data to convert, and procedures to write. There are countless tasks and details that must be appropriately coordinated and completed if the system is to be implemented on time and within budget—and widely accepted by users.

Along with attending to these activities, or tasks, it is equally important to address organizational and behavioral issues. Studies have shown that over half of all information system projects fail. Numerous political, cultural, and behavioral factors can affect the successful implementation and use of the new system (Ash, Anderson, & Tarczy-Hornoch, 2008; Ash et al., 2007). We devote a section of this chapter to the organizational and behavioral issues that can arise and other things that can go wrong during the system implementation process and offer strategies for avoiding these problems. The chapter concludes by describing the importance of supporting and maintaining information systems.

SYSTEM IMPLEMENTATION PROCESS

System implementation begins once the organization has acquired the system and continues through the early stages following the *go-live* date (the date when the system is put into general use for everyone). Like the system acquisition process, the system implementation process must have a high degree of support from the senior executive team and be viewed as an organizational priority. Sufficient staff, time, and resources must be devoted to the project. Individuals involved in rolling out the new system should have the resources available to them that will ensure a smooth transition.

The time and resources needed to implement a new health care information system can vary considerably based on the scope of the project, the needs and complexity of the organization, the number of applications being installed, and the number of user groups involved. There are, however, some fundamental activities that should occur during any system implementation, regardless of its size or scope:

- Organize the implementation team and identify a system champion.

- Determine project scope and expectations.

- Establish and institute a project plan.

Failing to appropriately plan for and manage these activities can lead to cost overruns, dissatisfied users, project delays, and even system sabotage. In today's environment, where capital is scarce and resources are limited, health care organizations cannot afford to mismanage implementation projects of this magnitude and importance.

Organize the Team and Identify a Champion

One of the first steps in planning for the implementation of a new system is to organize an *implementation team*. The primary role and function of the team is to plan, coordinate, budget, and manage all aspects of the new system implementation. Although the exact team composition will depend on the scope and nature of the new system, a team might include a project leader, system champion(s), key individuals from the clinical and administrative areas that are the focus of the system being acquired, vendor representatives, and information technology (IT) professionals (Figure 7.1). For large or complex projects, it is also a good idea to have someone skilled in project management principles on the team. Likewise, having a strong project leader and the right mix of people is critically important.

Implementation teams often include some of the same people involved in selecting the system; however, they may also include other individuals with knowledge and skills important to the successful deployment of the new system. For example, the implementation team will likely need at least one IT professional with technical database and network administration expertise. This person may have had some role in the selection process but is now being called on to assume a larger role in installing the software, setting up the data tables, and customizing the network infrastructure to adequately support the system and the organization's needs.

The implementation team should also include at least one *system champion*. A system champion is someone who is well respected in the organization, sees the new system as necessary to the organization's achievement of its strategic goals, and is passionate about implementing it. In many health care settings the system champion

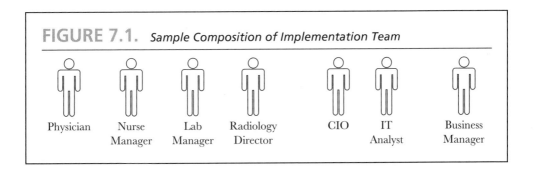

FIGURE 7.1. *Sample Composition of Implementation Team*

| Physician | Nurse Manager | Lab Manager | Radiology Director | CIO | IT Analyst | Business Manager |

is a physician, particularly when the organization is implementing a system that will directly or indirectly affect how physicians spend their time. The physician champion serves as an advocate of the system, assumes a leadership role in gaining buy-in from other physicians and user groups, and makes sure that physicians have adequate input into the decision-making process. Other important qualities of system champions are strong communication, interpersonal, and listening skills. The system champion should be willing to assist with pilot testing, to train and coach others, and to build consensus among user groups (Miller & Sim, 2004). Numerous studies have demonstrated the importance of the system champion throughout the implementation process (Miller, Sim, & Newman, 2003; Wager, Lee, White, Ward, & Ornstein, 2000; Ash, Stavri, Dykstra, & Fournier, 2003). When implementing clinical applications (such as computerized provider order entry [CPOE] or medication administration using bar coding) that span numerous clinical areas, such as nursing, pharmacy, and physicians, having a system champion from each division can be enormously helpful in gaining buy-in and in facilitating communication among staff.

Determine Project Scope and Expectations

One of the implementation team's first items of business is to determine the scope of the project and what the organization hopes the project will achieve. To set the tone for the project, a senior health care executive should meet with the implementation team to communicate how the project relates to the organization's overall strategic goals and to assure the team of administration's commitment to the project.

The goals of the project and what the organization hopes to achieve by implementing the new system should emerge from early team discussions. The system goals defined during the system selection process (discussed in Chapter Six) should be reviewed by the implementation team. Far too often health care organizations skip this important step and never clearly define the scope of the project or what they hope to gain as a result of the new system. At other times they define the scope of the project too broadly or scope creep occurs.

Let's look at two hypothetical examples, from two providers that we will call Mason Hospital and St. Luke's Medical Center. The implementation team at Mason Hospital defined its goal and the scope of the project and devised measures for evaluating the extent to which the hospital achieved this goal. The implementation team at St. Luke's Medical Center was responsible for completing phase 1 of a three-part project; however, the scope of the team's work was never clearly defined.

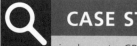

CASE STUDY

Mason Hospital   Mason Hospital decided that it wanted to implement a CPOE system. An implementation team was formed and charged with managing all aspects of the CPOE rollout. Mason Hospital's mission is to be "the premier academic community hospital in the United States." Considering how to achieve this mission, the team identified CPOE as the "building block" needed to improve quality of care, reduce errors, and create a far safer and more effective work environment for hospital medical staff. In addition to establishing this goal, the team went a step further to define what a successful CPOE implementation initiative would consist of. Team members then developed a core set of metrics (for example, physician CPOE adoption rate, use of telephone and verbal orders in nonemergency situations, reduction in adverse drug events, reduction in duplicate orders, improved quality of documentation, and increased compliance with practice-based guidelines) that were subsequently used to track the project's success in the defined areas.

St. Luke's Medical Center   St. Luke's Medical Center set out to implement an electronic medical record (EMR) system, planning to do so in three phases. Phase 1 would involve establishing a clinical data repository, a central database from which all ancillary clinical systems would feed. Phase 2 would consist of the implementation of CPOE and nursing documentation systems, and Phase 3 would see the elimination of all outside paper reports through the implementation of a document imaging system. St. Luke's staff felt that if they could complete all three phases, they would have, in essence, a "true" EMR. The implementation team did not, however, clearly define the scope of its work. Was it to complete phase 1 or all three phases? Likewise, the implementation team never defined what it hoped to accomplish or how implementation of the EMR fit into the medical center's overall mission or organizational goals. It never answered the question: How will we know if we are successful? The ambiguity of the implementation team's scope of work led to disillusionment and a sense of failing to ever finish the project.

Establish and Institute a Project Plan

Once the implementation team has agreed on its goals and objectives, the next major step is to develop and implement a project plan. The project plan should include

- Major activities (also called tasks)
- Major milestones
- Estimated duration of each activity
- Any dependencies among activities (so that, for example, one task must be completed before another can begin)
- Resources and budget available (including staff whose time will be allocated to the project)
- Individuals or team members responsible for completing each activity
- Target dates
- Measures for evaluating completion and success

These are the same components one would find in most major projects. What are the major activities, or tasks, that are unique to system implementation projects? Which tasks must be completed first, second, and so forth? How should time estimates be determined and milestones defined?

System implementation projects tend to be quite large, and therefore it can be helpful to break the project into manageable components. One approach to defining components is to have the implementation team brainstorm and identify the major activities that need to be done before the go-live date. Once these tasks have been identified, they can be grouped and sequenced based on what must be done first, second, and so forth. Those tasks that can occur concurrently should also be identified. A team may find it helpful to use a consultant to guide it through the implementation process. Or the health care IT vendor may have a suggested implementation plan; the team must make sure, however, that this plan is tailored to suit the unique needs of the organization in which the new system is to be introduced.

The subsequent sections describe the major activities common to most information system implementation projects (see the following list) and may serve as a guide. These activities are not necessarily in sequential order; the order used should be determined by the institution, based on its needs and resources.

Typical Components of an Implementation Plan

1. Workflow and process analysis
   - Analyze or evaluate current process and procedures
   - Identify opportunities for improvement and, as appropriate, effect those changes.
   - Identify sources of data, including interfaces to other systems.
   - Determine location and number of workstations needed.
   - Redesign physical location as needed.

2. System installation
   - Determine system configuration.
   - Order and install hardware.
   - Prepare computer room.
   - Upgrade or implement IT infrastructure.
   - Install software and interfaces.
   - Customize software.
   - Test, retest, and test again . . .

3. Staff training
   - Train staff.
   - Update procedure manuals.

4. Conversion
   - Convert data.
   - Test system.

5. Communications

    ■ Establish communication mechanisms for identifying and addressing problems and concerns.

    ■ Communicate regularly with various constituent groups.

6. Preparation for go-live date

    ■ Select date when patient volume is relatively low.

    ■ Ensure sufficient staff are on hand.

    ■ Set up mechanism for reporting and correcting problems and issues.

    ■ Review and effect process reengineering.

Conduct Workflow and Process Analysis   One of the first activities necessary in implementing any new system is to review and evaluate the existing workflow or business processes. Members of the implementation team might also observe the current information system (if there is one) in use. Does it work as described? Where are the problem areas? What are the goals and expectations of the new system? How do organizational processes need to change in order to optimize the new system's value and achieve its goals? Too often organizations never critically evaluate current business processes but plunge forward with implementing the new system while still using old procedures. The result is that they simply automate their outdated and inefficient processes.

Before implementing any new system, the organization should evaluate existing procedures and processes and identify ways to improve workflow, simplify tasks, eliminate redundancy, improve quality, and improve user (customer) satisfaction. Although describing them is beyond the scope of this book, many extremely useful tools and methods are available for analyzing workflow and redesigning business processes (see, for example, Whitten & Bentley, 2007). Simply observing the old system in use, listening to users' concerns, and evaluating information workflow can identify many of the changes needed.

Involving users at this early stage of the implementation process can gain initial buy-in to both the idea and the scope of the process redesign. In all likelihood the organization will need to institute a series of process changes as a result of the new system. Workflow and processes should be evaluated critically and redesigned as needed. For example, the organization may find that it needs to do away with old forms or work steps, change job descriptions or job responsibilities, or add to or subtract from the work responsibilities of particular departments. Getting users involved in this reengineering process can lead to greater user acceptance of the new system.

Let's consider an example. Suppose a multiphysician clinic is implementing a new patient scheduling system. Patients will be able to schedule their own appointments on line via the Internet, and receptionists will also be able to schedule patient appointments electronically. The clinic might wish to begin by appointing a small team of individuals knowledgeable about analyzing workflow and processes to work with staff in studying the existing process for scheduling patient appointments. This team might conduct a series of individual focus groups with schedulers, physicians and nurses, and patients and ask questions such as these:

- Who can schedule patient appointments?

- How are patient appointments made, updated, or deleted?

- Who has access to scheduling information? From what locations?

- How well does the current system work? How efficient is the process?

- What are the major problems with the current scheduling system and process? In what ways might it be improved?

The team should tailor the focus questions so they are appropriate for each user group. The answers can then be a guide for reengineering existing processes and workflow to facilitate the new system.

During the workflow analysis, the team should also examine where the new system's actual workstations will be located, how many workstations will be needed, and how information will flow between manual organizational processes and the electronic information system. Here are a few of the many questions that should be addressed in ensuring that physical layouts are conducive to the success of the new system:

- Will the workstations be portable or fixed? If users are given portable units, how will these be tracked and maintained (and protected from loss or theft)? If workstations are fixed, will they be located in safe, secure areas where patient confidentiality can be maintained?

- How will the user interact with the new system?

- Does the physical layout of each work area need to be redesigned to accommodate the new system and the new process?

- Will additional wiring be needed?

Install System Components   The next step, which may be done concurrently with the workflow analysis, is to install the hardware, software, and network infrastructure to support the new information system and build the necessary interfaces. IT staff play a crucial role in this phase of the project. They will need to work with the vendor in determining system specifications and configurations and in preparing the computer room for installation. It may be, for example, that the organization's current computer network will need to be replaced or upgraded. During implementation, having adequate numbers of computer workstations placed in readily accessible locations is critical. Those involved in the planning need to determine beforehand the maximum number of individuals likely to be using the system at the same time, and accommodate this scenario.

Typically when a health care organization acquires a system from a vendor, quite a bit of customization is needed. IT personnel will likely work with the vendor in setting up and loading data tables, building interfaces, and running pilot tests of the hardware and software using actual patient and administrative data. We recommend piloting the system in a unit or area before rolling out the system enterprise-wide. This test enables the implementation team to evaluate the system's effectiveness, address issues and concerns, fix bugs, and then apply the lessons learned to other units in the organization before most people even start using the system.

Consideration should be given to choosing an appropriate area (for example, department or location) or set of users to pilot the system. Some of the questions the implementation team should consider in identifying potential pilot sites are these:

- Which units or areas are willing and equipped to serve as a pilot site? Do they have sufficient interest, administrative support, and commitment?

- Are the staff and management teams in each of these units or areas comfortable with being system "guinea pigs"?

- Do staff have the time and resources needed to serve in this capacity?

- Is there a system champion in each unit or area who will lead the effort?

Plan, Conduct, and Evaluate Staff Training Training is an essential component of any new system implementation. Although no one would argue with this statement, the implementation team will want to consider many issues as it develops and implements a training program. Here are a few of the questions to be answered:

- How much training is needed? Do different user groups have different training needs?

- Who should conduct the training?

- When should the training occur? What intervals of training are ideal?

- What training format is best (for example, formal, classroom-style training; one-on-one or small-group training; computer-based training; a combination of methods)?

- What is the role of the vendor in training?

- Who in the organization will manage or oversee the training? How will training be documented?

- What criteria and methods will be used to monitor training and ensure that staff are adequately trained? Will staff be tested on proficiency?

There are various methods of training. One approach, commonly known as *train the trainer*, relies on the vendor to train selected members of the organization who will then serve as super-users and train others in their respective departments, units, or areas. These super-users should be individuals who work directly in the areas in which the system is to be used; they should know the staff in the area and have a good rapport with them. They will also serve as resources to other users once the vendor representatives have left. They may do a lot of one-on-one training, hand-holding, and other work with people in their areas until these individuals achieve a certain comfort level with the system. The main concern with this approach is that the organization may devote a great deal of time and resources to training the trainers only to have these trainers leave the institution (often because they've been lured away by career opportunities with the vendor).

Another method is to have the vendor train a pool of trainers who are knowledgeable about the entire system and who can rotate through the different areas of the organization working with staff. The trainer pool might include both IT professionals (including clinical analysts) and clinical or administrative staff such as nurses, physicians, lab managers, and business managers.

Regardless of who conducts the training, it is important to introduce fundamental or basic concepts first and allow people to master these concepts before moving on to new ones. Studies among health care organizations that have implemented clinical applications such as CPOE systems have shown that classroom training is not nearly as effective as one-on-one coaching, particularly among physicians (Metzger & Fortin, 2003). Most systems can track physician usage; physicians identified as low-volume users may be targeted for additional training.

Timing of the training is also important. Users should have ample opportunity to practice *before* the system goes live. For instance, when a nursing documentation system is being installed, nurses should have the chance to practice with it at the bedside of a typical patient. Likewise, when a CPOE system is going in, physicians should get to practice ordering a set of tests during their morning rounds. This just-in-time training might occur several times: for example, three months, two months, one month, and one week before the go-live date. Training might be supplemented with computer-based training modules that enable users to review concepts and functions at their own pace. Additional staff should be on hand during the go-live period to assist users as needed during the transition to the new system. In general the implementation team should work with the vendor to produce a thoughtful and creative training program.

Once the details of how the new system is to work have been determined, it is important to update procedure manuals and make the updated manuals available to the staff. Designated managers or representatives from the various areas may assume a leadership role in updating procedure manuals for their respective areas. When people must learn specific IT procedures such as how to log in, change passwords, and read common error messages, the IT department should ensure that this information appears in the procedure manuals and that the information is routinely updated and widely disseminated to the users. Procedure manuals serve as reference guides and resources for users and can be particularly useful when training new employees.

Effective training is important. Staff member need to be relatively comfortable with the application and need to know to whom they should turn if they have questions or concerns. We recommend having the users evaluate the training prior to go-live.

Convert Data and Test System   Another important task is to convert the data from the old system to the new system and then adequately test the new system. Staff involved in the data conversion must determine the sources of the data required for the new system and construct new files. It is particularly important that data be complete, accurate, and current before being converted to the new system. Data should be *cleaned* before being converted. Once converted, the data should run through a series of validation checkpoints or procedures to ensure the accuracy of the conversion.

IT staff knowledgeable in data conversion procedures should lead the effort and verify the results with key managers from the appropriate clinical and administrative areas. The specific conversion procedures used will depend on the nature of the old system and its structure as well as on the configuration of the new system.

Finally, the new system will need to be tested. The main purpose of the testing is to simulate the live environment as closely as possible and determine how well the system and accompanying procedures work. Are there programming glitches or other problems that need to be fixed? How well are the interfaces working? How does response time compare to what was expected? The system should be populated with live data and tested again. Vendors, IT staff, and user staff should all participate in the testing process. As with training, one can never test too much. A good portion of this work has to be done for the pilot testing. It may need to be repeated before going live. And the pilot lessons will guide any additional testing or conversion that needs to be done.

Communicate Progress or Status   Equally as important as successfully carrying out the activities discussed so far is having an effective plan for communicating the project's progress. This plan serves two primary purposes. First, it identifies how the members of the implementation team will communicate and coordinate their activities and progress. Second, it defines how progress will be communicated to key constituent groups, including but not limited to the board, the senior administrative team, the departments, and the staff at all levels of the organization affected by the new system. The communication plan may set up both formal and informal mechanisms. Formal communication may include everything from regular updates at board and administrative meetings to written briefings and articles in the facility newsletter. The purpose should be to use as many channels and mechanisms as possible to ensure that the people who need to know are fully informed and aware of the implementation plans. Informal communication is less structured but can be equally important. Implementing a new health care information system is major undertaking, and it is important that all staff (day, evening, and night shifts) be made aware of what is happening. The methods for communication may be varied, but the message should be consistent and the information presented up-to-date and timely. For example, do not rely on e-mail communication as your primary method only to discover later that your organization's nurses do not regularly check their e-mail or have little time to read your type of message.

Prepare for Go-Live Date   A great deal of work goes into preparing for the go-live date, the day the organization transitions from the old system to the new. Assuming the implementation team has done all it can to ensure that the system is ready, the staff are well trained, and appropriate procedures are in place, the transition should be a smooth one. Additional staff should be on hand and equipped to assist users as needed. It is best to plan for the system to go live on a day when the patient census is typically low or fewer patients than usual are scheduled to be seen. Disaster recovery plans should also be in place, and staff should be well trained on what to do should the system go down or fail. Designated IT staff should monitor and assess system problems and errors.

When organizations are implementing information systems with clinical decision support, we recommend that they adhere to these "ten commandments" for effective clinical decision support."

Ten Commandments for Effective Clinical Decision Support

- Speed is everything—this is what information system users value most.
- Anticipate needs and deliver in real time—deliver information when needed.
- Fit into user's work flow—integrate suggestions with clinical practice.
- Little things can make a big difference—improve usability to "do the right thing."
- Recognize that physicians will resist stopping—offer alternatives rather than insist on stopping an action.
- Changing direction is easier than stopping—changing defaults for dose, route, or frequency of a medication can change behavior.
- Simple interventions work best—simplify guidelines by reducing to a single computer screen.
- Ask for additional information only when you really need it—the more data elements requested, the less likely a guideline will be implemented.
- Monitor impact, get feedback and respond—if certain reminders are not followed, readjust or eliminate the reminder.
- Manage and maintain your knowledge-based systems—track users' response to decision support and update to coincide with changes in medical knowledge [Bates et al., 2003].

A great deal of planning and leadership is needed in implementing a new health care information system. Despite the best-made plans, however, things can and do go wrong. The next section describes some of the common organizational challenges associated with system implementation projects and offers strategies for anticipating and planning for them.

MANAGING THE ORGANIZATIONAL ASPECTS

Implementing an information system in a health care facility can have a profound impact on the organization, the people who work there, and the patients they serve. Individuals may have concerns and apprehensions about the new system. They may wonder: How will the new system affect my job responsibilities or productivity? How will my workload change? Will the new system cause me more or less stress? Even individuals who welcome the new system, see the need for it, and see its potential value may worry: What will I do if the system is down? Will the system impede my relationship with my patients? Who will I turn to if I have problems or questions? Will I be expected to type my notes into the system? With the new system comes change, and change can be difficult if not managed effectively.

The human factors associated with implementing a new system should not be taken lightly. A great deal of change can occur as a result of the new system. Some of the changes may be immediately apparent; others may occur over time as the system is used more fully. Many IT implementation studies have been done in recent years, and they reveal several strategies that may lead to greater organizational acceptance and use of a new system:

- Create an appropriate environment, one where expectations are defined, met, and managed.
- Do not underestimate user resistance.
- Allocate sufficient resources, including technical support staff and IT infrastructure.
- Provide adequate initial and ongoing training.
- Manage unintended consequences, especially those known to affect implementations such as CPOE.

More research is needed to explore the extent to which these and other strategies can lead to more widespread adoption of health care information systems, particularly clinical applications such as the CPOE and EMR systems.

Create an Appropriate Environment

If you ask a roomful of health care executives, physicians, nurses, pharmacists, or laboratory managers if they have ever experienced an IT system failure, chances are over half of the hands in the room would go up. In all likelihood the people in the room would have a much easier time describing a system failure than a system success. If you probed a little further and asked why the system was a failure, you might hear comments like these: "the system was too slow," "it was down all the time," "training was inadequate and nothing like the real thing," "there was no one to go to if you had questions or concerns," "it added to my stress and workload," and the list goes on. The fact is the system did not meet their expectations. You might not know whether those expectations were reasonable or not.

Earlier we discussed the importance of clearly defining and communicating the goals and objectives of the new system. Related to goal definition is the management of user expectations. Different people may have different perspectives on what they expect from the new system; in addition, some will admit to having no expectations, and others will have joined the organization after the system was implemented and consequently are likely to have expectations derived from the people currently using the system.

Expectations come from what people see and hear about the system and the way they interpret what the system will do for them or for their organization. Expectations can be formed from a variety of sources—they may come from a comment made during a vendor presentation, a question that arises during training, a visit to another site that uses the same system, attendance at a professional conference, or a remark made by a colleague in the hallway.

Furthermore, the main criterion used to evaluate the system's value or success depends on the individual's expectations and point of view. For example, the chief financial officer might measure system success in terms of the financial return on investment, the chief medical director might look at impact on physicians' time and quality of care, the nursing staff might consider any change in their workload, public relations personnel might compare levels of patient satisfaction, and the IT staff might evaluate the change in the number of help desk calls made since the new system was implemented. All these approaches are measures of an information system's perceived impact on the organization or individual. However, they are not all the same, and they may not have equal importance to the organization in achieving its strategic goals.

It is therefore important for the health care executive team not only to establish and communicate clearly defined goals for the new system but also to listen to needs and expectations of the various user groups and to define, meet, and manage expectations appropriately. Ways to manage expectations include making sure users understand that the first days or weeks of system use may be rocky, that the organization may need time to adjust to a new workflow, that the technology may have bugs, and that users should not expect problem-free system operation from the start. Clear and effective communication is key in this endeavor.

In managing expectations it can be enormously helpful to conduct formative assessments of the implementation process, in which the focus is on the process as well as the outcomes. Specific metrics need to be chosen and success criteria defined to determine whether or not the system is meeting expectations (McGowan, Cusack, & Poon, 2008). For example, if wide-scale usage is a priority, collection of actual numbers of transactions or usage logs may be meaningful information for the leadership team. Other categories of metrics that might be helpful are clinical outcome measures, clinical process measures, provider adoption and attitude measures, patient knowledge and attitude measures, workflow impact measures, and financial impact measures. The Agency for Healthcare Research and Quality recently published the *Health Information Technology Evaluation Toolkit*, which can serve as a guide for project teams involved in evaluating the system implementation process or project outcomes (Cusack & Poon, 2007).

Do Not Underestimate User Resistance

During the implementation process it is important to analyze current workflow and make appropriate changes as needed. Earlier we gave an example of analyzing a patient scheduling process. Patient scheduling is a relatively straightforward process. A change in this system may not dramatically change the job responsibilities of the schedulers and may have little impact on nurses' or physicians' time. Therefore these groups may offer little resistance to such a change. (This is not to guarantee a lack of resistance—if you mess up a practice's schedule, you can have a lot of angry people on your hands!) In contrast, changes in processes that involve the direct provision of patient care services and that do affect nurses' and physicians' time may be tougher for users to accept. The physician ordering process is a perfect example. Most physicians today are accustomed to picking up a pen and paper and handwriting an order or calling one in to the nurses' station from their phones. With CPOE, physicians may be expected to keyboard their orders directly into the system and respond to automated reminders and decision-support alerts. A process that historically took them a few seconds to do might now take several minutes, depending on the number of prompts and reminders. Moreover, physicians are now doing things that were not asked of them before—they are checking for drug interactions, responding to reminders and alerts, evaluating whether evidence-based clinical guidelines apply to the patient, again the list goes on. All these activities take time, but in the long run they will improve the quality of patient care. Therefore it is important for physicians to be actively involved in designing the process and in seeing its value to the patient care process.

Getting physicians, nurses, and other clinicians to accept and use clinical information systems such as CPOE or EMR can be challenging even when they are involved in the implementation. At times the incentives for using the system may not be aligned with their individual needs and goals. On the one hand, for example, if the physician is expected to see a certain number of patients per day and is evaluated on patient load and if writing orders used to take thirty minutes a day with the old system and now takes sixty to ninety minutes with the new CPOE system, the physician can either see fewer patients or work more hours. One should expect to see physician resistance. On the other hand, if the physician's performance and income is related to adherence to clinical practice guidelines, using the CPOE system might improve his or her income, creating a greater chance of acceptance.

The physician's workload or productivity goals might, however, be beyond the organization's control. They might be individual goals the physician has set for himself or herself. Can or should organizations mandate the use of clinical information systems like CPOE? In effect, the organization is stating that resistance is unacceptable. Several health care facilities have instituted policies mandating physician use of CPOE, with mixed results. Physicians' acceptance of such a mandate may have a lot to do with the organizational culture, the training they received, their confidence (or lack of confidence) in the system, how the mandate was imposed, and a host of other factors. Mandating use is most common in academic medical centers where residents and fellows are expected to enter orders in a computerized system. Mandating physician use can be taxing for community hospitals or other facilities that are not the physicians' employers. Community-based physicians often admit patients to more than one hospital and spend limited time at each facility. Trying to get these fairly independent physicians to buy into a facility's CPOE system and participate in the necessary training can be difficult.

To address this and related acceptance issues, the California HealthCare Foundation, in collaboration with First Consulting Group, conducted an in-depth study of ten community hospitals, throughout the United States, that have made significant progress in implementing CPOE (Metzger & Fortin, 2003). The study found that CPOE leaders tended to avoid the term *mandate* and instead recommended that health care executives work toward an enterprise-wide policy for universal CPOE. Key staff in participating hospitals recommended starting with a strong commitment to CPOE, delivering a consistent message that CPOE is the right thing to do, and working within the culture of the medical staff toward the goal of universal adoption. This goal might take years to achieve. Readiness for universal adoption occurred once (1) a significant number of physician CPOE adopters showed their peers what was possible, (2) sufficient progress was made toward achieving patient safety objectives, and (3) the medical staff came together with one voice to champion CPOE as the right thing to do.

Similarly, a study of five community hospitals in Massachusetts that had implemented CPOE found although all five hospitals started out with the intention that all physicians would use CPOE, only two had a formal policy to that effect (*Saving lives, reducing costs: CPOE lessons learned in community hospitals*, 2006), but all physicians were highly encouraged to do so. Tactics used for inducing or encouraging physician adoption included providing one-on-one training anywhere and anytime, making it easy to establish remote access from home and office, assigning high priority to enhancements that benefited ease of order completion, empowering nurses to serve as super-users and to encourage physician direct entry, investing in order sets and helping physicians build a personal favorites list and removing all paper order sheets from the floor (*Saving lives...*, 2006). In cases where the hospital had residents and employed physicians such as intensivists or hospitalists, these physicians were expected to use CPOE for all their orders. Every hospital, regardless of how it framed physician adoption, portrayed CPOE as a necessary change and made an enormous investment in ensuring the system was easy to learn and use.

Whether, and when, to mandate use or adopt a universal acceptance policy is a decision that should come with time. Experience has shown that a mandate should not be imposed until the organization has achieved a certain level of system use and medical staff overall have confidence in the system's functionality and have bought into the system. There may be a point in time where all orders will have to be entered directly by physicians or when paper medical records will no longer be pulled or maintained. However, that point in time should be clearly communicated, all efforts should be made to ensure users are trained and ready to make the change, and backup procedures should be in place when the day arrives.

System champions, particularly when they are also physicians, can be extremely helpful in preparing for the day of universal adoption. They can serve as coaches, listeners, teachers, and advocates for facility physicians and for the system. It is through their role and example that others will come along. Some medical staff may choose not to and may leave the organization; however, the great majority will stay and work toward the common goal.

It perhaps goes without saying that user acceptance occurs when users see or realize the value the health care information system brings to their work and the patients they serve. This value takes different forms. Some people may realize increased efficiency, less stress, greater organization, and improved quality of information, whereas others may find that the system enables them to provide better care, avoid medical mistakes, and make better decisions. In some cases an individual may not experience the value personally yet may come to realize the value to the organization as a whole.

Allocate Sufficient Resources

Sufficient resources are needed both during and after the new system has been implemented. User acceptance comes from confidence in the new system. Individuals want to know that the system works properly, is stable, and is secure and that someone is available to help them when they have questions, problems, or concerns. Therefore it is important for the organization to ensure that adequate resources are devoted to implementing and supporting the system and its users. At a minimum, adequate technical staff expertise should be available as well as sufficient IT infrastructure.

We have discussed the importance of giving the implementation team sufficient support as it carries out its charge, but what forms can this support take? Some methods of supporting the team are to make available release time, additional staff, and development funds. Senior managers might allocate travel funds so team members can view the system in use in other facilities. They might decide that all implementation team members or super-users will receive 50 percent release time for the next six months to devote to the project. This release time will enable those involved to give up some of their normal job duties so they can focus on the project. Senior leaders at one health care organization in South Carolina gave sixty-four full-time staff release time for one year to devote to the implementation of a facility-wide hospital information system. This substantial amount of release time was indicative of the high value the executive team members placed on the project. They saw it as critical to achieving the organization's strategic goals.

Providing sufficient time and resources to the implementation phase of the project is, however, only part of the overall support needed. Studies have shown that an information system's value to the organization is typically realized over time. Value is derived as more and more people use the system, offer suggestions for enhancing it, and begin to push the system to fulfill its functionality. If users are ever to fully realize the system's value, they must have access to local technical support—someone, preferably within the organization, who is readily available, is knowledgeable about the intricacies of the system, and is able to handle both hardware and software problems. This individual should be able to work effectively with the vendor and others to find solutions to system problems. Even though it is ideal to have local technical support in-house, that may be difficult in small physician office or community-based settings. In such cases the facility may need to consider such options as (1) devoting a significant portion of an employee's time to training so that he or she may assume a support role, (2) partnering with a neighboring organization that uses the same system to share technical support staff, or (3) contracting with a local computer firm to provide the needed assistance. The vendor may be able to assist the organization in identifying and securing local technical support.

In addition to arranging for local technical support, the organization will also need to invest resources in building and maintaining a reliable, secure IT infrastructure (servers, operating systems, and networks) to support the information system, particularly if it is a mission-critical system. Many patient information systems need to be available 24 hours a day, 7 days a week, 365 days a year. Health care professionals can come to rely on having access to timely, accurate, and complete information in caring for their patents, just as they count on having electricity, water, and other basic utilities. Failing to build the IT infrastructure that will adequately support the new clinical system can be catastrophic for the organization and its IT department.

An IT infrastructure's lifetime may be relatively short. It is reasonable to expect that within three to ten years, the hardware, software, and network will likely need to be replaced as advances are made in technology, the organization's goals and needs change, and the health care environment changes.

Provide Adequate Training

Earlier we discussed the importance of training staff on the new system prior to the go-live date. Having a training program suited to the needs of the various user groups is very important during the implementation process. People who will use the system should be relatively comfortable with it, have had ample opportunities to use it in a safe environment, and know where to turn should they have questions or need additional assistance. It is equally important to provide ongoing training months and even years after the system has been implemented. In all likelihood the system will go through a series of upgrades, changes will be made, and users will get more comfortable with the fundamental features and will be ready to push the system to the next level. Some users will explore additional functionality on their own; others will need prodding and additional training in order to learn more advanced features.

When implementing a new system, it important to view the system as a long-term investment rather than a one-time purchase. The resources allocated or committed to the system should include not only the up-front investment in hardware and software but also the time, people, and resources needed to maintain and support it.

Manage Unintended Consequences

Management expertise and leadership are important elements to the success of any system implementation. Effective leaders help build a community of collaboration and trust. However, effective leadership also entails understanding the unintended consequences that can occur during complex system implementations and managing them. Unintended consequences can be positive, negative, or both, depending on one's perspective. Ash and colleagues (2007) recently conducted interviews with key individuals from 176 U.S. hospitals that currently have CPOE. CPOE is one of the most complex and challenging of clinical information systems to implement. From their work, they identified eight types of unintended consequences that implementation teams should plan for and consider when implementing CPOE:

1. *More work or new work.* CPOEs can increase work due to the fact that systems may be slow, nonstandard cases may call for more steps in ordering, training may remain an issue, some tasks may become more difficult, the computer forces the user to complete "all steps," and physicians often take on tasks that were formerly done by others.

2. *Workflow.* CPOEs can greatly alter workflow, sometimes improving workflow for some and slowing or complicating it for others.

3. *System demands.* Maintenance, training, and support efforts can be significant for an organization, not only in building the system but also in making improvements and enhancements to it.

4. *Communication.* CPOE systems affect communication within the organization; they can reduce the need to clarify orders but also lead to people failing to adequately communicate with each other in appropriate situations.

5. *Emotions.* Clinician reactions to CPOE can run the gamut from positive to negative.

6. *New kinds of errors.* Although CPOE systems are generally designed to detect and prevent errors, they can lead to new types of errors such as juxtaposition errors, in which clinicians click on the adjacent patient name or medication from a list and inadvertently enter the wrong order.

7. *Power shifts.* Shifts in power may not be viewed as as much of a problem as some of the other unintended consequences, but CPOE can be used to monitor physician behavior.

8. *Dependence on the system.* Clinicians become dependent on the CPOE system, so managing downtime procedures is critical. Even then, while the system is down, CPOE users view the situation as managed chaos (adapted from Ash et al., 2007).

Health care executives and implementation teams should be aware of these unintended consequences, particularly those that can adversely affect the organization, and carefully plan for and manage them.

SYSTEM SUPPORT AND EVALUATION

Information systems evolve as an organization continues to grow and change. No matter how well the system was designed and tested, errors and problems will be detected and changes will need to be made. IT staff generally assume a major role in maintaining and supporting the information systems in the health care organization. When errors or problems are detected, IT staff correct the problem or work with the vendor to see that the problem is fixed. Moreover, the vendor may detect glitches and develop upgrades or patches that will need to be installed.

Many opportunities for enhancing and improving the system's performance and functionality will occur well after the go-live date. The organization will want to ensure that the system is adequately maintained, supported, and further developed over time. Selecting and implementing a health care information system is an enormous investment. This investment must be maintained, just as one would maintain one's home.

Like any other device, information systems have a life cycle and eventually need to be replaced. Health care organizations typically go through a process whereby they plan, design, implement, and evaluate their health care information systems. Too often in the past the organization's work was viewed as done once the system went live. It has since been discovered how vital system maintenance and support resources are and how important it is to evaluate the extent to which the system goals are being achieved.

Evaluating or accessing the value of the health care information system is increasingly important. Acquiring and implementing systems requires large investments, and stakeholders, including boards of directors, are demanding to know both the actual and future value of these projects. Evaluations must be viewed as an integral component of every major health information system project and not an afterthought. In fact we believe that assessing the value of a health IT investment is enormously important and thus have devoted Chapter Fifteen entirely to the subject.

SUMMARY

Implementing a new information system in a health care organization requires a significant amount of planning and preparation. The health care organization should begin by appointing an implementation team comprising experienced individuals, including representatives from key areas in the organization, particularly areas that will be affected by or responsible for using the new system. Key users should be involved in analyzing existing processes and procedures and making recommendations for changes. A system champion should be part of the implementation team and serve as an advocate in soliciting input, representing user views, and spearheading the project. When implementing a clinical application, it is important that the system champion be a physician or clinician, someone who is able to represent the views of the care providers.

Under the direction of a highly competent implementation team, a number of important activities should occur during the system rollout. This team should assume a leadership role in ensuring that the system is effectively incorporated into the day-to-day operations of the facility. This generally requires the organization to (1) analyze workflow and processes and perform any necessary process reengineering, (2) install and configure the system, (3) train staff, (4) convert data, (5) adequately test the system, and (6) communicate project progress using appropriate forums at all levels throughout the organization. Attention should be given to the countless details associated

with ensuring that backup procedures are in place, security plans have been developed, and the organization is ready for the go-live date.

During the days immediately following system implementation, the organization should have sufficient staff on hand to assist users and provide individual assistance as needed. A stable and secure IT infrastructure should be in place to ensure minimal, ideally zero, downtime and adequate response time. The IT department or other appropriate unit or representative should have a formal mechanism in place for reporting and correcting errors, bugs, and glitches in the system.

Once the system has gone live, it is critical for the organization to have in place the plans and resources needed to adequately maintain and support the new system. Technical staff and resources should be available to the users. Ongoing training should be an integral part of the organization's plans to support and further develop the new system. In addition, the leadership team should have in place a thoughtful plan for evaluating the implementation process and assessing the value of the health care information system.

Beyond taking ultimate responsibility for completion of the activities needed to implement and to support and evaluate the new system, the health care executive should assume a leadership role in managing the organizational and human aspects of the new system. Information systems can have a profound impact on health care organizations, the people who work there, and the patients they serve.

Acquiring a good product and having the right technical equipment and expertise is not enough to ensure system success. Health care executives must also be attuned to the human aspects of introducing new IT into the care delivery process.

KEY TERMS

Implementation team
System champion
System implementation
Train the trainer

Unintended consequences
User resistance
Workflow and process analysis

LEARNING ACTIVITIES

1. Visit a health care organization that has recently implemented a health care information system. What process did it use to implement the system? How does that process compare with the one described in this chapter? How successful was the organization in implementing the new system? To what do staff attribute this success?

2. Search the literature for a recent article on a system implementation project. Briefly describe the process used to implement the system and the lessons learned. How might this particular facility's experiences be useful to others? Explain.

3. Physician acceptance and use of clinical information systems is often cited as a challenge. What do you think the health care leadership team can or should do to foster acceptance by physicians? Assume a handful of physicians in your organization are actively resisting a new clinical information system. How would you approach and address their resistance and concerns?

4. Assume you are working with an implementation team in installing a new nursing documentation system for a home health agency. Historically, all its nursing documentation was recorded in paper form. The home health agency has little computerization beyond basic registration information and has no IT staff. What recommendations might you offer to the implementation team as it begins the work of installing the new nursing documentation system?

5. Discuss the risks to a health care organization in failing to allocate sufficient support and resources to a newly implemented health care information system.

6. Assume you are the CEO of a large group practice (seventy-five physicians) that implemented an EMR system two years ago. The physicians are asking for an evaluation of the system and its impact on quality, costs, and patient satisfaction. Devise a plan for evaluating the EMR system's impact on the organization in these three areas.

PART

3

INFORMATION
TECHNOLOGY

CHAPTER

8

TECHNOLOGIES THAT SUPPORT HEALTH CARE INFORMATION SYSTEMS

LEARNING OBJECTIVES

- To gain a basic understanding of the core technologies behind health care information systems:

    System software

    Data management

    Networks and data communications

    Information processing distribution schemes

    Internet, intranets, and extranets

    Clinical and managerial decision support

- To be able to discuss emerging trends in information technology (such as mobility, Web services, Internet, wireless).

- To be able to identify some of the major issues in the adoption of information technologies in health care organizations.

- To be able to discuss why it is important for a health care organization to adopt an overall information systems architecture.

Thus far in this book we have explored a variety of health care information systems. These systems have been presented with minimal discussion of the technology behind them. We have focused instead on how the various applications are adopted, implemented, and used. Although we do not believe that health care executives need to become information technology (IT) experts in order to make informed decisions about which health care information systems to employ in their organizations, we do believe that an exposure to some of the core technologies used to develop and implement common health care information systems is quite useful. This knowledge will help health care executives be more informed decision makers.

This chapter provides a broad view of several categories of core, or base, technologies. They are not unique to health care but are frequently found in health care organizations. We discuss technologies used in each of the following categories:

- System software
- Data management and access
- Networks and data communications
- Information processing distribution schemes
- The Internet, intranets, and extranets
- Clinical and managerial decision support
- Trends in user interactions with systems

We end with a discussion of the concept of system architecture, that is, how all the technologies *fit together* within an organization to support health care applications. Like many other fields, IT has its own language. It is helpful for health care executives to learn IT terminology and concepts so they can communicate effectively with IT staff and vendors.

SYSTEM SOFTWARE

Up to this point we have discussed health care information system applications without looking at the technologies on which they run. In this section we will begin with a general discussion of software and then define programming languages, operating systems, and interface engines.

There are two basic types of software, *systems software* and *applications software*. These two types of software have a common characteristic: both represent a series of computer programs. Remember that at its most basic level of functioning the computer recognizes two things, an electrical impulse that is on and an electrical impulse that is off; these signals are often represented as 0 and 1 (or *bits*). A human programmer must write programming code to translate the desires of the user into computer actions. There are many different programming languages in use today, and they are continuing to evolve.

Machine languages are the oldest computer programming languages. Machine language programmers had to literally translate each character or operator into binary code, displayed as groups of 0s and 1s. Machine languages are often referred to as *first-generation languages*. Fortunately, by the 1950s, *assembly languages*, the *second-generation languages*, were developed, which simplified machine language programming. The *procedural programming languages* (*third generation*), for example, FORTRAN and COBOL, came along shortly after the assembly languages, allowing programmers to write computer programs without being as concerned with manually producing the machine language. Today, *fourth-generation languages* (4GLs), which have many preprogrammed functions, allow individuals to develop applications without writing a single line of program code themselves. The software creates the code in the background, invisibly from the developer's point of view. In the data management section we will discuss *structured query language* (SQL), which is an example of a 4GL.

Two other types of programming frequently used today are *visual programming* and *object-oriented programming*. The most common type of visual programming is Microsoft's Visual Basic, which allows developers to see the final visual appearance of an application, such as the buttons, scroll-down menus, and windows, as they develop the application. The object-oriented languages differ from traditional procedural languages in that they allow the programmer to create *objects* that include the operations (methods) linked to the data. For example, a *master patient index* (MPI) object would contain both the MPI data, such as each patient's medical record number, last name, first name, and so forth, and the procedures that use this data, such as assigning the medical record number, retrieving patient names by medical record number, and so forth. Object-oriented languages allow *chunks* of code to be reused and facilitate program maintenance. Common object-oriented programming languages are C++ and Java. A full discussion of programming languages is beyond the scope of this book, but as health care executives you may hear the IT professionals talk about different types of programming languages such as C++, Visual Basic, or Java.

Operating Systems

System software is a series of programs that carry out basic computing functions: for example, managing the user interface, files, and memory. System software also operates any peripherals linked to the computer, such as printers, monitors, and other devices. System software is what allows developers to create applications without having to manually code basic computer instructions. The most important component of system software is the *operating system*. The operating system is loaded when a computer is turned on, and it is responsible for managing all other programs subsequently used by the computer. Common types of operating systems are Windows (in several different versions), Mac OS, Unix, and Linux.

Operating systems may be *proprietary* or *open source*. Proprietary operating systems, such as Windows and Mac OS, are purchased, and the actual source code (programs) is not made available to purchasers. The most popular operating systems are proprietary. However, in the 1990s, open source (or nonproprietary) operating systems became viable when a Finnish graduate student, Linus Torvald, developed a variant of the operating system Unix, called Linux. Torvald never claimed rights to that operating system, and it is widely available via the Internet. Linux has gained popularity as commercial software companies have begun to support it (Oz, 2006).

Interface Engines

An *interface engine* is "a software program designed to simplify the creation and management of interfaces between application systems" (Altis, 2004). Interfaces between applications became increasingly important as health care systems moved from best of breed to more integrated architectures. (These architecture distinctions will be discussed at the end of the chapter.) Users wanted their various applications to be able to talk to one another. They wanted to eliminate the need for entering patient demographic information multiple times into separate systems, for example. In fact, users began to ask for a *single sign-on system* so they could access all the information they needed through a single user interface.

Interface engines are actually a form of *middleware*, a class of software that works "between" or "in the middle" of applications and operating systems. Other examples of middleware are applications that check for viruses, medical logic processors, and data encryption software. A typical interface engine operates in three basic steps. Figure 8.1 illustrates a typical one-to-many transaction involving a hospital admission, discharge, and transfer (ADT) system. Here, the ADT system needs to communicate to the lab and pharmacy systems that a patient has been admitted. The ADT system sends

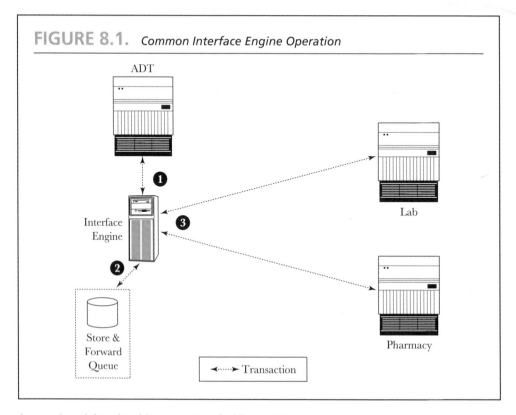

FIGURE 8.1. *Common Interface Engine Operation*

ADT

Interface
Engine

Store &
Forward
Queue

Lab

Pharmacy

◄┈┈► Transaction

a message with the relevant demographic and account detail to the interface engine. The interface engine receives the message, processes it as necessary, and places it in a *queue*, or wait line, for delivery to the lab and pharmacy systems. The message is subsequently forwarded from the queue to those systems. Some interface engines can handle many-to-many transactions as well as one-to-many transactions. Messages are received by the interface engine from multiple systems and are then forwarded to multiple systems.

DATA MANAGEMENT AND ACCESS

All the health care applications discussed thus far require data. The electronic medical record (EMR) system relies on comprehensive databases, as do other clinical applications. Data must be stored and maintained so that they can be retrieved and used within these applications. In this section we discuss common types of databases and the database management systems with which they are associated. The majority of our discussion centers on the *relational database* because it is the type of database most commonly developed today. Two older types of databases, hierarchical and network (not to be confused with a computer network), may still exist in health care organizations as components of older, legacy applications, but because they no longer have a significant presence in the database market, they are not discussed here. A fourth type of database, the *object-oriented database*, has received a lot of attention in the literature during the past few years. Although a "pure" object-oriented database is not yet common in the health care market, there are applications with object-oriented components built upon relational databases. This hybrid database type is referred to as an *object-relational database*.

Relational Databases

Relational databases were first developed in the early 1970s (Rob & Coronel, 2004). These early relational databases were not practical, however, because of the large amount of processing power they required. As computers became more powerful in the 1980s and 1990s, the role of relational databases became more significant. Today the relational database is the predominant type used in health care and business. A relational database is implemented through a *relational database management system* (RDBMS). Microsoft Access is an example of an RDBMS for desktop computing; Oracle, Sybase, and Microsoft SQL Server are examples of the more robust RDBMS that are used to develop larger applications.

An application developed using a RDBMS has three distinct components, or layers (Figure 8.2). The interface is developed using software such as Visual Basic or Java. In Microsoft Access this layer is created with Visual Basic for Applications (VBA), which is built into the Access package and used to create the forms and reports that make up the majority of the user interface. The bottom layer of the RDBMS is created with a special type of software, a *data definition language* (DDL). The DDL creates the database table structure and the relationships among the various tables. Each table can be thought of as a file, with each row in the table being a record and each column being a

---

FIGURE 8.2. *Relational Database Management System Layers*

Interface
Variety of computer languages (VBA, Java, Delphi, and so forth)
Data Manipulation
Data Manipulation Language (DML)
Tables
Data Definition Language (DDL)

---

field or piece of data. In between the data tables and the interface an RDBMS has a *data manipulation layer*. The functions of this layer are performed by a *data manipulation language* (DML). The DML is the software that allows the user to retrieve, query, update, and edit the data in the underlying tables.

The language most widely used for both the DLL and DML functions in relational databases is *structured query language* (SQL). SQL is an example of a 4GL. The user or programmer specifies what must be done but not *how* it must be done. In other words the programmer does not need to design the complex actions the computer takes when an SQL command is executed. SQL is recognized as a de facto standard for relational database functioning. The common RDBMS products support some type of SQL, but many of them also employ extensions to the basic language.

To further support interoperability among databases using different management systems, the *Open Database Connectivity* (ODBC) standard was developed for the database *application program interface* (API). This standard is closely aligned with SQL, was developed by the SQL Access Group, and was first released in 1992. ODBC allows programs to use SQL requests without having to know the proprietary interfaces to the databases (Whatis?.com, 2002). Using databases that comply with the ODBC standard allows a health care organization to more easily integrate its databases. The organization can move data from ODBC-compliant PC-based application programs or databases to larger databases and vice versa, for example.

PERSPECTIVE

RELATIONAL DATA MODELING

Figure 8.3 is an example of an *entity relationship diagram* (ERD), which graphically depicts the tables and relationships in a simple relational database. Data modeling is an important tool for database designers. Although a complete discussion of

FIGURE 8.3. *Entity Relationship Diagram*

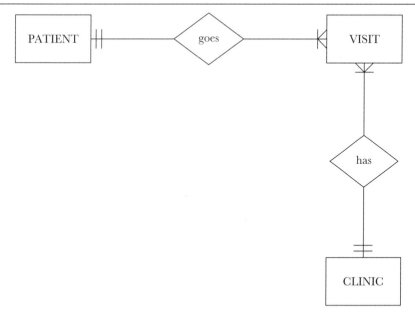

ERDs (and data modeling in general) is beyond the scope of this book, we will point out several key components here because these models are frequently used not only as "blueprints" for building databases but also as tools for communication between the designers and the eventual users. Therefore it may be necessary for the health care executive to have a cursory understanding of their components.

Entities. The rectangles in the ERD represent entities. An entity is a person, place, or thing about which the organization wishes to store data. The entities depicted in the final version of the ERD will be transformed into tables in the relational database. Figure 8.4 shows an example of a table structure that might be created from the entity CLINIC. (Please note that these examples are quite simplistic and meant to illustrate general concepts rather than represent actual database design practices.)

Attributes. The attributes of an ERD can be shown as oval shapes extending from the entities; however, it is more common to see the entities listed separately or within the entity rectangle (see Figure 8.4). Attributes transform to data fields. Each entity in the ERD must have a unique identifier, called its *primary key*. The primary key cannot be duplicated within a table and cannot contain a null value. The primary key is also used to link entities together in order to form relationships.

FIGURE 8.4. *Partial Attribute Lists for Patient, Clinic, and Visit*

PATIENT ENTITY ATTRIBUTES

```
PATIENT_MRN (PK)
PATIENT_LNAME
PATIENT_FNAME
PATIENT_MNAME
PATIENT_SSN
PATIENT_STREET
PATIENT_CITY
PATIENT_STATE
PATIENT_ZIPCODE
PATIENT_PHONE
PATIENT_DOB
...
```

VISIT ENTITY ATTRIBUTES

```
VISIT_ID (PK)
VISIT_DATE
VISIT_REASON
PATIENT_MRN (FK)
CLINIC_ID(FK)
...
```

CLINIC ENTITY ATTRIBUTES

```
CLINIC_ID (PK)
CLINIC_NAME
CLINIC_STREET
CLINIC_CITY
CLINIC_STATE
CLINIC_ZIPCODE
CLINIC_PHONE
CLINIC_FAX
...
```

Relationships. Relationships within ERDs may be shown as diamond shapes. The name of the relationship is usually a verb. There are three possible relationships among any two entities: one-to-one, one-to-many, or many-to-many. Many-to-many relationships must be converted to one-to-many before a relational database can be implemented. In our ERD example (Figure 8.3), the one side of a relationship is shown by a single mark across the line and the many side is shown by a three-pronged crow's foot. To decipher the relationship between PATIENT and VISIT as shown in Figure 8.3, you would say, "for each instance of PATIENT there are many possible instances of VISIT, and for each instance of VISIT there is only one possible instance of PATIENT."

Preparing a data model to include only those relationships that can and should be implemented in the resulting database is called *normalization*. Normalizing the database ensures that data are stored in only one location in the database (except for planned redundancy). Storing each piece of data in only one location decreases the possibility of data anomalies as a result of additions and deletions. This reduction in data redundancy and decreased potential for data anomalies is the hallmark of a relational database. It is what distinguishes it from the flat file, an older database model.

Object-Oriented Databases

A newer database structure is the *object-oriented database* (OODB). The basic component in the OODB is an object rather than a table. An object includes both data and the relationships among the data in a single conceptual structure. An *object-oriented database management system* (OODBMS) uses *classes* and *subclasses* that inherit characteristics from one another in a hierarchical manner. Think, for example, of mammals as one class of animals in the physical world (with reptiles being another class) and humans as one subclass of mammals. Because all mammals have hair, humans "inherit" this characteristic. Object subclasses "inherit" properties from an object class in a similar manner. If a "person" object is defined as having a last name and a first name variable, then any subclass objects, such as "patient," will "inherit" these definitions. The "patient" object may also have additional characteristics. A pure OODB is not common in the health care market, but products are beginning to incorporate elements of OODB and object-oriented programming with relational databases (Lee, 2002).

The *object-relational database management system* (ORDBMS) is a product that has relational database capabilities plus the ability to add and use objects. One example on the market today is ObjectStore. The advantage of an ORDBMS is that many of the newer health care applications use video and graphical data, which an ORDBMS can handle better than a traditional RDBMS can. An ORDBMS also has the capability of incorporating hypermedia and spatial data technology. Hypermedia technology allows data to be connected in *web* formations, with hyperlinks. Spatial data technology allows data to be stored and accessed according to locations (Stair & Reynolds, 2003).

Data Dictionaries

One very important step in developing a database to use in a health care application is the development of the *data dictionary*. The data dictionary gives both users and developers a clear understanding of the data elements contained in the database. Confusion about data definitions can lead to poor-quality data and even to poor decisions based on data misconceptions. A typical data dictionary allows for the documentation of

- Table names
- All attribute or field names
- A description or definition of each data element
- The data type of the field (text, number, date, and so forth)
- The format of each data element (such as DD-MM-YYYY for the date)
- The size of each field (such as 11 characters for a Social Security Number, including the dashes)
- An appropriate range of values for the field (such as integers 000000 to 999999 for a medical record number)
- Whether or not the field is required (is it a primary key or a linking key?)
- Relationships among fields

The importance of a well thought out data dictionary cannot be overstated. When an organization is trying to link or combine databases, the data dictionary is a vital tool. Think, for example, how difficult it might be to combine information from databases with different definitions for fields with the same name.

Clinical Data Repositories

Many health care organizations, particularly those moving toward electronic medical records, develop *clinical data repositories*. Although these databases can take different forms, in general the clinical data repository is a large database that gets data from various data stores within application systems across the organization. There is generally a process by which data are *cleaned* before they are moved from the source systems into the repository. Once the clean data are in the repository, they can be used to produce reports that integrate data from two or more data stores.

Data Warehouses and Data Marts

A *data warehouse* is a type of large database designed to support decision making in an organization. Traditionally, health care organizations have collected data in a variety of *online transactional processing* (OLTP) systems, such as the traditional relational database and clinical data repository. OTLP systems are well suited for supporting the daily operations of a health care organization but less well suited for decision support. Data stored in a typical OLTP system are always changing, making it difficult to track trends over time, for example. The data warehouse, in contrast, is specifically designed for decision support. It differs from the traditional OLTP database in several key areas, summarized in Table 8.1.

Like a clinical data repository, a data warehouse stores data from other database sources. Creating a data warehouse involves extracting and cleaning data from a variety of organizational databases. However, the underlying structure of a data warehouse is

TABLE 8.1. **Differences Between OLTP Databases and Data Warehouses**

Characteristic	OLTP Database	Data Warehouse
Purpose	Support transaction processing	Support decision support
Source of data	Business transactions	Multiple files, databases—data internal and external to the firm
Data access allowed to users	Read and write	Read only
Primary data access mode	Simple database update and query	Simple and complex database queries with increasing use of data mining to recognize patterns in the data
Primary database model employed	Relational	Relational
Level of detail	Detailed transactions	Often summarized data
Availability of historical data	Very limited—typically a few weeks or months	Multiple years
Update process	On-line, ongoing process as transactions are captured	Periodic process, once per week or once per month
Ease of update	Routine and easy	Complex, must combine data from many sources; data must go through a data cleanup process
Data integrity issues	Each individual transaction must be closely edited	Major effort to clean and integrate data from multiple sources

Source: *Principles of Information Systems*, 6th Edition, by STAIR/REYNOLDS. © 2004. Reprinted with permission of Course Technology, a division of Thomson Learning: www.thomsonrights.com. Fax 800-730-2215.

different from the table structure of a relational database. This different structure allows data to be extracted along such dimensions as time (by week, month, or year), location, or diagnosis. Data in a data warehouse can often be accessed via *drill-down* menus that allow you to see smaller and smaller units within the same dimension. For example, you could view the number of patients with a particular diagnosis for a year, then a month in that year, then a day in that month. Or you could see how many times a procedure was performed at all locations in the health system, then see the total by region, then by facility. Even though the same data might be available in a relational database, its normalized structure makes the queries you would have to use to get at the information quite complex and difficult to execute. Data warehouses help organizations transform large quantities of data from separate transactional files into a single decision-support database. *Data marts* are structurally similar to data warehouses but generally not as large. The typical data mart is developed for a particular purpose or unit within an organization.

Data Mining

Data mining is another concept closely associated with large databases such as clinical data repositories and data warehouses. However, data mining (like several other IT concepts) means different things to different people. Health care application vendors may use the term data mining when referring to the user interface of the data warehouse or data repository. They may refer to the ability to drill down into data as data mining, for example. However, more precisely used, data mining refers to a sophisticated analysis tool that automatically discovers patterns among data in a data store. Data mining is an advanced form of decision support. Unlike passive query tools, the data mining analysis tool does not require the user to pose individual specific questions to the database. Instead, this tool is programmed to look for and extract patterns, trends, and rules. True data mining is currently used in the business community for marketing and predictive analysis (Stair & Reynolds, 2003). This analytical data mining is, however, not currently widespread in the health care community.

NETWORKS AND DATA COMMUNICATIONS

The term *data communications* refers to the transmission of electronic data within or among computers and other related devices. In this section we will take a cursory look at many of the components that go into building computer networks for the purpose of data communications. (Although the Internet is certainly a part of the overall data communications system that health care organizations use, we believe it is significant enough to warrant its own section, which follows this one.)

Devices that make up computer networks must be compatible. They must be able to communicate with one another. Much of what we introduce in this section takes the form of definitions and examples of different types of network components whose compatibility and interoperability might be an issue. Specifically, we cover the following topics as they relate to data communications, particularly in health care settings:

- Network communication protocols
- Network types and configurations
- Network media and bandwidth
- Network communication devices

Network Communication Protocols

Data communication across computer networks is possible today because of *communication protocols and standards*. Without the common *language* of protocols, networked computers and other devices would not be able to connect with and talk to one another.

The distinction between protocols and standards is often misunderstood. On the one hand the English language is a protocol for communication. It is also a standard. People taught English by different instructors in different parts of the globe will learn (more or less) the same thing and be able to communicate with each other because there is a standard vocabulary and standards for such things as verb tense. On the other hand the plugs for appliances are protocols—there is a specification for the two flat prongs that form the plug. But the plug is not a standard. Appliances in Switzerland use two round prongs and an American appliance cannot be plugged into a Swiss outlet.

The need for standard network protocols has been evident since the first computer networks were built. To this end the International Organization for Standardization developed the *Open Standards Interconnection* (OSI) model. Work on OSI was begun in the 1980s. Although this model has been well accepted as a conceptual, or reference, model for network protocols, it is important to be aware that it has not evolved into detailed specifications, as was once anticipated (Whatis?.com, 2002). OSI is not a set of protocols. Rather, it is a model, or scheme, for describing network protocols that have been or will be developed and adopted by the industry. A general introduction to OSI is useful as a point of reference when discussing other aspects of computer networks. Table 8.2 provides a brief description of each of the layers of the OSI model. Figure 8.5 depicts the conceptual framework, showing how data would flow from one computer to another on the network.

To date, the network model most commonly adopted for creating software for network communications has been the Internet model, which employs *Transmission Control Protocol/Internet Protocol* (TCP/IP). TCP/IP was first introduced in the 1970s by the U.S. government to support defense activities (Stair & Reynolds, 2003). However, it was not until the boom of the World Wide Web that this set of protocols began to dominate the computer network industry. Like the OSI model, the Internet model is a layered model (Figure 8.6). However, the Internet model has fewer layers, and unlike the OSI reference model, it represents actual protocol specifications at each layer (White, 2001).

A few other standard network protocols are also worth mentioning, although the following list is by no means all inclusive. Each layer of a network requires specific protocols, which must then work together to make sure that data flow from the sender to the receiver.

- *Ethernet* is the most popular *local area network* (LAN) technology in use today, both in health care and in business. Ethernet is specified as an IEEE standard (802.3). It was originally developed as a joint effort by several prominent vendors: Xerox, Digital Equipment Corporation, and Intel. Ethernet systems are offered by many different network vendors and come in a variety of *speeds*. 10-BASE-T Ethernet provides transmission speeds of up to 10 megabits per second (Mbps), Fast Ethernet provides up to 100 Mbps, and Gigabit Ethernet provides up to 1,000 Mbps. (We will discuss transmission speed a little later in this section.)

- *Asynchronous Transfer Mode* (ATM) is a switching technology protocol designed to be implemented with hardware devices allowing faster transmission speeds—up to 10 Gbps.

TABLE 8.2. **Seven-Layer OSI Model**

Application (Layer 7)	This layer supports application and end-user processes. Communication partners are identified, quality of service is identified, user authentication and privacy are considered, and any constraints on data syntax are identified. Everything at this layer is application specific. This layer provides application services for file transfers, e-mail, and other network software services.
Presentation (Layer 6)	This layer provides independence from differences in data representation (for example, encryption) by translating from application to network format and vice versa. It works to transform data into the form that the application layer can accept. It formats and encrypts data to be sent across a network, providing freedom from compatibility problems.
Session (Layer 5)	This layer establishes, manages, and terminates connections between applications. It sets up, coordinates, and terminates conversations, exchanges, and dialogues between the applications at each end. It deals with session and connection coordination.
Transport (Layer 4)	This layer provides transparent transfer of data between end systems, or hosts. It ensures complete data transfer.
Network (Layer 3)	This layer provides switching and routing technologies, creating logical paths, known as virtual circuits, for transmitting data from node to node. Routing and forwarding are functions of this layer, as well as addressing, Internet working, error handling, congestion control, and packet sequencing.
Data Link (Layer 2)	At this layer, data packets are encoded and decoded into bits. It furnishes transmission protocol knowledge and management and handles errors in the physical layer, flow control, and frame synchronization. The data link layer is divided into two sublayers: the media access control (MAC) layer and the logical link control (LLC) layer. The MAC sublayer controls how a computer on the network gains access to the data and permission to transmit it. The LLC layer controls frame synchronization, flow control, and error checking.
Physical (Layer 1)	This layer conveys the bit stream—electrical impulse, light, or radio signal—through the network at the electrical and mechanical level. It provides the hardware means of sending and receiving data on a carrier, including defining cables, cards, and physical aspects. Fast Ethernet and ATM are protocols with physical layer components.

Source: Based on webopedia.com, 2004b.

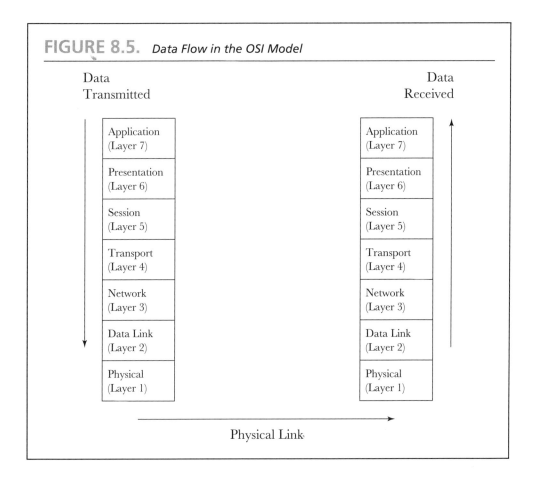

FIGURE 8.5. *Data Flow in the OSI Model*

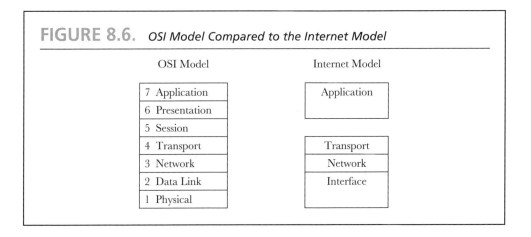

FIGURE 8.6. *OSI Model Compared to the Internet Model*

■ *Bluetooth* is a developing communication standard that was first introduced in 1994. It is designed to support communications among cellular phones, handheld computers, and other wireless devices. Health care organizations might employ Bluetooth technology in wireless keyboards, mice, headsets, or PDAs.

■ *IEEE 802.11* standards apply to wireless Ethernet LAN technology. Standard 802.11a applies to wireless ATM systems and high-speed switching devices. Standards 802.11b, 802.11g, and 802.11n (or Wi-Fi specifications), are used by wireless computer networks.

Network Types and Configurations

Computer networks used in health care and elsewhere are described with a variety of terms. In this section you will be introduced to many of these terms. Again, this is not an exhaustive list. As you read these sections, keep in mind that a computer network is a collection of devices (sometimes called *nodes*) that are connected to one another for the purpose of transmitting data. A *network operating system* (NOS) is a special type of system software that controls the devices on a network and allows the devices to communicate with one another. Some of the most common network operating systems on the market today are Microsoft's Windows and Novell's NetWare (Stair & Reynolds, 2003).

LAN Versus WAN The first distinction that is often made when describing a network is to identify it as either a *local area network* (LAN) or a *wide area network* (WAN.) LANs typically operate within a building or sometimes across several buildings belonging to a single organization and located in the same general vicinity. The actual distance a LAN covers can vary greatly. One common way to distinguish a LAN from a WAN is that the LAN will have its network hardware and software under the control of a single organization. As the Internet and its related technologies are used more by organizations, the line between LANs and WANs may be becoming somewhat blurred. For our purposes, we will think of the LAN as being confined to a single geographical area and controlled by a single organization. A WAN is any network that extends beyond the LAN. WANs may be public (like the Internet) or private. They may be connected by dedicated lines, a satellite, or other media.

Each device and computer within a LAN has a *network interface card* (NIC). These cards are generally specific to the type of LAN transmission technology being employed, such as Ethernet or Wi-Fi. (This is why you may hear the term *Ethernet card* or *Wi-Fi card* used to refer to your computer's NIC.) Clearly, most health care organizations today operate one or more LANs and use WANs as well.

Topology A second way that wired networks are described is by their *topology*, or layout. There are two types of network topology: *physical* and *logical*. The physical topology is how the wires are physically configured. The logical topology is the way data flow from node to node in the network. Various arrangements and standards dictate this movement.

Ethernet employs a *logical bus topology*, so this topology is the one most commonly found in health care networks. The bus topology in its simplest form consists of computers and other devices operating along a single *line*. This arrangement allows each device on the network to communicate directly with any other device on the network, without having to pass through interim devices or nodes. It is called a bus topology because the data signals travel up and down the single line (like buses on a commuter bus line) until they reach their designation (Webopedia, 2004c).

Physical topology, the manner in which the network cables are arranged, may be a *bus* or *star* arrangement. Figure 8.7 shows an Ethernet network, which is a logical bus, in a physical star layout. Note that the wiring from the various computer devices on the network comes together in another device, which is called a *hub*.

The physical layout for wireless LANs differs from the layout for wired LANS, because the wireless networks use radio frequency transmissions rather than cables to transmit data. Wireless LANs allow health care organizations greater flexibility and portability than wired LANs do. The 802.11 standard defines two types of wireless networks, the *infrastructure network* and the *ad hoc network*.

The infrastructure network relies on fixed *access points* (APs) with which the mobile devices (such as laptops, smart phones, and the like) can communicate. These fixed APs are then connected to a wired Ethernet LAN. APs typically have wireless coverage of up to 100 meters. Each coverage area is referred to as a *range*, or *cell*. Users can move from one range to another within the wireless LAN.

Ad hoc networks, such as those that employ Bluetooth technology, are generally designed to dynamically connect remote devices, such as laptops, cell phones, PDAs, or smart phones. The ad hoc network does not have the range of the infrastructure

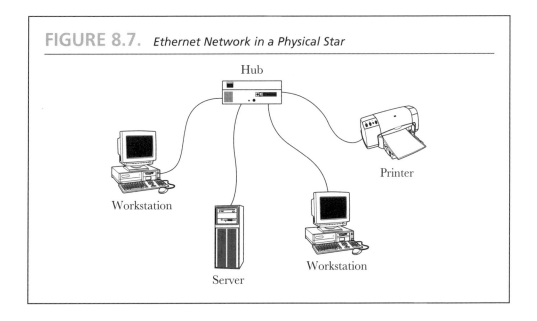

FIGURE 8.7. *Ethernet Network in a Physical Star*

network and it relies on a *master-slave* system of wireless links to connect the devices (Karygiannis & Owens, 2002).

Network Media and Bandwidth

Two frequently discussed aspects of a network are its media and its bandwidth. *Media* refers to the physical "wires" or other transmission devices used on the network. *Bandwidth* is a measure of media capacity.

Media   Data may be transmitted on a network through several types of media. Common types of conducted media for LANs include *twisted pair wire, coaxial cable*, and *fiber-optic cable*. Common wireless media include *terrestrial* and *satellite microwave transmissions* as well as *spread spectrum radio transmissions*. Mobile phone technology and infrared technology are also being used for wireless computer data transmission (White, 2001).

> *Twisted pair.* Twisted pair wire comes in categories, ranging from the "slowest," Category 1, to the "fastest," Category 7 (Categories 6 and 7 are currently considered developing technologies, with draft standards). Traditional telephone wire is Category 1 twisted pair. Typical LAN wire is Category 5 or 5e.

> *Coaxial cable.* Coaxial cable is the cable used to transmit cable television signals. The use of coaxial cable in LANs has decreased in recent years due to the availability of high-quality twisted pair and fiber-optic cable.

> *Fiber-optic cable.* Fiber-optic cable is made of thin glass fibers only a little bigger in diameter than a human hair. These glass "wires" are encased in insulation and plastic. The big advantage of fiber-optic cable is its ability to transmit data over longer distances than traditional twisted pair can. However, fiber-optic cable is more expensive to use.

> *Microwaves.* Microwaves are a type of radio wave with very short wavelengths. Terrestrial microwave transmission occurs between two microwave antennas. In order to receive and send microwave signals, the sending and receiving antennas must be in sight of one another. Satellite microwave transmission sends microwave signals from an antenna on the ground to an orbiting satellite and then back to another antenna on the ground.

> *Spread spectrum.* Spread spectrum wireless transmission uses another type of radio wave. Unlike conventional radio broadcasting, which uses a specific, consistent wave frequency, spread spectrum technology employs a deliberately varied signal, resulting in greater bandwidth. The popular Wi-Fi (802.11) standard for wireless computing is based on spread spectrum technology (Whatis?.com, 2002).

Service Carriers   Communications across a WAN may involve some type of telecommunications carrier. These carriers provide the telephone lines, satellites, modems, and other services that allow data to be transmitted across distances. They can be either *common carriers*, primarily the long-distance telephone companies, or *special-purpose* *carriers*. Common carriers can provide either a traditional switched line, sometimes referred to as *plain old telephone service* (POTS), or a *dedicated* or *leased line*, which offers a permanent connection between two locations. Telephone companies also offer *integrated services digital network* (ISDN) services. ISDN uses existing phone lines to transmit not only voice but also video and image data in digital form. A purchased *T-1 line* may be another option for transmitting integrated voice, data, and images for large health care organizations, depending on their needs.

Bandwidth   *Bandwidth* is another name for the capacity of a transmission medium. Generally, the greater the capacity, or bandwidth, of the medium, the greater the speed of transmission. Multiple factors influence transmission speed, and bandwidth is only one of them, but a low bandwidth can impede transmission rates across the network. Transmission rates are expressed as *bits per second* (bps). In other words, a medium's capacity is determined by the maximum number of bps it can carry. Category 1 twisted pair wire has a relatively low transmission speed, 56 Kbps typically, whereas satellite microwave can have speeds exceeding 200 Gbps (Oz, 2004). With some media, a signal that must travel a long distance may have to be enhanced along the way in order to maintain its speed of transmission. Devices that accomplish this task are called *repeaters*.

Network Communication Devices

If you think about how computers are used in the health care organization today, they rarely depend on a single LAN to access all the information needed. At the least a computer will be connected to one LAN and the Internet. Often a single computer in a health care organization will be connected to multiple LANs and several WANs, including the Internet. LANs employ combinations of software and hardware in order to communicate with other networks.

There are several types of devices that allow networks to communicate with another. We describe a few of the common devices in this section, including *hubs, bridges, routers, gateways*, and *switches*.

Hub. As its name implies, a hub is a device in which data from a network come together. On a schematic a hub may appear as the box where all the Ethernet lines come together for a LAN or a segment of a LAN. Today single devices may serve as hubs and switches or even routers (Whatis?.com, 2002).

Bridge. A bridge connects networks that use the same communication protocol. In the OSI reference model (Figure 8.5), a bridge operates at the data link layer, which is fairly low in the model, which means that it cannot translate signals between networks using different protocols.

Router. A router operates at a higher level, the network layer of the OSI model. Routers are more sophisticated devices than bridges. Whereas bridges send on all data they receive, routers are able to help determine the actual destination of specific data.

Gateway. A gateway can connect networks that have different communication protocols. These devices operate at the transport level of the OSI model, or higher.

Switch. A switch may either be a gateway or a router. In other words, it may operate at the router level or at a higher level. There are many types of switches available on the market today. All switches will route, or *switch*, data to their destination (Stair & Reynolds, 2003).

INFORMATION PROCESSING DISTRIBUTION SCHEMES

Networks and databases are often described in terms of the method through which the organization distributes their information processing. Three common distribution methods are *terminal-to-host, file server*, and *client/server*. All three types are found in health care information networks. A single health care organization may in fact employ one, two, or all three methods of processing distribution, depending on its computing needs and its strategic decisions regarding architecture.

In *terminal-to-host* schemes the application and database reside on a host computer, and the user interacts with the computer using a dumb terminal, which is a workstation with no processing power. In some terminal-to-host setups the user may interact with the host computer from his or her personal computer (which obviously has computing power), but special software, called *terminal emulation* software, is used to make the PC act as if it were a dumb terminal when connecting to a specified host computer. *Thin client* schemes are a variation of the host-to-terminal type. The major advantage cited for using this type of distribution is the centralized control. The individuals who support the network and databases no longer have to worry about PC maintenance or how the user might inadvertently modify the configuration of the workstation.

File server systems have the application and database on a single computer. However, the end-user's workstation runs the database management system. When the user needs the data that reside on the file server, the file server will send the entire file to the computer requesting it.

Client/server systems differ from traditional file server systems in that they have multiple servers, each of which is dedicated to one or more specialized functions. For example, servers may be dedicated to database management, printing, or other program execution. The servers are accessible from other computers in the network, either all computers in the network or a designated subset. The client side of the network usually runs the applications and sends requests from the applications to the server side, which returns the requested data.

THE INTERNET, INTRANET, AND EXTRANETS

Think of how health care organizations use the Internet today. They maintain informational Web pages for patients, providers, and insurers. They use Internet technologies to facilitate communications and transactions internally and with suppliers and customers. Some health care organizations have developed health information Web applications or have contracted with third parties to maintain patient records electronically.

Telemedicine and *electronic data interchange* (EDI) functions may be Web based. The list of examples goes on. This is truly an amazing phenomenon when you consider that the vast majority of this Internet and Web application development has occurred in the last decade. Although the Internet has its early roots in an effort that began in the late 1960s, it was not until the development of the *World Wide Web (WWW)* that businesses, including health care organizations, began to see the benefit of online communications and online business transactions (e-commerce). Internet use is one of the most rapidly growing aspects of health information technology. In this section we will examine the technologies that make Web-based e-commerce possible for health care organizations. We will describe the fundamentals of Internet and WWW technologies and explore a few of the more recent developments.

The Internet

What, exactly, is the Internet? The image that today's user has of the Internet is the multimedia world of the WWW; however, this is only one part of the vast network of networks known as the Internet. The WWW is the means by which the majority of users interact with the Internet, but the WWW and the Internet are not the same.

The Internet began in 1969 as a government project to improve defense communications. This precursor to today's Internet was known as the Advanced Research Projects Agency Network (ARPANET). The goal of the Advanced Research Projects Agency was to establish a network that could survive a nuclear strike; therefore it was intentionally developed without a central point of control. This is a characteristic of the Internet that still exists today. Believe it or not, ARPANET began as a network of four computers. In the beginning ARPANET was open only to academic institutions and portions of the national defense infrastructure. As it grew, the network divided into a civilian branch and a government branch. The civilian branch became known as the Internet. In 1991, the government decided to allow businesses to link to the Internet, but not many businesses were interested in this until the WWW was introduced a couple of years later. The WWW is what brought multimedia and ease of use to the Internet and its applications. Since the introduction of the WWW, Internet use among all types of businesses (including health care) has exploded.

The backbone of the Internet today is owned and maintained by multiple organizations in many countries. The Internet backbone is made up of many high-speed networks linked together. These networks use multiple types of communication media, such as optical fiber, satellite, and microwave transmission. Think of the components of this backbone as the major highways of the Internet. The Internet, like its predecessor, ARPANET, has no single point of control. Specific segments of the Internet backbone are owned and maintained by telecommunications companies and Internet service providers (ISPs), such as Sprint, MCI, Verizon, and America Online (AOL), to name just a few (Oz, 2004; Stair & Reynolds, 2003; Whatis?.com, 2002).

How the Internet Works Every computer and device that operates within the Internet has a unique identifier known as an *Internet protocol* (IP) number, or address. Specific Internet protocols (discussed earlier in this chapter) allow each computer or device on the Internet to use these IP addresses to locate other computers or devices. The IP address is a four-part number, with each part separated by a period. All Web sites have an IP address; however, most are also associated with a character-based address, which is easier for people to remember. The process of associating the numerical IP address with the character-based name is accomplished by a *Domain Name System* (DNS) server, which is maintained by an ISP. IP addresses may be static or dynamic. Static addresses are permanently assigned to a computer or device. A dynamic address is assigned "as needed" by a special server that recognizes when a computer or device needs an address. Dynamic IP addressing gives an organization flexibility in using its allotted IP addresses.

Blocks of IP addresses are assigned to organizations by one of several domain name registrars. Again, remember that one of the hallmarks of the Internet is the absence of a central point of control. The companies that register domain names and IP addresses are for-profit organizations that sell their name registration services. There is also one database that contains all domain names, IP addresses, and "owners"; it is maintained by Network Solutions, Inc. (Oz, 2004; Stair & Reynolds, 2003; Whatis?.com, 2002).

World Wide Web   The use of the Internet changed dramatically when a British scientist invented the software protocol *Hypertext Transfer Protocol* (HTTP). HTTP allows full-color graphics, tables, forms, video, and animation to be shared over the Internet. The code used for displaying files on the WWW is called a *markup language*. The most common markup language today is HTML (*hypertext markup language*). HTML defines how pages look on the Web by using *tags*, special codes that inform a Web browser how text or other content should look. A newer markup language that many think will change the way data are captured and stored is the *extensible markup language* (XML). Unlike HTML, which defines only how pages look, XML also defines what the data enclosed in the tags are. XML holds a lot of promise as a messaging standard in health care applications. Figure 8.8 presents examples of HTML and XML code.

Think about using the WWW. How do you get to the Web page you want? Typically, you type the URL (uniform resource locator) for the page (for example, http://www.musc.edu/chp/facstaff.htm) into an application known as a *Web browser*. The best-known Web browsers are Internet Explorer and Netscape. However, interest is increasing in the open-source browser Mozilla. Browser software allows Web users to search for and retrieve specific Web sites. Today, browsers also allow the user to use additional software components, known as *plug-ins*, to perform functions such as viewing videos or listening to audio.

Figure 8.9 shows the various components of a URL. The HTTP part of the address indicates that Hypertext Transfer Protocol is being used. HTTP is one of the protocols that make up TCP/IP. (Another TCP/IP protocol, HTTPS, is a secure variation of HTTP that employs encryption to protect the site.) The next component, www.musc.edu, is the domain name (a domain name may or may not include www). The *edu* section of the address in Figure 8.9 is the *top-level domain* (TLD), which often indicates the type of organization that registered the domain name. Some TLDs, such as *edu, mil*, and *gov*, are restricted to use by qualified organizations. However, some, such as *com, org*, and *net*,

FIGURE 8.8. *XML and HTML Code*

XML

```
<patient>
<patient.id>12345</patient.id>
<patient.name>John Doe</patient.name.
<patient.date.of.birth>November 21, 1953</patient.date.of.birth>
</patient>
```

Tags define the actual data elements.

HTML

```
<p>MRN: 12345<br>
Name: John Doe<br>
Date of Birth: November 21, 1953</p>
```

Tags define how the text will look and not the data the text represents.

FIGURE 8.9. *URL Components*

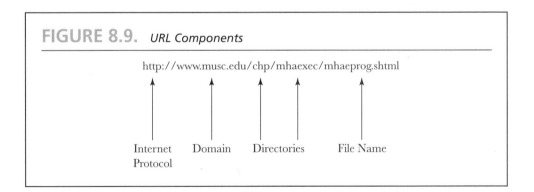

are less restricted and can be used by any individual or organization in the appropriate generic category. The next section of the URL indicates the specific directory, or folder, where the Web page resides. In our example there are two directories, but there could be several or only one. The final component of the URL is the actual name of the file to be located. In this example the file ends with the extension *shtml*, which shows that it was created, or coded, using a specific version of HTML (Oz, 2004; Stair & Reynolds, 2003; Whatis?.com, 2002).

Other Internet Applications   As mentioned earlier, most of us associate the Internet with the WWW, but Web browsers are not the only Internet applications that are used by health care organizations. Some other common applications are e-mail, file transfer, and Internet telephoning.

> *E-mail.* E-mail is one of the most popular uses of the Internet. The TCP/IP set of protocols include e-mail protocols that allow point-to-point, text-based communications. The basic form of e-mail is encoded text, but graphic and sound files can be sent as attachments. The most common protocol for outgoing e-mail is *Simple Mail Transfer Protocol* (SMTP). *Post Office Protocol 3* (POP3) and *Internet Message Access Protocol* (IMAP) are common protocols for receiving e-mail (Whatis?.com, 2002).

> *File transfer. File Transfer Protocol* (FTP) is the TCP/IP protocol that allows point-to-point transfer of files from one computer to another. FTP is incorporated into Web sites and e-mail to allow the downloading of files. Files transferred using FTP can be text, graphics, animation, or sound files.

> *Internet telephoning.* Internet telephoning is gaining popularity in the business community and in health care organizations. The protocol that allows Internet telephoning is *Voice over Internet Protocol* (VoIP). Organizations that want to use Internet telephoning must have the appropriate software and microphones attached to computers. They must either purchase software or use a company that provides Internet telephone services. As this technology continues to improve over time, organizations are finding it to be a viable, and less expensive, option to traditional long distance. According to one estimate, the cost of a VoIP telephone conference will be about 25 percent that of a traditional telephone conference (Oz, 2006).

Intranets and Extranets

An *intranet* is a computer network that is internal to an organization and that uses Internet technologies. Intranets can be used for virtually any type of internal network application. The network designers develop Web applications that are accessible via Web browsers. Although an intranet uses both "public" Internet routes and internal network lines, it is generally a secure network that is protected from outside users. For example, a hospital may set up an intranet site with employee benefits and forms that can be accessed only from authorized computers within the organization or by employees entering the organization's network through a secure mechanism. The secure path established between the Internet and an intranet, using a combination of software and hardware protections, is sometimes referred to as a *tunnel*.

An *extranet* is similar to an intranet except that the network of users includes business partners of the health care organization, such as suppliers, customers, or other health care providers. Again, extranets are generally secure, limiting access to their sites (Oz, 2004).

Web 2.0

Web 2.0 is an umbrella term that covers a range of Web-based communities, services, and technologies, including *social-networking* sites, *wikis, blogs*, and messaging capabilities.

The "2.0" part of Web 2.0 reflects the view that this collection represents the second generation of Web technologies and capabilities. Although the transformational potential of Web 2.0 can be debated—ranging from a view that this is all hype to a view that this is a radical step forward—there is no doubt that these technologies and capabilities materially extend the power of the Web.

Web-based communities such as Facebook and MySpace provide a means for individuals to share information with other people with whom they have a common bond. This bond might, for example, be a school class or type or place of employment, a chronic disease, a specific hobby, or an interest in some aspect of politics or religion.

A *wiki* incorporates software that allows users to easily create, edit, and link pages together. Wikis are generally used to enable individuals to create and maintain knowledge. For example, Wikipedia is a collection of user-contributed knowledge on a range of topics, and a hospital-sponsored wiki could be used by care providers to create knowledge on the best way to treat a particular disease.

Blogs, or Web logs, provide the means for an author to create a diary or running commentary on topics of his or her choosing. Blog readers can post their reactions to and comments on the material entered by the blog author and by other readers.

Messaging capabilities such as RSS (*Really Simple Syndication*) enable Web users to receive a message when new material has been added to Web sites.

Web 2.0 advances the ability of the Web to be used to support communities and the sharing of information between people. Hospitals and other health care facilities have adopted Web 2.0 to create opportunities for patients and other consumers. The impact of Web 2.0 in the future is unclear but likely to be potent.

CLINICAL AND MANAGERIAL DECISION SUPPORT

Health care executives and providers are faced with decisions every day, multiple times per day. The success of any health care organization literally depends on these large and small decisions. In this section we will describe technologies that support decision making in health care today, for both clinical and managerial decisions. The types of systems that we examine are

- Decision-support systems (DSS)
- Artificial intelligence systems, including expert systems, natural language processing, fuzzy logic, and neural networks

Nobel Prize–winning economist Herbert Simon described decision making as a three-step process (Oz, 2004; Stair & Reynolds, 2003). The steps involve

1. Intelligence: collecting facts, beliefs, and ideas. In health care these facts may be stored as data elements in a variety of data stores.

2. Design: designing the methods with which to consider the data collected during intelligence. These methods may be models, formulas, algorithms, or other analytical tools. Methods are selected that will reduce the number of viable alternatives.

3. Choice: making the most promising choice from the limited set of alternatives.

Problems that face health care executives and clinicians may be *structured, unstructured*, or *semistructured*. Structured problems are also referred to as *programmable* problems, because a computer program can be written with relative ease to solve this kind of problem. Transaction-based applications can be used to solve structured, or programmable, problems. For example, a payroll system is based on known facts about each employee's salary, deductions, and so on. The "decision" of how much to write the monthly paycheck for is fairly straightforward. The unstructured and semistructured problems present much more of a challenge for computer application developers.

Decision-Support Systems

How do we harness the power of a computer to solve a problem or make a decision about a solution when the situation is not easily structured with a simple algorithm (sequence of logical steps)? The computer systems developed to tackle the unstructured or semistructured problem are called *decision-support systems* (DSS). Decision-support system is another term that can mean slightly different things to different vendors or users. In this section we are referring primarily to the traditional, stand-alone DSS: in other words, an application that is designed for the purpose of supporting decisions. This is not the only form of decision support available to health care executives and providers today. For example, patient care or administrative applications may have components, such as data mining, that aid in decision making, but these applications might not be classified as full-blown DSS. An electronic spreadsheet, such as Excel, can also be used as a decision-support tool. Spreadsheets have built-in functions as well as the ability to use what-if statements.

The stand-alone DSS generally has three distinct components:

■   The data management module, which is an existing or built-in transactional database or data warehouse. In a clinical DSS, the data module could be a clinical data repository.

■   The model management module, which allows the user to select a model to be applied to the problem at hand. Models can be mathematical, statistical, or based on expert knowledge. The model management module of a DSS is its most complex component and may seem like a "black box" to the health care executive.

■   The dialog module, which is the user interface. This module allows the user to pose the problem to the system by selecting the data and the decision model to use on the data. The dialog module also displays results, generally in text and graphical formats.

Executive information systems (EIS) are decision-support systems specifically designed for the higher-level manager. Most of these systems have drill-down capability to allow the executive to examine a problem at different levels of granularity, and many are tied to data warehouses (Oz, 2004).

Artificial Intelligence

Artificial intelligence (AI) is a branch of computer science devoted to emulating the human mind. One very common use of AI today is incorporated into the Google search engine. When the user types a misspelled word in a string of keywords, Google will suggest alternative keywords based on the context of the query (Oz, 2004). AI is a broad field with many different types of technology. Most AI is quite complex and describing the underlying technology is beyond the scope of this text. However, we will introduce a few types of AI that may be found in health care settings.

Expert Systems   The hallmark of expert systems is that they use *heuristics*, or "rules of thumb," collected from experts in the particular field for which the system was built. Expert systems comprise

- A *knowledge base*, which stores all the relevant information, data, rules, and cases that will be used by the system. It is similar to a database, but the relationships are designed to match those dictated by the human experts. One of the challenges of building the knowledge base is getting the expert knowledge. Experts, being people, do not always agree on the way to approach a problem.

- An *inference engine*, which provides the expert advice from the knowledge base.

- An *explanation facility*, which allows the user to understand how the inference engine arrived at the advice it is presenting.

- A *knowledge acquisition facility*, which allows the user to update the knowledge base with new or additional expert information (Stair & Reynolds, 2003).

Natural Language Processing   *Natural language processing* (NLP) programs take human language (typed as text or input as voice) and translate it into a standard computer instructions, such as SQL. Suppose you typed this text into an application:
List the names of all drugs that will treat shingles for less than $60 per month.
Or:
What are the names of the drugs that will treat shingles for less than $60 per month?
    A NLP program might recognize either form of this sentence in context and convert it to an SQL statement similar to this:

> SELECT NAME FROM DRUGS
> WHERE DISEASE = "SHINGLES"
> AND COST ¡ 60

So far NLP programs have met with limited success. The difficulty is in identifying all of the possible meanings of words or combination of words based on context. This problem is magnified in the health care community by medical terminology that is both complex and seems to be ever changing.

Neural Networks   *Neural networks*, or *neural nets*, may be used by sophisticated expert systems. They are software programs that attempt to mimic the way the human brain operates. This is in contrast to the traditional, step-by-step process used in other computer programming languages. Neural networks involve a very sophisticated level of programming, but they are employed in both business and health care applications today.

Fuzzy Logic   *Fuzzy logic* is based on rules that may have overlapping boundaries. This logic is designed to help the expert system deal with ambiguity and uncertainty (Oz, 2006).

TRENDS IN USER INTERACTIONS WITH SYSTEMS

This section of this technology chapter is devoted to describing some of the new and not-so-new devices that enhance the user interface with the health care information system. There have been many developments in input and output devices, along with personal computing devices, in the past few years. These developments are likely to continue and will affect the way in which users expect to interact with health information systems. The list of devices discussed in this section is by no means all inclusive. Each coming year will likely see new or improved devices on the market. However, these discussions will give you an overview of the various types of devices that are available at the time of this writing. We examine four categories of devices:

- Input devices
- Output devices
- External storage devices
- Mobile personal computing devices

Input Devices

The most common computer input devices in use today are the standard keyboard and the mouse. These devices have undergone a few changes since their introduction with personal computers, such as ergonomic improvements in shape and size and the addition of wireless technologies. Both the keyboard and the mouse are now available in wireless forms, which employ infrared or radio frequency technologies.

Other commonly used input devices and methods include trackballs, trackpads, touch screens, source data input devices such as bar-code scanners, and systems for imaging and speech recognition. *Trackballs* and *trackpads* work like the standard mouse. The computer detects the movement of the ball or the user's touch on the pad and translates it into digital coordinates on the computer screen. *Touch screens* (Figure 8.10) allow the user to choose operations by touching the surface of the computer screen. The technology of touch screens comes in two basic forms. In one, the pressure of the touch results in an electrical contact between two layers of the screen, causing an electrical current to move through the screen to a sensing device. In the other, acoustical

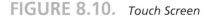

FIGURE 8.10. *Touch Screen*

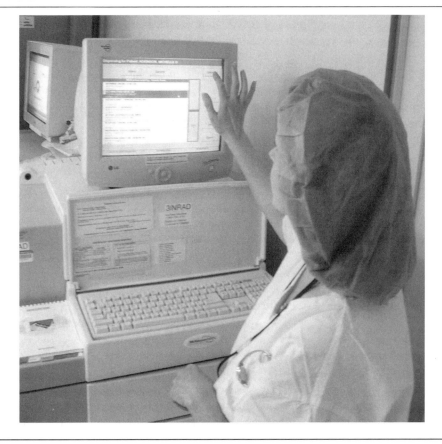

Source: Courtesy of Medical University of South Carolina.

waves are converted to electrical signals. Touch screens are used in handheld computing devices as well as in PCs (Oz, 2004; Stair & Reynolds, 2003).

A special class of input devices known as *source data input* devices includes optical mark recognition, optical character recognition, and bar-coding devices, among others. Although bar coding has been commonplace in retail venues for many years, it has recently received a lot of attention in the health care community as a means of improving patient safety. *Optical bar-code recognition* devices recognize data encoded as a series of thick and thin *bars*. As with other technologies, the success of bar coding in health care stems from the development of standards, in this case the Health Industry Bar Code (HIBC) standard. The HIBC standard was developed for applications such as medical product and drug identification and device tracking. It is approved by the American National Standards Institute (a standards-governing organization discussed in the next chapter) and administered by the Health Industry Business Communications Council

(HIBCC). The standard specifies a primary label and an optional secondary label. The primary label bar code includes the labeler's unique identification code, the product or catalogue number, and the packaging level. The secondary label bar code allows the inclusion of such data as expiration date, lot number, quantity, batch number, and serial number, which are important when dealing with medical products and devices (Hankin, 2002). As mentioned in Chapter Five, a common health care use of bar coding is in medication administration systems that employ bar-code-enabled point of care (BPOC) functions.

Many health care organizations have looked to *document imaging* systems as a means of getting data into health care information systems. Document imaging systems scan documents and convert them to digital images. These images are then stored in databases for later retrieval. The disadvantage of imaging systems is that they require a great deal of storage capacity, but their greatest advantage is that a digitized document, such as a patient record, is available to multiple users simultaneously. With the availability of inexpensive, high-capacity storage media, such as compact disks (CDs) and digital video disks (DVDs), imaging systems became feasible alternatives for integrating documents into health care information systems. Think back to our discussion of the Medical Records Institute's levels of automation and computerization of medical records; Level 2 systems rely on this form of imaging.

Speech recognition, or *voice recognition*, is another input method used in health care. It is particularly suited for situations or work environments where using a keyboard, mouse, or touch screen is not practical, such as the pathology lab or surgical suite. Speech recognition systems today vary in level of sophistication. The simplest systems are designed to "learn" a person's speech pattern. A user speaks into a microphone, and the speech recognition software learns the particular intonations, vocabulary, and patterns associated with that user. Once the user's speech pattern is learned, the voice is converted to computer-readable data. The disadvantage of these systems is the time it takes to "train" the computer to recognize the speech. This is a particular challenge in an area with many users. Higher-end systems are designed to understand any person's speech, but most of these systems have fairly limited built-in vocabularies. Most would agree that speech recognition is still under development and its use is most likely in certain segments of health care, such as radiology, pathology, and emergency medicine. However, it does have the potential to be used with many other types of health care applications. An example of a voice recognition system marketed to health care providers is Dragon Naturally Speaking Medical Solutions (Oz, 2004).

Output Devices

The most commonly used computer output devices are the computer monitor and the printer. There are two basic types of monitors: traditional monitors that use *cathode ray tube* (CRT) technology and flat panel monitors, such as those that use *liquid crystal display* (LCD) technology. Notebook and handheld computing devices rely on flat screen technology, and they have also become a popular alternative to the CRT for desktop computers. Printers are either *impact* or *nonimpact*. Nonimpact printers use laser, ink jet, electrostatic, and electrothermal methodologies. They print without a printhead that touches the paper. They can produce a very high quality printed document. Impact printers include dot matrix printers, in which pins strike an inked ribbon to produce the print. Impact printers have become less popular as the cost of nonimpact printers has dropped considerably.

Speech output is another form of computer output that is becoming more commonplace. Automated telephone answering systems employ computer speech output, for example. There are two approaches to speech output: in one, phrases prerecorded by a person are strung together to form the output desired; in the other, *synthesized speech*, a machine produces the speech sounds (Oz, 2004).

External Storage Devices

Health care information systems require the extensive use of external storage devices. Critical systems must be backed up regularly, and data must be frequently archived for permanent or nearly permanent storage. What are some of the options available for external storage of computer data? There are two basic types of storage media, *sequential* and *direct access*.

In sequential storage, data are stored one record after another, in some logical order, such as by patient identification number or date. When the computer is asked to locate a record, it must read through all the stored data that precede the record it is seeking. This makes retrieval from sequential storage slower than retrieval from direct access devices. Magnetic tape is the most common sequential storage medium. Data are stored as magnetic *spots*, or points, on magnetic tapes. The data are then read via a device called a *tape drive*. Magnetic tapes are inexpensive and frequently are used to store large amounts of backup data.

Direct access storage media allow the data of interest to be accessed without first going through previously stored data. Common forms of direct access storage media are magnetic disks (including external hard drives), floppy disks, and zip drives. Information is coded in a manner similar to that used for magnetic tape, with magnetized spots, or points, on the disk surface. Data are read by a compatible *disk drive*. A special form of disk technology called *redundant array of independent disks* (RAID) can be used by health care organizations to protect their information by creating redundancy: in other words, they can still reproduce data even if one disk fails. RAID systems have groups of hard disks, which can number in the hundreds, controlled through a software application. RAID systems come in a variety of capacity levels, but all are designed to enable data restoration in a timely manner (Oz, 2004).

Among the newer types of external storage is optical disk technology, which is available in such forms as *compact disks* (CDs), *digital video disks* (DVDs), and *optical tape*. The technology behind optical storage media is that the medium's surface is altered by a laser so that it reflects light in two different ways. These two ways are then interpreted by the computer as the 1s and 0s needed for digitizing. CDs come in several forms, read-only memory (CD-ROM), recordable (CD-R), and rewritable (CD-RW). CDs are less expensive than magnetic storage media and they can hold more data per unit of surface area. Newer CD drives allow CD users to read, write, edit, and delete data as they would on a magnetic disk. DVDs hold even more data than CDs and are particularly well suited for storing multimedia. Personal computers now come equipped with drives that will read and write to both DVDs and CDs. Optical tape uses the same technology as optical disks, but data are stored sequentially and the storage capacity is very large (one cassette can hold about nine gigabytes of data) (Oz, 2004; Stair & Reynolds, 2003).

Flash memory is another form of external storage (and internal storage in many handheld computer devices) that is gaining popularity as its costs come down. Flash memory consists of a computer memory chip that can be rewritten and does not lose its data when the power source is removed. Portable flash memory devices take several forms, but one of the most popular is a *thumb drive* (Figure 8.11). This device plugs into an USB port and can provide over 2 GBs of memory. Compared to other external storage, flash memory can be accessed more rapidly, consumes less power, and is smaller in size. The disadvantage is its comparative cost (Oz, 2004; Stair & Reynolds, 2003).

Mobile Personal Computing Devices

Many types of mobile personal computing and handheld devices are used in health care today. In fact many health care organizations have had to respond to providers who have adopted *personal digital assistants* (PDAs) and *pocket PCs* and who subsequently

---

FIGURE 8.11. *Thumb Drive*

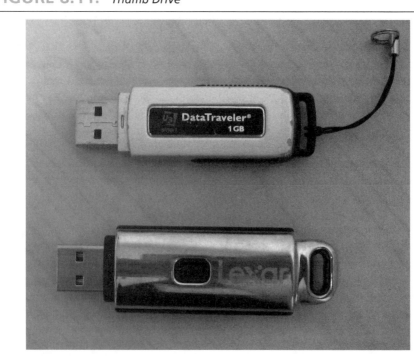

want and expect to be able to access health care applications from these devices. In this section we will look at several types of personal computing devices, including laptop computers, tablet computers, PDAs, and so-called smart phones. All of these devices have two things in common—they are portable and they are wireless or, in the case of laptop computers, have wireless operation as an option. This feature creates special security issues for health care organizations (discussed in more detail in Chapter Ten). The use of mobile devices to access sensitive health care data must be addressed and ultimately controlled.

A *laptop* (or *notebook*) *computer* (Figure 8.12) is a compact, lightweight personal computer. The screen and keyboard are built in. Although they still lag somewhat behind desktop computers in speed, memory, and capacity, today's laptops are powerful enough to replace traditional desktop computers. The *tablet computer* (Figure 8.13) is a relative new comer to the PC market. It was introduced by Microsoft in 2001. It is a full-power PC that is the size of a thick writing tablet. Although the tablet computer can be connected to a mouse and keyboard, the user may instead use a stylus to navigate (Oz, 2004). This increases the mobility of the tablet computer. Laptops and tablet computers are being adopted by health care organizations for point-of-care or bedside systems.

PDAs began to be marketed to the general public in the early 1990s. Since that time their use has steadily increased. PDAs generally use a stylus for data input and most can recognize handwriting to some extent (though not yet perfectly) (Oz, 2004). Newer

FIGURE 8.12. *Laptop Computer*

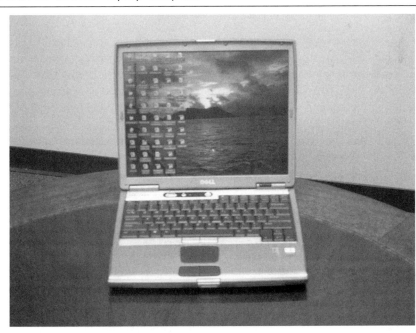

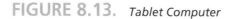

FIGURE 8.13. *Tablet Computer*

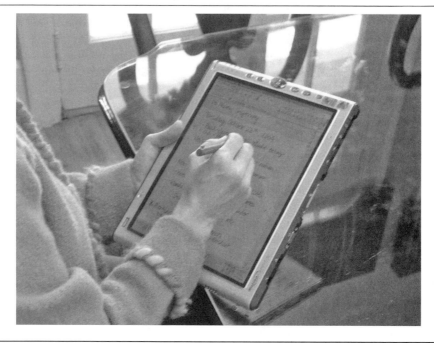

PDAs allow users not only to store data, such as calendars and personal notes, but also to connect to the Internet to browse Web pages and send or receive e-mail. These devices are becoming more powerful and less expensive, which will likely increase their popularity. More software applications are being developed specifically for PDAs. In the health care community, resources such as medical dictionaries, formularies, and clinical coding systems can be installed on PDAs.

As PDAs and cellular phones both gained popularity, the market recognized the potential for incorporating aspects of both into a single device, sometimes called a *smart phone*. These devices are evolving rapidly and are being employed in health care organizations.

INFORMATION SYSTEMS ARCHITECTURE

In the preceding sections we introduced many specific technologies that can be used in health care organizations. However, a huge question remains: How does the organization choose among these technologies and ultimately bring them together into a cohesive set of health care information systems? This section answers these questions by examining health care information system architecture.

An organization's information systems require that a series of core technologies *come together*, or work together as whole, to meet the IT goals of the organization. Up to this point we have discussed the core technologies but have not discussed how they work together as a cohesive information system. The way that core technologies, along with the application software, come together should be the result of decisions about what information systems are implemented and used within the organization and how they are implemented and used. For example, the electronic medical record system or the patient accounting system with which users ultimately interact involves not just the application software but also the network, servers, security systems, and so forth that all come together to make the system work effectively. This coming together should never be a haphazard process. It should be engineered.

In discussing health care information system architecture, we will cover several topics:

- A definition of architecture
- Architecture perspectives
- Architecture examples
- Observations about architecture

A Definition of Architecture

A design and a blueprint guide the coming together of a house. The coming together of information systems is guided by information systems *architecture*. For the house, the development of the blueprint and the design is influenced by the builder's objectives for the house (is it to be a single-family house or an apartment building, for example), and the desired properties of the house (energy efficient or handicap accessible, for example). For an organization's information systems, the development of an architecture is influenced by the organization's objectives (electronic medical records that span multiple hospitals, for example) and the systems' desired properties (efficient to support and having a high degree of application integration, for example).

Following the design and the blueprints, the general contractor, plumbers, carpenters, and electricians use building materials to create the house. Following the architecture for the organization's information systems, the IT staff and the organization's vendors implement the core technologies and application software and integrate them to create the information systems.

Information systems architecture consists of concepts, strategies, and principles that guide an organization's technology choices and the manner in which the organization integrates and manages these choices. For example, an organization's architecture discussion concludes that the organization should use industry standard technology. This decision reflects an organizational belief that standard technology will have a lower risk of obsolescence, be easier to support, and be available from a large number of information technology vendors that use standard technology. Guided by its architecture decision, the organization chooses to implement networks that conform to a specific standard network protocol and decides to use the Windows operating system for its workstations.

Two additional terms are sometimes used either as synonyms for or in describing architecture, *platform* and *infrastructure*. In this text, however, we adhere to accepted distinctions among these three terms. For example, you might hear IT personnel say that "our systems run on a Microsoft, HP, and Cisco platform." *Platforms* are the specific vendors and technologies that an organization chooses for its information systems. You might hear of a Windows platform or Web-based platform. Platform choices should be guided by architecture discussions. You might also hear IT personnel talk about the infrastructure of the health care information system. *Infrastructure* as we use it refers primarily to the organization's computer networks and, perhaps, to the applications running on those networks. Although *infrastructure* is not vendor or technology specific, it is not quite as broad a term as *architecture*, which encompasses much more than specific technologies and networks.

Architecture Perspectives

Organizations adopt various frames of reference as they approach the topic of architecture. This section will illustrate two approaches, one based on the characteristics and capabilities of the desired architecture and the other based on application integration.

Characteristics and Capabilities   Glaser (2002, p. 62) defines architecture as "the set of organizational, management, and technical strategies and tactics used to ensure that the organization's information systems have critical, organizationally defined characteristics and capabilities." For example, an organization can decide that it wants an information system that has characteristics such as being agile, efficient to support, and highly reliable. In addition, the organization can decide that its information systems should have capabilities such as being accessible by patients from their homes or being able to incorporate clinical decision support. If it wants high reliability, it will need to make decisions about fault-tolerant computers and network redundancy. If it wants users to be able to customize their clinical information screens, this will influence its choice of a clinical information system vendor. If it wants providers to be able to structure clinical documentation, it will need to make choices about natural language processing, voice recognition, and templates in its electronic medical record.

Application Integration   Another way of looking at information systems architecture is to look at how applications are integrated across the organization. One often hears vendors talk about architectures such as best of breed, monolithic, and visual integration. *Best of breed* describes an architecture that allows each department to pick the best application it can find and that then attempts to integrate these applications by means of an interface engine that manages the transfer of data between these applications—for example, it can send a transaction with registration information on a new patient from the admitting system to the laboratory system.

Monolithic describes the architecture of a set of applications that all come from one vendor and that all use a common database management system and common user interface.

Visual integration architecture wraps a common browser user interface around a set of diverse applications. This interface enables the user, for example, a physician, to use one set of screens to access clinical data even though those data may come from several different applications.

This view of architecture is focused on the various approaches to the integration of applications; integration by sharing data between applications, integration by having all applications use one database, and integration by having an integrated access to data. This view does not address other aspects of architecture: for example, the means by which the organization might get information to mobile workers.

Architecture Examples

A few examples will help to illustrate how architecture can guide information technology choices. Each example begins with an architecture statement and then shows some choices about core technologies and applications and the approach to implementing them that might result from this statement.

Statement: We would like to deliver an electronic medical record to our small physician practices that is inexpensive, reliable, and easy to support. To do this we will

- Run the application from our computer room, reducing the need for practice staff to manage their own servers and do tasks such as backups and applying application enhancements.
- Run several practices on one server to reduce the cost.
- Obtain a high-speed network connection, and a backup connection, from our local telephone company to provide good application performance and improve reliability.

Statement: We would like to have decision-support capabilities in our clinical information systems. To do this we will

- Purchase our applications from a vendor whose product includes a very robust rules engine.
- Make sure that the rules engine has the tools necessary to author new decision support and maintain existing clinical logic.
- Ensure that the clinical information systems use a single database with codified clinical data.

Statement: We want all of our systems to be easy and efficient to support. To do this we will

- Adopt industry standard technology, making it easier to hire support staff.
- Implement proven technology, technology that has had most of the bugs worked out.

■ Purchase our application systems from one vendor, reducing the support problems and the finger-pointing that can occur between vendors when problems arise.

Observations About Architecture

Organizations will often bypass the architecture discussion in their haste to "get the IT show on the road and begin implementing stuff." Haste makes waste, as people say. It is terribly important to have thoughtful architecture discussions. There are many organizations, for example, that never took the time to develop thoughtful plans for integrating applications and that then discovered, after millions of dollars of IT investments, that this oversight meant that they could not integrate these applications or that the integration would be both expensive and limited.

As we will see in Chapter Thirteen, organizations that have been very effective in their applications of IT over many years have had a significant focus on architecture. They have realized that thoughtful approaches to agility, cost efficiency, and reliability have a significant impact on their ability to continue to apply technology to improve organizational performance. For example, information systems that are not agile can be difficult (or impossible) to change as the organization's needs evolve. This ossification can strangle an organization's progress. In addition, information systems that have reliability problems can lead an organization to be hesitant to implement new, strategically important applications—how can they be sure that this new application will not go down too often and impair their operations? In Chapter Twelve, we will discuss planning the system architecture as a component of strategic IT planning.

Organizational leadership must take time to engage in the architecture discussion. The health care executive does not need to be involved in deciding which vendor to choose to provide network switches. But he or she does need a basic understanding of the core technologies in order to help guide the formation of the principles and strategies that will direct that decision. In the following example, the application integration perspective on architecture (choosing among best of breed, monolithic, and visual integration) illustrates a typical architecture challenge that a hospital might face.

PERSPECTIVE

CHOOSING THE SYSTEM ARCHITECTURE

A hospital has adopted a best-of-breed approach and, over the course of several years, has implemented separate applications that support the registration, laboratory, pharmacy, and radiology departments and the transcription of operative notes and discharge summaries. An interface engine has been implemented that enables registration transactions to flow from the registration system to the other systems.

However, the physicians and nurses have started to complain. To retrieve a patient's laboratory, pharmacy, and radiology records and transcribed materials, they have to sign into each of these systems, using a separate user name and password. To obtain an overall view of a patient's condition, they have to print out the results from each of these systems and assemble the different print-outs. All of this takes too much time, and there are too many passwords to remember.

Moreover, the hospital would like to analyze its care, in an effort to improve care quality, but the current architecture does not include an integrated database of patient results.

The hospital has two emerging architectural objectives that the current architecture cannot meet:

1. Provide an integrated view of a patient's results for caregivers.

2. Efficiently support the analysis of care patterns.

To address these objectives, the hospital decides to implement a browser-based application that

■ Gathers clinical data from each application and presents it in a unified view for the caregivers

■ Supports the entry of one user ID and password that is synchronized with the user ID and password for each application

In addition the hospital decides to implement a database that receives clinical results from each of the applications and stores these data for access by query tools and analysis software.

To achieve its emerging objectives, the hospital has migrated from best-of-breed architecture to visual integration architecture. The hospital has also extended to visual integration architecture by adding an integrated database for analysis purposes.

In analyzing what would be the best architecture to meet its new objectives, the hospital considered monolithic architecture. It could meet its objectives by replacing all applications with one integrated suite of applications from one vendor. However, the hospital decided that this approach would be too expensive and time consuming. Besides, the current applications (laboratory, pharmacy, and radiology) worked well; they just weren't integrated. The monolithic architecture approach to integration was examined and discarded.

SUMMARY

The value of this chapter to the health care executive is that it provides a broad overview of health care information architecture and several categories of specific information technologies. Although these technologies are not unique to health care, health care organizations use them for their information systems. We discussed various technologies used for system software; data management and access; networks and data communications; information processing distribution schemes; the Internet, intranets, and extranets; and clinical and managerial decision support; and we also looked at trends in user interactions with systems.

We ended our discussion with the concept of system architecture, the way in which all the technologies in an organization fit together to support health care applications. Like many fields, IT has its own language. It is helpful for health care executives to learn IT terminology so they can to communicate effectively with IT staff and vendors. The overall goal of this chapter was to provide information to support an understanding of the many components that go into health care information systems.

KEY TERMS

Ad hoc network
Applications software
Artificial Intelligence
Asynchronous Transfer Mode (ATM)
Bandwidth
Bits per second (bps)
Blog
Bluetooth
Bridge
Client/server
Clinical data repository
Clinical decision support systems
Coaxial cable
Data communication
Data dictionary
Data management
Data mart
Data mining
Data warehouse
Decision support systems
Domain Name System (DNS) server
Electronic data interchange
Entity relationship diagram (ERD)
Ethernet

Executive Information systems
Expert systems
Extensible markup language (XML)
External storage devices
Extranet
Fiber-optic cable
File server
Fuzzy logic
Gateway
Hub
Hypertext markup language (HTML)
Hypertext transfer Protocol (HTTP)
IEEE 802.11 standards
Information processing distribution schemes
Information systems architecture
Infrastructure
Infrastructure network
Input devices
Interface engine
Internet
Internet protocol (IP) address
Intranet

Local area network (LAN)
Logical bus topology
Managerial decision support systems
Microwave transmissions
Middleware
Natural language processing
Network
Network interface card (NIC)
Network media
Network operating system
Neural networks
Object oriented database
Object-oriented programming
Object-relational database
Online transactional processing (OLTP)
Open database connectivity (ODBC)
Open source
Open standards Interconnection (OSI)
  model
Operating system
Output devices
Personal digital assistants (PDA)
Physical bus topology
Physician start topology
Platform
Proprietary

Really Simple Syndication (RSS)
Relational database
Router
Single sign-on system
Smart phone
Spread spectrum radio transmissions
Structured query language
  (SQL)
Switch
System software
Systems software
Terminal emulation
Terminal-to-host
Thin client
Transmission control Protocol/Internet
  Protocol (TCP/IP)
Twisted pair wire
Uniform resource locator (URL)
Visual programming
Voice over Internet Protocol (VoIP)
Web 2.0
Web browser
Wide area network (WAN)
Wiki
Wireless network
World Wide Web

LEARNING ACTIVITIES

1. Technology is changing and evolving. Conduct a search of the Internet or print literature to identify several new or emerging technologies. Describe each technology, and discuss its potential use in the management of health care information or the development of health care information systems.

2. Visit a small health care facility or physician's office. Describe the computer network that is used. Does this location use both a LAN and a WAN? What functions are limited to the LAN? Which use a WAN? Discuss the topology (physical and logical) of the LAN, the hardware components, and the specific protocols employed. Ask for a copy of the LAN diagram for the office (if one exists) or create one from your visit.

3. Do an Internet search and find at least one site that offers a decision-support product to health care executives. Describe the product. Can you tell from the site whether or not the product employs artificial intelligence? Can you tell which type? How useful would the product be to you as a health care executive?

4. Meet with the chief information officer or director or the IT manager in a health care organization. Ask him or her to describe the architecture used for the clinical component of the organization's health care information system. Based on this conversation, describe how this IT professional views the architecture. What process did this organization use to determine its architecture design? Does it have plans to move to a different architecture?

5. Do an Internet search of health care organizations. Which ones are using Web 2.0 technologies to establish connections with patients or other consumers?

CHAPTER

HEALTH CARE INFORMATION SYSTEM STANDARDS

LEARNING OBJECTIVES

- To be able to identify the major types of health care information standards and the organizations that develop or approve them, including

  Messaging standards

  Content and coding standards

  Network standards

  Standards for electronic data interchange

  Electronic health record standards

- To be able to give examples of the four major methods by which standards are developed—ad hoc, de facto, government mandate, and consensus.

- To be able to identify and discuss the role of organizations that currently have a significant impact on the adoption of health care information standards in the United States.

- To be able to discuss the relationships among health information exchanges, regional health information networks, and the Nationwide Health Information Network.

In order to achieve interoperability, portability, and data exchange, health care information systems must employ standards. Systems that conform to different standards cannot communicate with one another. For a simple analogy, think about traveling to a country where you do not speak the language. You would not be able to communicate with that country's citizens without a common language or translator. Think of the common language as the standard to which all parties agree to adhere. Once you and others agree on a common language, you and they can communicate. You may still have some problems, but generally these can be overcome.

A plethora of information technology (IT) standards, including standards for messaging, content and coding, networks, electronic data interchange, and electronic health records, are important to health care information systems. Some of these standards compete with one another. By 2004, the National Alliance for Health Information Technology (NAHIT) had identified 450 voluntary and mandated standards from 150 organizations (Bazzoli, 2004), and this number has increased over the past few years. It is important to recognize that many IT standards that do not specifically address health care also have a tremendous impact on health care information systems. In Chapter Eight we reviewed basic communication protocols and extensible markup language (XML), which is emerging as a messaging standard not only in business-related Internet transactions but also in health care transactions and communications. In discussing system software we mentioned the emergence of Linux, and in examining data management we commented on structured query language (SQL) and Open Database Connectivity (ODBC) as standards. These are but a few examples of general IT standards that have had a real impact on the development and use of health care information systems.

In the sections that follow we provide an overview of the standards development process and introduce several key initiatives, some formal and some less so, that have led to the development of standards to facilitate interoperability among health care information systems. These standards will be reviewed in three main categories:

- Classification, vocabulary, and terminology standards
- Data interchange standards
- Health record content standards

We will conclude this chapter with a discussion of the impact of the recent HIPAA regulations and the efforts of the Office of the National Coordinator for Health Information Technology on the adoption of health care information standards to facilitate interoperability. We will also discuss the relationship among health information exchanges, regional health information networks, and the Nationwide Health Information Network.

STANDARDS DEVELOPMENT PROCESS

When seeking to understand why so many different IT and health care information standards exist, it is helpful to look first at the basic standards development process that exists in the United States (and internationally) and the changes that have occurred in this process over the past decade. Four methods have been used to establish health care IT standards (Hammond & Cimino, 2001):

- *Ad hoc.* A standard is established by the ad hoc method when a group of interested people or organizations agrees on a certain specification, without any formal adoption process. The Digital Imaging and Communications in Medicine (DICOM) standard for health care imaging came about in this way.

■ *De facto.* A de facto standard arises when a vendor or other commercial enterprise controls such a large segment of the market that its product becomes the recognized norm. SQL and the Windows operating system are examples of de facto standards. Some individuals predict that XML will become a de facto standard for health care messaging.

■ *Government mandate.* Standards are also established when the government mandates that the health care industry adopt them. Examples are the transaction and code sets mandated by the Health Insurance Portability and Accountability Act (HIPAA) regulations.

■ *Consensus.* Consensus-based standards come about when representatives from various interested groups come together to reach a formal agreement on specifications. The process is generally open and involves considering comment and feedback from the industry. This method is employed by the *standards development organizations* (SDOs) accredited by the American National Standards Institute (ANSI). Most health care information standards are developed by this method, including Health Level 7 (HL7) standards and Accredited Standards Committee (ASC) X12N standards.

Libicki, Schneider, Frelinger, and Slomovic (2000) outline a two-by-two matrix topology for IT standard-setting organizations. They classify the organizations that set IT standards by membership type (open to all or members only) and by process (democratic or dependent on "a strong leader"). The organizations with the most formal standard-setting processes, such as the International Organization for Standardization (ISO), ANSI, and the ANSI-accredited SDOs, fall into the member-only, democratic classification. The relationships among the various standard-setting organizations can be confusing. Not only do many of the acronyms sound similar, but the organizations themselves, as voluntary, member-based organizations, can set their own missions and goals. Therefore, although there is a formally recognized relationship among ISO, ANSI, and the SDOs, there is also some overlap in activities. Table 9.1 outlines the relationships among these formal standard-setting organizations and for each one gives a brief overview of important facts and a current Web site.

All the ANSI-accredited SDOs must adhere to the guidelines established for accreditation; therefore they have similar standard-setting processes. According to ANSI, this process includes

■ Consensus on a proposed standard by a group or "consensus body" that includes representatives from materially affected or interested parties;

■ Broad-based public review and comment on draft standards;

■ Consideration of and response to comments submitted by voting members of the relevant consensus body and by public review commenters;

■ Incorporation of approved changes into a draft standard; and

■ Right to appeal by any participant that believes that due process principles were not sufficiently respected during the standards development in
accordance with the ANSI-accredited procedures of the standards developer
[ANSI, 2004].

TABLE 9.1. Organizations Responsible for Formal Standards Development

Organizations	Facts
International Organization for Standardization (ISO), www.iso.org	■ Members are national standards bodies from many different countries around the world. ■ ANSI is the U.S. national body member. ■ Oversees the flow of documentation and international approval of standards developed under the auspices of its member bodies.
American National Standards Institute (ANSI), www.ansi.org	■ U.S. member of ISO ■ Accredits standards development organizations (SDOs) from a wide range of industries, including health care ■ Oversees the work of the SDOs, technical committees, subcommittees, and working groups ■ Does *not* develop standards itself, but accredits the organizations that develop standards ■ Publishes the 10,000+ American National Standards developed by accredited SDOs
Standards development organizations (SDOs)	■ Must be accredited by ANSI ■ Develop standards in accordance with ANSI criteria
SDOs that develop health care related standards discussed in this chapter: ASTM International (formerly American Society for Testing and Materials), www.astm.org Health Level 7 (HL7), www.hl7.org ANSI Accredited Standards Committee (ASC) X12, www.x12.org	■ Can use the label "Approved American National Standard" ■ Currently, there are 270+ ANSI-accredited SDOs representing many industries, including health care

In the last decade the IT industry in general has experienced a movement away from the process of establishing standards via the SDOs. The Internet and World Wide Web standards, for example, were developed by groups with much less formal structures. The emergence of the Linux operating system has been cited as an example of a standard developed with minimal formal input. In fact in Libicki et al.'s typology (2000), the Linux development process would be furthest from the formal SDO process, as it was spearheaded by a strong leader with input from all.

CLASSIFICATION, VOCABULARY, AND TERMINOLOGY STANDARDS

One of the most difficult problems in exchanging health care information and building longitudinal electronic health records (EHRs) is coordinating the vast amount of health information that is generated in diverse locations for patients and populations. To date, no single vocabulary has emerged to meet all the information exchange needs of the health care sector. The most widely recognized coding and classification systems, ICD-9-CM, Current Procedural Terminology (CPT), and diagnosis related groups (DRGs), were discussed in Chapter One. Although these systems do not meet the criteria for full clinical vocabularies, they are used to classify diagnoses and procedures and are the basis for information retrieval in health care information systems.

The National Committee on Vital and Health Statistics (NCVHS) has the responsibility, under a HIPAA mandate, to recommend uniform data standards for patient medical record information (PMRI). Although no single vocabulary has been recognized by NCVHS as "the" standard, in a November 2003 letter to the then Department of Health and Human and Services secretary Tommy Thompson, NCVHS (2003) identified a core set of PMRI terminology standards:

- Systematized Nomenclature of Medicine—Clinical Terms (SNOMED CT)
- Logical Observation Identifiers Names and Codes (LOINC) laboratory subset
- Several federal drug terminologies, including RxNorm

In this section we will describe SNOMED CT and LOINC, along with the National Library of Medicine's Unified Medical Language, which has become the standard for bibliographical searches in health care and has the potential for other uses as well.

Systematized Nomenclature of Medicine—Clinical Terms

Systematized Nomenclature of Medicine—Clinical Terms (SNOMED CT) is a comprehensive clinical terminology developed specifically to facilitate the electronic storage and retrieval of detailed clinical information. It is the result of collaboration between the College of American Pathologists (CAP) and the United Kingdom's National Health Service (NHS). SNOMED CT merges CAP's SNOMED Reference Terminology, an older classification system used to group diseases, and the NHS's Clinical Terms Version 3 (better known as Read Codes), an established clinical terminology used in Great Britain and elsewhere. As a result, SNOMED CT is based on decades of research. As of April 2007 SNOMED is owned, maintained, and distributed by the International

Health Terminology Standards Development Organisation (IHTSDO), a nonprofit association based in Denmark. The National Library of Medicine is the U.S. member of the IHTSDO and distributes SNOMED at no cost within the United States (NLM, 2008).

Logical Observation Identifiers Names and Codes

The Logical Observation Identifiers Names and Codes (LOINC) system was developed to facilitate the electronic transmission of laboratory results to hospitals, physicians, third-party payers, and other users of laboratory data. Initiated in 1994 by the Regenstrief Institute at Indiana University, LOINC provides a standard set of universal names and codes for identifying individual laboratory and clinical results. These standard codes allow users to merge clinical results from disparate sources (LOINC, 2008a).

LOINC codes have a fixed length field of seven characters. Current codes range from three to seven characters long. There are six parts in the LOINC name structure: component/analyte, property, time aspect, system, scale type, and method. The syntax for a name follows this pattern:

<component/analyte> :<kind of property> :<time aspect> :
<system type> :<scale> :<method>

Here are some sample names (LOINC, 2008b):

Examples of Fully Specified LOINC Names

Sodium:SCnc:Pt:Ser/Plas:Qn

Sodium:SCnc:Pt:Urine:Qn

Sodium:SRat:24H:Urine:Qn

Creatinine renal clearance:VRat:24H:Ur+Ser/Plas:Qn

Glucose^2H post 100 g glucose PO:MCnc:Pt:Ser/Plas:Qn

Gentamicin^trough:MCnc:Pt:Ser/Plas:Qn

ABO group:Type:Pt:Bld^donor:Nom

Body temperature:Temp:8H^max:XXX:Qn

Chief complaint:Find:Pt:^Patient:Nar:Reported

Physical findings:Find:Pt:Abdomen:Nar:Observed

Binocular distance:Len:Pt:Head^fetus:Qn:US.measured

Unified Medical Language System

The National Library of Medicine (NLM), an agency of the National Institutes of Health, began the Unified Medical Language System (UMLS) project in 1986, and it is ongoing today. The purpose of the UMLS project is to "aid the development of systems that help health professionals and researchers retrieve and integrate electronic biomedical information from a variety of sources and make it easy for users to link disparate information systems, including computer-based patient records, bibliographic databases, factual databases and expert systems" (NLM, 2003, p. 1).

The UMLS has three basic components, called *knowledge sources:*

- *UMLS Metathesaurus.* Annual editions of the metathesaurus have been distributed by the NLM since 1990. The November 2003 edition included 975,354 concepts and 2.4 million concept names. All the common health information vocabularies, including SNOMED CT, ICD, and CPT, along with approximately 100 other vocabularies, are incorporated into the metathesaurus. The metathesaurus project's goal is to incorporate and map existing vocabularies into a single system.

- *SPECIALIST Lexicon.* The lexicon contains information for many terms, component words, and English language words that do not appear in the metathesaurus.

- *UMLS Semantic Network.* The semantic network contains information about the categories (such as "Disease or Syndrome" and "Virus") to which metathesaurus concepts are assigned. The semantic network also outlines the relationships among the categories (for example, "Virus" causes "Disease or Syndrome").

The UMLS products are widely used in NLM's own applications, such as PubMed. They are available to other organizations free of charge, provided the users submit a license agreement (NLM, 2008).

Data Interchange Standards

The ability to exchange and integrate data among health care applications is critical to the success of any overall health care information system, whether an organizational, regional, or national level of integration is desired. Much of the health care information standards development activity has been in the area of standards for data interchange or integration. In this section we will look at a few of the standards that have been developed for this purpose. There are others, and new needs are continually being identified. However, the following groups of standards are recognized as important to the health care sector, and together they provide examples of both broad standards addressing all types of applications and specific standards addressing one type of application.

- Health Level Seven standards
- Digital Imaging and Communications in Medicine (DICOM)
- National Council for Prescription Drug Programs (NCPDP)
- ANSI X12N standards

Health Level Seven Standards   Health Level Seven (HL7) is an ANSI-accredited standards organization that was founded as an ad hoc group in 1987. HL7 was founded with a purpose of developing a messaging standard (see Figure 9.1 for an example of a HL7 message) to support the "exchange, management, and integration of data

FIGURE 9.1. *HL7 Encoded Message*

This message is sent when a new patient arrives at the hospital. The patient's demographics are entered into the HIS (hospital information system) and then the information is communicated to all the other systems to avoid multiple entries of the patient's demographic information.

```
MSH|^~\&|EPIC|EPICADT|SMS|SMSADT|199912271408|CHARRIS|ADT^A04|1817457|D|2.3|
EVN|A04|199912271408|||CHARRIS
PID||0493575^^^2^ID 1|454721||DOE^JOHN^^^^|DOE^JOHN^^^^|19480203|M||B|254
E238ST^^EUCLID^OH^44123^USA||(216)731-4359|||M|NON|400003403~1129086|999-|
NK1||CONROY^MARI^^^^|SPO||(216)731-4359||EC|||||||||||||||||||||||||||
PV1||O|168  ~219~C~PMA^^^^^^^^^||||277^ALLEN FADZL^BONNIE^^^^||||||||||
||2688684|||||||||||||||||||||||||||199912271408||||||002376853
```

Source: Health Level Seven Canada, 2004.

that support clinical patient care" (Marotta, 2000). Since its inception, HL7 has grown from a small group of 14 individuals to a large organization with nearly 2,000 health care provider, vendor, and consultant members. The HL7 messaging standard set of protocols has been widely adopted and used since Version 2.0 was released in the late 1980s. By the time Version 2.4 was released, the standard had expanded to require 1,500 pages of detailed interfacing information (Kurtz, 2002). (Version 2.5 is the most recently approved version of the standard, but 3.0 is in active development at this time.)

The name HL7 refers to the highest level in the OSI network reference model, the seventh layer. The HL7 set of messaging protocols is designed to deal with the network issues that occur at this level. They are

1. The data to be exchanged

2. The timing of the exchange

3. The communication of errors between applications

Digital Imaging and Communications in Medicine   The growth of digital diagnostic imaging (such as CAT scans and MRIs) gave rise to the need for a standard for the electronic transfer of these images between devices manufactured by different vendors. The American College of Radiology (ACR) and the National Electrical Manufacturers Association (NEMA) published the first standard, a precursor to the current Digital Imaging and Communications in Medicine (DICOM) standard, in 1985. The stated purpose for the standard was to

■   Promote communication of digital image information, regardless of device manufacturer

- Facilitate the development and expansion of picture archiving and communication systems (PACS) that can also interface with other systems of hospital information
- Allow the creation of diagnostic information data bases that can be interrogated by a wide variety of devices distributed geographically [NEMA, 2003, p. 5].

The current DICOM standard accomplishes these purposes by specifying (NEMA, 2003)

- A set of protocols for network communications
- The syntax and semantics of commands that can be used with these protocols
- A set of media storage services to be followed, including a file format and medical directory structure

National Council on Prescription Drug Programs The mission of the National Council for Prescription Drug Programs (NCPDP) states that "NCPDP creates and promotes standards for the transfer of data to and from the pharmacy services sector of the healthcare industry. The organization provides a forum and support wherein our diverse membership can efficiently and effectively develop and maintain these standards through a consensus building process. NCPDP also offers its members resources, including educational opportunities and database services, to better manage their businesses." To this end the NCPDP, an ANSI-accredited SDO, has developed a set of standards for the electronic submission of third-party drug claims. Current standards include the following (Chamberlain, 2007):

- Batch Transaction Standard
- Billing Unit Standard
- Manufacturer Rebates, Utilization, Plan, Formulary, Market Basket, and Reconciliation Flat File Standard
- Payment Reconciliation Payment Tape Format
- Pharmacy ID Card
- SCRIPT Standard for e-Prescribing
- Telecommunication Standard
- Medicaid Subrogation
- Formulary and Benefit
- Universal Claim Form

ASC X12N Standards The ANSI Accredited Standards Committee (ASC) X12 develops standards, in both X12 and XML formats, for the electronic exchange of business

TABLE 9.2. X12 TG2 Work Groups

Work Group Number	Work Group Name
WG1	Health Care Eligibility
WG2	Health Care Claims
WG3	Claim Payments
WG4	Enrollment/Premium Payment
WG5	Claims Status
WG9	Patient Information
WG10	Health Care Services Review
WG12	Interactive Claims
WG15	Provider Information
WG20	Insurance Transaction Acknowledgement

Source: Accredited Standards Committee X12, 2008.

information. One ASC X12 subcommittee, X12N, has been specifically designated to deal with electronic data interchange (EDI) standards in the insurance industry, and this subcommittee has a special health care task group, known as TG2. According to the X12/TG2 Web site: "the purpose of the Health Care Task group shall be the development and maintenance of data standards (both national and international) which shall support the exchange of business information for health care administration. Health care data includes, but is not limited to, such business functions as eligibility, referrals and authorizations, claims, claim status, payment and remittance advice, and provider directories." To this end ASC X12N has developed a set of standards that are monitored and updated through ASC X12N work groups. Table 9.2 lists the current X12 work group areas.

HEALTH RECORD CONTENT STANDARDS

In this section we will look at two set of standards currently being developed. The first is the HL7 EHR Functional Model and the second is the ASTM Healthcare Informatics subcommittee's Continuity of Care Record (CCR) standard. Although these standards are being developed for different purposes, both address the content of the patient's electronic health record.

HL7 EHR Functional Model

The HL7 EHR System Functional Model provides a reference list of over 160 functions that may be present in an EHR system. This functional model "is not a list of specifications for messaging, implementation or conformance"(Wise & Mon, 2004). Instead, the model enables standardized descriptions of functions by health care setting. Each setting, such as intensive care, office practice, emergency room, and so forth, is described in a specific *functional profile*. Figure 9.2 shows the basic structure of the HL7 EHR Functional Model.

Continuity of Care Record Standard

The ASTM Continuity of Care Record (CCR) standard is designed as a standard health care data summary. Its purpose is to aggregate essential health care data from multiple sources, such as patient records and other health care–related documents in order to provide an overall clinical picture of a patient's current and past health status. The CCR was developed jointly by ASTM International, the Massachusetts Medical Society, the Healthcare Information and Management Systems Society, the American Academy of Family Physicians, the American Academy of Pediatrics, and other health care organizations.

FIGURE 9.2. *HL7 EHR Functional Model Outline*

Direct Care	DC1.0	Care Management
	DC2.0	Clinical Decision Support
	DC3.0	Operations Management and Communication
Supportive	S1.0	Clinical Support
	S2.0	Measurement, Analysis, Research, Reporting
	S3.0	Administrative and Financial
Information Infrastructure	I 1.0	EHR Security
	I 2.0	EHR Information and Records Management
	I 3.0	Unique Identity, Registry, and Directory Services
	I 4.0	Support for Health Informatics & Terminology Standards
	I 5.0	Interoperability
	I 6.0	Manage Business Rules
	I 7.0	Workflow

Source: Wise & Mon, 2004, slide 16.

Here are some key features of the CCR, as described in a summary on the CCR standard specification Web site.

> 1.1 The Continuity of Care Record (CCR) is a core data set of the most relevant administrative, demographic, and clinical information facts about a patient's health care, covering one or more health care encounters. It provides a means for one health care practitioner, system, or setting to aggregate all of the pertinent data about a patient and forward it to another practitioner, system, or setting to support the continuity of care.
> 1.1.1 The CCR data set includes a summary of the patient's health status (for example, problems, medications, allergies) and basic information about insurance, advance directives, care documentation, and the patient's care plan. It also includes identifying information and the purpose of the CCR. . . .
> 1.1.2 The CCR may be prepared, displayed, and transmitted on paper or electronically, provided the information required by this specification is included. When it is prepared in a structured electronic format, strict adherence to an XML schema and an accompanying implementation guide is required to support standards-compliant interoperability. The Adjunct to this specification contains a W3C XML schema and contains an Implementation Guide for such representation.
> 1.2 The primary use case for the CCR is to provide a snapshot in time containing the pertinent clinical, demographic, and administrative data for a specific patient. . . .
> 1.3 To ensure interchangeability of electronic CCRs, this specification specifies XML coding that is required when the CCR is created in a structured electronic format. . . . [ASTM International, 2008]:

Federal Initiatives on Health Care IT Standards

The federal government has several important initiatives related to health care information standards, including HIPAA transaction standards, e-prescribing, and the development of the Office of the National Coordinator for Health Information Technology. These key initiatives are discussed in the following sections.

HIPAA In August 2000, the U.S. Department of Health and Human Services published the final rule outlining the standards to be adopted by health care organizations for electronic transactions, and announced the *designated standard maintenance organizations* (DSMOs). Modifications to this final rule were subsequently published in 2002. In publishing this rule the federal government mandated that health care organizations adopt certain standards for electronic transactions and identified the standards organizations that would oversee the adoption of standards for HIPAA compliance.

The majority of the HIPAA transaction standards were taken from ASC X12N standards. Specifically, the transaction standards cited in the HIPAA regulations (42 C.F.R. Part 162, 2003) were

■ Health Care Claims or equivalent encounter information (X12N 837)

■ Eligibility for a Health Plan (X12N 270/271)

■ Referral Certification and Authorization (X12N 278, or NCPDP for retail pharmacy)

■ Health Care Claim Status (X12N 276/277)

■ Enrollment and Disenrollment in a Health Plan (X12N 834)

■ Health Care Payment and Remittance Advice (X12N 835)

■ Health Plan Premium Payments (X12N 820)

■ Coordination of Benefits (X12N 837, or NCPDP for retail pharmacy)

In addition to these transaction standards, several standard code sets were established for use in electronic transactions. These code sets (a topic discussed in earlier chapters) include

■ International Classification of Diseases, Ninth Revision, Clinical Modification (ICD-9-CM)

■ Code on Dental Procedures and Nomenclature (CDT)

■ Healthcare Common Procedure Coding System (HCPCS)

■ Current Procedural Terminology, Fourth Edition (CPT-4).

The role of the DSMOs, as outlined in the regulations, is to take responsibility for the development, maintenance, and modification of relevant electronic data interchange standards. Currently, the following organizations are recognized by the federal government as DSMOs. All except the Dental Content Committee have been discussed in this book. All are significant players in the establishment of health care information standards.

■ Accredited Standards Committee X12 (ANSI ASC X12)

■ Dental Content Committee of the American Dental Association (ADA DCC)

■ Health Level Seven (HL7)

■ National Council for Prescription Drug Programs (NCPDP)

■ National Uniform Billing Committee (NUBC)

■ National Uniform Claim Committee (NUCC)

Centers for Medicare and Medicaid e-Prescribing   The Centers for Medicare and Medicaid (CMS) required the adoption of standards for e-prescribing (defined as the prescriber's ability to electronically send an accurate, error-free, and understandable prescription directly to a pharmacy for the point of care) as a part of the Medicare Modernization Act of 2003. This mandate applies to Medicare Part D transactions. In its final rule, published in April 2008, CMS outlines tools to be used for (Department of Health and Human Services [HHS], 2008a):

■ *Formulary and benefit transactions:* gives prescribers information about which drugs are covered by a Medicare beneficiary's prescription drug benefit plan.

- *Medication history transactions:* provides prescribers with information about medications a beneficiary is already taking, including those prescribed by other providers, to help reduce the number of adverse drug events.

- *Fill status notifications:* allows prescribers to receive an electronic notice from the pharmacy telling them that a patient's prescription has been picked up, not picked up, or has been partially filled, to help monitor medication adherence in patients with chronic conditions.

The final rule adopts existing health care IT standards, including NCPDP's SCRIPT Standard for e-Prescribing and ASC X12N standards.

Office of the National Coordinator for Health Information Technology   In April 2004, President Bush established the Office of the National Coordinator for Health Information Technology (ONC) and charged the office with providing "leadership for the development and nationwide implementation of an interoperable health information technology infrastructure to improve the quality and efficiency of health care." In its strategic plan for 2008–2012, the ONC identified two major goals (HHS, 2008d).

- "*Patient-focused health care:* Enable the transformation to higher quality, more cost-efficient, patient-focused health care through electronic health information access and use by care providers, and by patients and their designees."

- "*Population health:* Enable the appropriate, authorized, and timely access and use of electronic health information to benefit public health, biomedical research, quality improvement, and emergency preparedness."

In achieving these goals, four themes are important: privacy and security, collaborative governance, adoption, and interoperability. The ONC recognizes the need for health care IT standards in order to achieve objectives related to each theme and ultimately reach these goals.

Healthcare Information Technology Standards Panel   The Office of the National Coordinator established the Healthcare Information Technology Standards Panel (HITSP), a public-private partnership with broad participation across more than 300 health care–related organizations, "to identify and harmonize data and technical standards for healthcare. HITSP operates with an inclusive governance model established through the American National Standards Institute (ANSI)" (HHS, 2008b).

HITSP endeavors to

- Harmonize standards to use for specific priorities advanced by the American Health Information Community (AHIC).

- Work with standard development organizations (SDOs) to ensure that standards exist to meet health needs.

- Ensure specific guidance exists to unambiguously implement harmonized standards.

- Foster the availability and use of health information technology standards nationally.

In its first year, the HITSP developed three sets of interoperability specifications that included thirty consensus standards and more than 800 pages of specific implementation guidance describing how these thirty standards need to be used. These interoperability specifications include existing standards such as HL7, NCPDP, ASC X12N and others. The HITSP purpose is not to write standards but rather to identify and publish the specifications for how to use approved standards.

Nationwide Health Information Network   The Nationwide Health Information Network (NHIN) is another significant component of the ONC health care IT plan. It was conceived as a "secure, nationwide, interoperable health information infrastructure that will connect providers, consumers, and others involved in supporting health and health care" (HHS, 2008b).

The NHIN seeks to achieve these goals by

- Developing capabilities for standards-based, secure data exchange nationally

- Improving the coordination of care information among hospitals, laboratories, physicians offices, pharmacies, and other providers

- Ensuring appropriate information is available at the time and place of care

- Ensuring that consumers' health information is secure and confidential

- Giving consumers new capabilities for managing and controlling their personal health records (PHRs) as well as providing access to their health information stored in EHRs and other sources

- Reducing risks from medical errors and supporting the delivery of appropriate, evidence-based medical care

- Lowering health care costs resulting from inefficiencies, medical errors, and incomplete patient information

- Promoting a more effective marketplace, greater competition, and increased choice through access to accurate information on health care costs, quality, and outcomes

The NHIN is being advanced by the ONC as a "network of networks" that will include various types of health information exchange.

Health Information Exchanges, Regional Health Information Networks, and the Nationwide Health Information Network   Health information exchange (HIE) refers to the technology, standards, and governance that enables the exchange of data between the information systems of various health care stakeholders. In this chapter we examined multiple standards that promote HIE, and as we have seen, there are diverse types of HIEs. An HIE can be dedicated to moving medication-related transactions (new prescription requests and prescription renewals and refills) between EHR systems and pharmacies. An HIE can be used to exchange a patient's health data between two or more providers. A freestanding radiology center can use an HIE to move images and reports between its PACS and providers' electronic health records.

A regional health information organization (RHIO) is an organization that provides an HIE to health care stakeholders in a specific region, for example, a city or multicounty area. The RHIO is seen as governed by regional stakeholders, for example, providers, health plans, and diagnostic centers. The HIE, sponsored and supported by the RHIO, is traditionally viewed as enabling the broad exchange of data between stakeholders. A *broad* exchange is one that supports the full set of patient data that could be contained in an EHR.

The Nationwide Health Information Network (NHIN), therefore, is the technology, standards, and governance that could connect all HIEs. The NHIN would connect RHIOs in cities such as San Antonio, Cleveland, and Seattle with HIEs that focused on medication transactions and clinical laboratory transactions. The NHIN can be viewed as similar to the interstate highway system that connects the roads in individual towns and cities. Figure 9.3, from the ONC strategic plan for 2008–2012, provides a graphic representation of the NHIN.

HIEs, RHIOs, and the NHIN are in their infancy. These efforts face daunting challenges of developing sustainable business models, managing patient privacy, ensuring effective governance, implementing data standards and creating scalable technologies. Although establishing health IT interoperability across the country is a logical and necessary goal, achieving that goal will be a multiyear and complex undertaking.

FIGURE 9.3. *Nationwide Health Information Network*

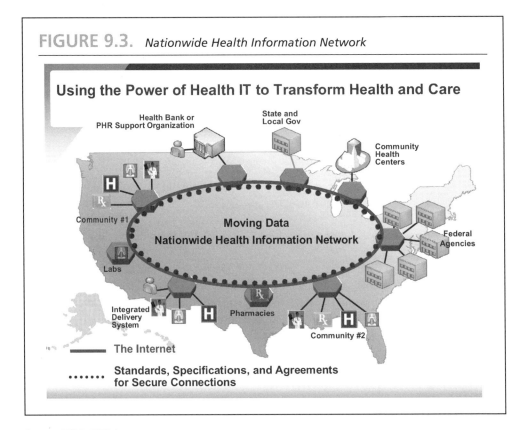

Source: HHS, 2008d.

SUMMARY

In this chapter we reviewed the processes by which health care information standards are developed, and looked at some of the common standards that exist today, including standards in three main categories: classification, vocabulary, and terminology standards; data interchange standards; and health record content standards.

Multiple standard-setting organizations and health care professional organizations play a role in standards development. Standards can be developed through a formal process or by less formal mechanisms, including de facto designation.

The standards discussed in this chapter and other general IT standards enable health care information systems to be interoperable and portable and to exchange data. Without such standards the EMR system and other health care information systems would have limited functionality.

The future of health care information systems is unknown; however, it is clear that the goal of having functional EHRs will not be realized until national standards are adopted. The government, as well as the private sector, plays a role in the development of national standards. HIPAA, for example, has had an impact on the development of health care information standards through designating the transaction and code sets required to be used. In addition, the creation of the Office of the National Coordinator for Health Information Technology and of the Healthcare Information Technology Standards Panel has contributed to the movement toward true health care IT interoperability.

KEY TERMS

Accredited Standards Committee (ASC)
Ad hoc standard development
American National Standards Institute (ANSI)
Consensus standards
Content and coding standards
Continuity of Care Record (CCR)
De facto standard development
Dental Content Committee of the American Dental Association (ADA DCC)
Designated standard maintenance organizations (DSMOs)
Digital Imaging and Communications in Medicine (DICOM)
Electronic data interchange standards
Electronic health record standards
E-prescribing
Government mandated standards

Health information exchange
Health information exchange (HIE)
Health Level 7 (HL7)
Healthcare Information Technology Standards Panel (HITSP)
HIPAA transaction standards
HL7 EHR System Functional Model
International Health Terminology Standards Development Organisation (IHTSDO)
Logical Observation Identifiers Names and Codes (LOINC)
Messaging standards
National Alliance for Health Information Technology (NAHIT)
National Committee on Vital and Health Statistics (NCVHS)
National Council for Prescription Drug Programs (NCPDP)

National health information network

National Library of Medicine (NLM)

National Uniform Billing Committee (NUBC)

National Uniform Claim Committee (NUCC)

Nationwide Health Information Network (NHIN)

Network standards

Office of the National Coordinator for Health Information Technology (ONC)

Regional health information network

Regional health information organization (RHIO)

Standards development organizations (SDOs)

Systematized Nomenclature of Medicine—Clinical Terms (SNOMED CT)

Unified Medical Language (UMLS)

X12N standards

 ## LEARNING ACTIVITIES

1. Standards development is a dynamic process. Select one or more of the standards listed in this chapter, and conduct an Internet search for information on that standard. Has the standard changed? What are the current issues surrounding the standard?

2. Visit a hospital IT department, and speak with a clinical analyst or other person who works with clinical applications. Investigate the standards that the hospital's applications use. Discuss any issues surrounding these standards.

3. Interview the chief information officer (CIO) of a health care organization. Find out his or her views on the current state of health care IT standards or on the need for standards as the United States moves toward broader adoption of EMR systems.

4. Visit the ONC Web site: http://www.dhhs.gov/healthit/onc/mission. Discuss the efforts of the ONC as they relate to the adoption of health care IT standards.

CHAPTER

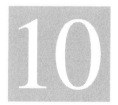

10

SECURITY OF HEALTH CARE INFORMATION SYSTEMS

LEARNING OBJECTIVES

- To be able to understand the importance of establishing a health care organization-wide security program.
- To be able to identify significant threats—internal, external, intentional, and unintentional—to the security of health care information.
- To be able to outline the components of the HIPAA security regulations.
- To be able to give examples of administrative, physical, and technical security safeguards currently in use by health care organizations.
- To be able to discuss the impact and the risks of using wireless networks and allowing remote access to health information, and describe ways to minimize the risks.

By now it should be clear that much of the information in today's health care organizations is transmitted, maintained, and stored electronically. Electronic medical record (EMR) systems are becoming more common, but as we have seen, even primarily paper-based health care information systems contain data and information that have been created and transmitted electronically.

In this chapter we define security, examine the need for establishing an organization-wide security program, and discuss a variety of security-related topics. We also look at the various existing threats to health care information. In addition, we outline the components of the Health Insurance Portability and Accountability Act (HIPAA) security regulations. Although security concerns certainly predate the implementation of the HIPAA Security Rule, the standards in this rule provide an excellent and comprehensive outline of the components necessary for securing health information and, to some extent, provide a framework for establishing a viable health care information security program. The chapter then continues with a look at the following topics, including examples of actual practices and procedures:

- Administrative safeguards
- Physical safeguards
- Technical safeguards

The chapter concludes with a discussion of the special security issues associated with increased use of wireless networks and related devices in health care organizations, along with a discussion of the security issues raised when employees have remote access to health care organizations' computer networks.

THE HEALTH CARE ORGANIZATION'S SECURITY PROGRAM

Health care organizations must protect their information systems from a range of potential threats. Among these threats are viruses, fire in the computer room, untested software, and employee theft of clinical and administrative data. Threats may also involve intentional or unintentional damage to hardware, software, or data or misuse of the organization's hardware, software, or data. The realization of any of these threats can cause significant damage to the organization. Resorting to manual operations if the computers are down for days can lead to organizational chaos. Theft of organizational data can lead to litigation by the individuals harmed by the disclosure of the data. Viruses can corrupt databases, corruption from which there may be no recovery. Health care organizations must have programs in place to combat security breaches.

The function of the health care organization's security program is to identify potential threats and implement processes to remove these threats or mitigate their ability to cause damage. For example, the use of antivirus software is designed to reduce the threat from viruses; the installation of fire protection systems in computer rooms is intended to reduce the damage that might be caused by a fire.

It is important to understand how patient privacy is related to security. The intentional or unintentional release of patient-identifiable information constitutes a misuse of the organization's information systems. Security in a health care organization should be designed, however, to protect not only patient-specific information but also the organization's IT assets—such as the networks, hardware, software, and applications that make up the organization's health care information systems—from potential threats, both threats that come from human beings and those that come from natural and environmental causes.

The primary challenge of developing an effective security program in a health care organization is balancing the need for security with the cost of security. An organization does not know how to calculate the likelihood that a hacker will cause serious damage or a backhoe will cut through network cables under the street. The organization may not fully understand the consequences of being without its network for four hours or four days. Hence, it may not be sure how much to spend to remove or reduce the risk. This dilemma is similar to the one posed when individuals consider obtaining long-term care insurance. None of us know whether we will or will not need this insurance, how long we might live in a long-term care facility, or the acuity of the care we may need. How much insurance should we buy?

One aspect of this challenge is maintaining a satisfactory balance between health care information system security and health care data and information availability. As we saw in Chapter One, the major purpose of maintaining health information and health records is to facilitate high-quality care for patients. On the one hand, if an organization's security measures are so stringent that they prevent appropriate access to the health information needed to care for patients, this important purpose is undermined. On the other hand, if the organization allows unrestricted access to all patient-identifiable information to all its employees, the patients' rights to privacy and confidentiality would certainly be violated and the organization's IT assets would be at considerable risk.

As health care organizations develop their security programs they should be sure to seek input from a wide range of health care providers and other system users as well as legal counsel and technical experts. The balance between access and security should be reasonable—protecting patients' rights while allowing appropriate access.

THREATS TO HEALTH CARE INFORMATION

What are the threats to health care information systems? In general, threats to health care information systems fall into one of these three categories:

- Human threats, which can result from intentional or unintentional human tampering
- Natural and environmental threats, such as floods, fires, and power outages
- Technology malfunctions, such as a drive that fails and has no backup

Within these categories are multiple potential threats. Threats to health care information systems from human beings can be *intentional* or *unintentional*. They can be *internal*, caused by employees, or *external*, caused by individuals outside the organization. Intentional threats include theft, intentional alteration of data, and intentional destruction of data. The culprit could be a disgruntled employee, a computer hacker, or a prankster. In a Florida case several years ago, for example, the daughter of a hospital employee accessed confidential information through an unattended computer workstation in the facility's emergency room. She wrote down names and addresses of recent patients and then called to tell them that they had tested positive for HIV. Several of the recipients of these prank calls became extremely distraught (Associated Press, 1995a, 1995b).

Computer viruses are among the most common and virulent forms of intentional computer tampering. They pose a serious threat to computerized patient data and health care applications. (See the section on virus checking later in this chapter for more information on viruses.) Some of the causes of unintentional damage to health care information systems are lack of training in proper use of the system or human error. When users share passwords or download information from a nonsecure Internet site, for example, they create the potential for a breach in security.

Internal breaches of security are far more common than external breaches. Some of the more common forms of internal breaches of security across all industries are the installation or use of unauthorized software, use of the organization's computing resources for illegal or illicit communications or activities (porn surfing, e-mail harassment, and so forth), and the use of the organization's computing resources for personal profit.

Computer hardware used in health care information systems must also be protected from loss. In recent years there have been multiple instances of computer thefts from health care organizations, resulting in exposure of confidential patient information (Health Privacy Project, 2007).

Electronic health care information is vulnerable to internal and external threats. Whether intentional or unintentional, these threats pose serious security risks. To minimize the risk and protect patients' sensitive health care information, well-established and well-implemented administrative, physical, and technical security safeguards are essential for any health care organization, regardless of size.

The security standards established by the Department of Health and Human Services under the terms of the Health Insurance Portability and Accountability Act (HIPAA) provide an excellent framework for developing an overall security plan and program for a health care institution. The regulations are designed to be flexible and scalable and are not reliant on specific technologies for implementation, making it possible for health care organizations of all sizes to be compliant.

OVERVIEW OF HIPAA SECURITY RULE

The final rule on the HIPAA security standards, known generally as the Security Rule, was published in the Federal Register on February 20, 2003 (68 Fed. Reg. 34, 8333–8381). (In Chapter Three we looked at the various components of the far-reaching HIPAA legislation. In this section we discuss the security component in greater detail. You may wish to refer back to Chapter Three for a description of how the Security Rule fits into the overall Act.) Covered entities (CEs) had two years to comply with the rules. The HIPAA Security Rule is closely connected to the HIPAA Privacy Rule (also discussed in Chapter Three). However, whereas the Privacy Rule governs all protected health information (PHI), the Security Rule governs only ePHI. *EPHI* is defined as protected health information maintained or transmitted in electronic form. The Security

Rule does not distinguish between electronic forms of information or between transmission mechanisms. EPHI may be stored in any type of electronic media, such as magnetic tapes and disks, optical disks, servers, and personal computers. Transmission may take place over the Internet, on local area networks (LANs), or by disks, for example.

The HIPAA Security Rule was first published, in draft form, in August 1998. At that time one of the complaints was that the standards were too prescriptive and not flexible enough. As a result the standards in the final rule are defined in general terms, focusing on what should be done rather than on how it should be done. According to the Centers for Medicare and Medicaid Services (CMS, 2004), the final rule specifies "a series of administrative, technical, and physical security procedures for covered entities to use to assure the confidentiality of electronic protected health information. The standards are delineated into either required or addressable implementation specifications" (see also Quinsley, 2004; American Health Information Management Association, 2003a; Gue, 2003).

There are few key terms to be defined before we examine the content of the HIPAA Security Rule. What is a covered entity? What is the difference between a required implementation specification and an addressable one?

The HIPAA standards govern *covered entities* (CEs), which are defined as

- A health plan.
- A health care clearinghouse.
- A health care provider who transmits protected health information in electronic form. This includes practically every type of health care organization imaginable, including hospitals, clinics, physicians' offices, nursing homes, and so forth.

The specifications contained in the Security Rule are designated as either *required* or *addressable*. A required specification must be implemented by a CE for that organization to be in compliance. However, the CE is in compliance with an addressable specification if it does any one of the following:

- Implements the specification as stated.
- Implements an alternative security measure to accomplish the purposes of the standard or specification.
- Chooses not to implement anything, provided it can demonstrate that the standard or specification is not reasonable and appropriate and that the purpose of the standard can still be met. Because the Security Rule is designed to be technology neutral, this flexibility was granted for organizations that employ nonstandard technologies or have legitimate reasons not to need the stated specification (AHIMA, 2003a; Gue, 2003).

The standards contained in the HIPAA Security Rule are divided into five sections, or categories, the specifics of which we outline here. You will notice overlap among the sections. For example, contingency plans are covered under both administrative and physical safeguards, and access controls are addressed in several standards and specifications. In subsequent sections of this chapter we will look at some actual practices that might be employed by health care organizations in each of the first four categories.

As you read through this outline, consider how it would work as a framework or model for a health care organization's security program.

OUTLINE OF HIPAA SECURITY RULE

The Administrative Safeguards section of the Final Rule contains nine standards:

1. *Security management functions.* This standard requires the CE to implement policies and procedures to prevent, detect, contain, and correct security violations. There are four implementation specifications for this standard:

   - *Risk analysis* (required). The CE must conduct an accurate and thorough assessment of the potential risks to and vulnerabilities of the confidentiality, integrity, and availability of ePHI.

   - *Risk management* (required). The CE must implement security measures that reduce risks and vulnerabilities to a reasonable and appropriate level.

   - *Sanction policy* (required). The CE must apply appropriate sanctions against workforce members who fail to comply with the CE's security policies and procedures.

   - *Information system activity review* (required). The CE must implement procedures to regularly review records of information system activity, such as audit logs, access reports, and security incident tracking reports.

2. *Assigned security responsibility.* This standard does not have any implementation specifications. It requires the CE to identify the individual responsible for overseeing development of the organization's security policies and procedures.

3. *Workforce security.* This standard requires the CE to implement policies and procedures to ensure that all members of its workforce have appropriate access to ePHI and to prevent those workforce members who do not have access from obtaining access. There are three implementation specifications for this standard:

   - *Authorization and/or supervision* (addressable). The CE must have a process for ensuring that the workforce working with ePHI has adequate authorization and supervision.

   - *Workforce clearance procedure* (addressable). There must be a process to determine what access is appropriate for each workforce member.

   - *Termination procedures* (addressable). There must be a process for terminating access to ePHI when a workforce member is no longer employed or his or her responsibilities change.

4. *Information access management.* This standard requires the CE to implement policies and procedures for authorizing access to ePHI. There are three implementation specifications within this standard. The first (not shown here) applies to health care clearinghouses, and the other two apply to health care organizations:

   - *Access authorization* (addressable). The CE must have a process for granting access to ePHI through a workstation, transaction, program, or other process.

- *Access establishment and modification* (addressable). The CE must have a process (based on the access authorization) to establish, document, review, and modify a user's right to access to a workstation, transaction, program, or process.

5. *Security awareness and training.* This standard requires the CE to implement awareness and training programs for all members of its workforce. This training should include periodic security reminders and address protection from malicious software, log-in monitoring, and password management. (These items to be addressed in training are all listed as addressable implementation specifications.)

6. *Security incident reporting.* This standard requires the CE to implement policies and procedures to address security incidents.

7. *Contingency plan.* This standard has five implementation specifications:

   - *Data backup plan* (required).
   - *Disaster recovery plan* (required).
   - *Emergency mode operation plan* (required).
   - *Testing and revision procedures* (addressable). The CE should periodically test and modify all contingency plans.
   - *Applications and data criticality analysis* (addressable). The CE should assess the relative criticality of specific applications and data in support of its contingency plan.

8. *Evaluation.* This standard requires the CE to periodically perform technical and nontechnical evaluations in response to changes that may affect the security of ePHI.

9. *Business associate contracts and other arrangements.* This standard outlines the conditions under which a CE must have a formal agreement with business associates in order to exchange ePHI.

   The Physical Safeguards section contains four standards:

1. *Facility access controls.* This standard requires the CE to implement policies and procedures to limit physical access to its electronic information systems and the facilities in which they are housed to authorized users. There are four implementation specifications with this standard:

   - *Contingency operations* (addressable). The CE should have a process for allowing facility access to support the restoration of lost data under the disaster recovery plan and emergency mode operation plan.
   - *Facility security plan* (addressable). The CE must have a process to safeguard the facility and its equipment from unauthorized access, tampering, and theft.
   - *Access control and validation* (addressable). The CE should have a process to control and validate access to facilities based on users' roles or functions.

■ *Maintenance records* (addressable). The CE should have a process to document repairs and modifications to the physical components of a facility as they relate to security.

2. *Workstation use.* This standard requires the CE to implement policies and procedures that specify the proper functions to be performed and the manner in which those functions are to be performed on a specific workstation or class of workstation that can be used to access ePHI, and that also specify the physical attributes of the surroundings of such workstations.

3. *Workstation security.* This standard requires the CE to implement physical safeguards for all workstations that are used to access ePHI and to restrict access to authorized users.

4. *Device and media controls.* This standard requires the CE to implement policies and procedures for the movement of hardware and electronic media that contain ePHI into and out of a facility and within a facility. There are four implementation specifications with this standard:

   ■ *Disposal* (required). The CE must have a process for the final disposition of ePHI and of the hardware and electronic media on which it is stored.

   ■ *Mediareuse* (required). The CE must have a process for removal of ePHI from electronic media before the media can be reused.

   ■ *Accountability* (addressable). The CE must maintain a record of movements of hardware and electronic media and any person responsible for these items.

   ■ *Data backup and storage* (addressable). The CE must create a retrievable, exact copy of ePHI, when needed, before movement of equipment.

The Technical Safeguards section has five standards:

1. *Access control.* This standard requires the CE to implement technical policies and procedures for electronic information systems that maintain ePHI in order to allow access only to those persons or software programs that have been granted access rights as specified in the administrative safeguards. There are four implementation specifications with this standard:

   ■ *Unique user identification* (required). The CE must assign a unique name or number for identifying and tracking each user's identity.

   ■ *Emergency access procedure* (required). The CE must establish procedures for obtaining necessary ePHI in an emergency.

   ■ *Automatic log-off* (addressable). The CE must implement electronic processes that terminate an electronic session after a predetermined time of inactivity.

   ■ *Encryption and decryption* (addressable). The CE should implement a mechanism to encrypt and decrypt ePHI as needed.

2. *Audit controls.* This standard requires the CE to implement hardware, software, and procedures that record and examine activity in the information systems that contain ePHI.

3. *Integrity.* This standard requires the CE to implement policies and procedures to protect ePHI from improper alteration or destruction.

4. *Person or entity authentication.* This standard requires the CE to implement procedures to verify that a person or entity seeking access to ePHI is in fact the person or entity claimed.

5. *Transmission security.* This standard requires the CE to implement technical measures to guard against unauthorized access to ePHI being transmitted across a network. There are two implementation specifications with this standard:

   ■ *Integrity controls* (addressable). The CE must implement security measures to ensure that electronically transmitted ePHI is not improperly modified without detection.

   ■ *Encryption* (addressable). The CE should encrypt ePHI whenever it is deemed appropriate.

The Policies, Procedures, and Documentation section has two standards:

1. *Policies and procedures.* This standard requires the CE to establish and implement policies and procedures to comply with the standards, implementation specifications, and other requirements.

2. *Documentation.* This standard requires the CE to maintain the policies and procedures implemented to comply with the Security Rule in written form. There are three implementation specifications:

   ■ *Time limit* (required). The CE must retain the documentation for six years from the date of its creation or the date when it was last in effect, whichever is later.

   ■ *Availability* (required). The CE must make the documentation available to those persons responsible for implementing the policies and procedures.

   ■ *Updates* (required). The CE must review the documentation periodically and update it as needed.

This section has provided an outline of the key components of the HIPAA security standards (68 Fed. Reg. 34, 8333–8381, Feb. 20, 2003). In the next sections we will examine some of the practices that can be employed to address the regulations and ensure that an organization has an effective security program.

ADMINISTRATIVE SAFEGUARDS

As you have seen from the HIPAA standards outline, administrative safeguards cover a wide range of organizational activities. We do not attempt in this section to give a comprehensive, detailed view of all possible administrative safeguards but rather to present a few practices that can be used as part of a total administrative effort to improve the health care organization's information security program. We will discuss the following topics:

■ Risk analysis and management

■ Chief security officer

■ System security evaluation

Risk Analysis and Management

One of the key components of applying administrative safeguards to protect the organization's health care information is risk analysis. It is impossible to establish an effective risk management program if the organization is not aware of the risks or threats that exist. Risk analysis is relatively new to health care. Few organizations had implemented formal security risk assessment prior to the publication of the HIPAA rules. This in no way minimizes its importance. However, health care has had to look to other industries for examples of risk assessment processes (Walsh, 2003; Reynolds, 2009).

Steve Weil (2004), on the HIPAAdvisory.com Web site, defines risk as the "likelihood that a specific threat will exploit a certain vulnerability, and the resulting impact of that event." He introduces a risk analysis process with eight parts, or steps:

1. *Boundary definition.* During the boundary definition step the organization should develop a detailed inventory of all health information and information systems. This review can be conducted using interviews, inspections, questionnaires, or other means. The important thing in this step is to identify all the patient-specific health information, health care information systems (both internal and external), and users of the information and systems.

2. *Threat identification.* Identifying threats will result in a list of all potential threats to the organization's health care information systems. The three general types of threats that should be considered are

    a. Natural, such as floods and fires

    b. Human, which can be intentional or unintentional

    c. Environmental, such as power outages

3. *Vulnerability identification.* In this step the organization identifies all the specific vulnerabilities that exist in its own health care information systems. Generally, vulnerabilities take the form of flaws or weaknesses in system procedures or design. Software packages are available to assist with identifying vulnerabilities, but the organization may also need to conduct interviews, surveys, and the like. Some organizations may employ external consultants to help them identify the vulnerabilities in their systems.

4. *Security control analysis.* The organization also needs to conduct a thorough analysis of the security controls that are currently in place. These include both preventive controls, such as access controls and authentication procedures, and controls designed to detect actual or potential breaches, such as audit trails and alarms.

5. *Risk likelihood determination.* This step in the process involves assigning a risk rating to each area of the health care information system. There are a variety of rating systems that may be employed. Weil recommends using a fairly straightforward high-risk, medium-risk, and low-risk system of rating.

6. *Impact analysis.* This is the step in which the organization determines what the actual impact of specific security breaches would be. A breach may affect

confidentiality, integrity, or availability. Impact too can be rated as high, medium, or low.

7. *Risk determination.* The information gathered up to this point in the risk analysis process is now brought together in order to determine the actual level of risk to specific information and specific information systems. The risk determination is based on

    a. The likelihood that a certain threat will attempt to exploit a specific vulnerability (high, medium, or low)

    b. The level of impact should the threat successfully exploit the vulnerability (high, medium, or low)

    c. The adequacy of planned or existing security controls (high, medium, or low)

    Each specific system or type of information can be assessed for each of these three factors, and then these assessments can be combined to produce an overall risk rating of high—needing immediate attention, medium—needing attention soon, or low—existing controls are acceptable.

8. *Security control recommendations.* The final step of the process is to compile a summary report on the findings of the analysis and recommendations for improving security controls.

The risk analysis should lead to the development of policies and procedures outlining risk management procedures and sanctions or consequences for employees and other individuals who do not follow the established procedures. All health care organizations should have a formal security risk management program in place. In general, this program is administered by the organization's security officer.

Chief Security Officer

Each health care organization must have a single individual who is responsible for overseeing the information security program. Generally, this individual is identified as the organization's *chief security officer*. The chief security officer may report to the chief information officer (CIO) or to another administrator in the health care organization. The role of security officer may be 100 percent of an individual's job responsibilities or only a fraction, depending on the size of the organization and the scope of its health care information systems. Regardless of the actual reporting structure, it is essential that the chief security officer be given the authority to effectively manage the security program, apply sanctions, and influence employees. As Tom Walsh (2003, p. 15) stated in identifying the importance of the security officer, "influence can leverage the right people to get the job done."

System Security Evaluation

Chief security officers must periodically evaluate their organization's health care information systems and networks for proper technical controls and processes. Clearly, an established set of health information technical standards for security would facilitate this evaluation process. Unfortunately, there are currently no widely adopted technical security standards designed for health care information systems (and recall from our earlier discussion that the HIPAA standards are technology neutral). There are, however, general standards for security techniques across all types of organization, which were developed by the International Organization for Standardization (ISO), as ISO Standard 15408 (titled Information Technology—Security Techniques—Evaluation Criteria for IT Security). These standards, updated in 2005, allow an organization to use a common set of requirements and thus to compare the results of independent security evaluations (ISO, 2005).

PHYSICAL SAFEGUARDS

A security program must address physical as well as technical and administrative safeguards. Physical safeguards involve protecting the actual computer hardware, software, data, and information from physical damage or loss due to natural, human, or environmental threats. Several specific issues related to physical security are addressed in this section

- Assigned security responsibility
- Media controls
- Physical access controls
- Workstation security

Assigned Security Responsibility

Each component of the health care information system should be secure, and one easily identifiable employee should be responsible for that security. These individuals are in turn accountable to the chief security officer. For example, in a nursing department the department manager might be responsible for ensuring that all employees have been trained to understand and use security measures and that they know the importance of maintaining the security of patient information. The network administrator, however, might be the person responsible for assigning initial passwords and removing access from terminated employees or employees who transfer to other departments (Reynolds, 2009).

Media Controls

The physical media on which health information is stored must be physically protected. Media controls are the policies and procedures that govern the receipt and removal of hardware, software, and computer media such as disks and tapes into and out of the organization and also their movements inside the organization.

Media controls also encompass data storage. Backup tapes, for example, must be stored in a secure area with limited access. The final disposition of electronic media is another aspect of media controls. Policies for the destruction of patient information must address the electronic media and hardware (workstations and servers) that contain patient information. As organizations gather old computers, all patient data must be removed before this equipment goes to surplus or is otherwise disposed of (Reynolds, 2009).

Physical Access Controls

Physical access controls are designed to limit physical access to health information to persons authorized to see that information. Locks and keys are examples of physical access controls. However, it is obvious that all workstations cannot be kept under lock and key. This might create a secure system, but it would not be readily available to the health care providers who need patient information. Some of the physical access control components that can be employed are equipment control; a facility security plan; procedures that verify user identity before allowing physical access to an area; a procedure for maintaining records of repairs and modifications to hardware, software, and physical facilities; and a visitor sign-in procedure. Organizations should have a system, such as an inventory control system, that tells them exactly what equipment is currently in use in their health care information system. An inventory control system generally involves marking or tagging each piece of equipment with a unique number and assigning each piece to a location and a responsible person. When equipment is moved, retired, or destroyed, that action must be documented in the inventory control system. Another form of equipment control is to install antitheft devices, such as chains that attach computers to desks, alarms, and other tools that deter thieves.

A facility security plan is a plan that ensures that the individuals in a certain area are authorized to have access to that area. The main computer operations of a health care organization will generally be under tight security, including video surveillance and personal security checks. Badges with photographs are common in health care facilities to help identify personnel who are authorized to access certain buildings and facilities. Some secure areas require individuals to punch a code into a keypad or swipe an identification card over a card reader before entry is allowed. The facility security plan should also have procedures for admitting visitors. Each visitor might sign in and be issued a temporary identification badge, for example. There may be areas of the organization that are not open to visitors at all (Reynolds, 2009).

Workstation Security

Workstations that allow access to patient information should be placed in areas that are secure or monitored at all times. The workstations in the reception area or other public areas should be situated so that visitors or others cannot read the screens. Devices can be placed over workstation monitors that prevent people from reading a screen unless they are directly in front of it. Another aspect of workstation security is developing clear policies for workstation use. These policies should delineate, among other things, the appropriate functions to perform on the workstation and rules for sharing workstations.

Organizations that allow personnel to work from home have additional workstation security issues. Employees working from home must be given clear guidance on appropriate use of the organization's computer resources, whether these resources involve hardware, software, or Web access. Employees should access any patient-identifiable information through a secure connection, with adequate monitoring to ensure that the user is in fact the authorized employee.

All the aspects of physical security require adequate training of all personnel with potential access to the health care information systems. Employees, agents, and contractors with access to locations that house patient information must all participate in security and confidentiality awareness education (Reynolds, 2009).

TECHNICAL SAFEGUARDS

Many different technical safeguards can be used to help secure health care information systems and the networks on which they reside. Again, we will not provide a comprehensive list of all available safeguards but will present a few representative examples. We will discuss technical safeguards related to the following topics:

- Access control
- Entity authentication
- Audit trails
- Data encryption
- Firewall protection
- Virus checking

Access Control

Only individuals with a *need to know* should have access to patient-identifiable health information. Modern computer systems, including databases and networks, allow users to access a variety of resources such as individual files, database files, and tapes and to use printers and other peripheral devices. This sharing of resources is an important component of effective health care information systems, but it requires that network administrators and database administrators set appropriate access rights for each resource. Often users of a health care information system have to be assigned network access rights and separate application access rights before they can use the system.

Control over access to health data may involve any of the following methods:

- User-based access
- Role-based access
- Context-based access

Before we discuss each of these options, a brief explanation of access rights is necessary. Traditional user-based and role-based access rights have two parameters—who and how. The *who* is a list of the users with rights to access the information or computer resource in question. This list, called an *access control list*, may be organized by individual users or by groups of users. These groups are generally defined by role or job function. For example, all coders in the health information management department would be granted the same access rights, all registered nurses in a particular job classification would be granted the same access, and so forth.

The *how* parameter of the access control scheme specifies how a user may access the resource. Typical actions users might be allowed to take are read, write, edit, execute, append, and print. Only so-called owners and administrators will be granted full rights so that they can modify or delete or create new components for the resource. Clearly, owner and administrative privileges for the use of health care information systems should be carefully monitored.

User-based access control is defined as "a security mechanism used to grant users of a system access based upon the identity of the user." With *role-based access* control (RBAC), access decisions are based on the roles individual users have within the organization. "With RBAC, rather than attempting to map an organization's security policy to a relatively low-level set of technical controls (typically, access control lists), each user is assigned to one or more predefined roles, each of which has been assigned the various privileges needed to perform the role" (63 Fed. Reg. 155, August 12, 1998). One of the benefits of role-based over user-based access is that as new applications are added, privileges are more easily assigned. Discretionary assignment of access by an administrator is limited with RBAC. Users must be assigned to a specific role in order to be assigned access to a specific application.

Context-based access control is the most stringent of the three options. Harry Smith (2001) describes it this way: "A context-based access control scheme begins with the protection afforded by either a user-based or role-based access control design and takes it one step further. . . . Context-based access control takes into account the person attempting to access the data, the type of data being accessed and the *context* of the transaction in which the access attempt is made." In other words the context-based access has three parameters to consider—the who, the how, and the context in which the data are to be accessed. The following example illustrates the differences among the three types of access control (Reynolds, 2009).

CASE STUDY

Three Types of Access Control Mary Smith is the director of the Health Information Management Department in a hospital. Under a user-based access control scheme, Mary would be allowed read-only access to the hospital's laboratory information system because of her personal identity—that is, because she is Mary Smith and uses the proper log-in and password(s) to get into the system. Under a role-based control scheme, Mary would be allowed read-only access to the hospital's lab system because she is part of the Health Information Management Department and all department employees have been granted read-only privileges for this system. If the hospital were to adopt a context-based

(Continued)

CASE STUDY (*Continued*)

control scheme, Mary might be allowed access to the lab system only from her own workstation or another workstation in the Health Information Services Department, provided she used her proper log-in and password. If she attempted to log in from the Emergency Department or another administrative office, she might be denied access. The context control could also involve time of day. Because Mary is a daytime employee, she might be denied access if she attempted to log in at night.

Entity Authentication

Access control mechanisms are effective means of controlling who gains entry to a health care information system only when there is a system for ensuring the identity of the individual attempting to gain access. *Entity authentication* is defined in the HIPAA Security Rule as "the corroboration that a person is the one claimed." Entity authentication associated with health care information systems should include at least (1) automatic log-off and (2) a unique user identifier (Reynolds, 2009).

Automatic log-off is a security procedure that causes a computer session to end after a predetermined period of inactivity, such as ten minutes. Multiple software products are available that allow network administrators to set automatic log-off parameters. Once installed, these log-off systems act like any other screen saver on a typical workstation, coming on after a set period of inactivity. Users are then required to enter a network password to deactivate the log-off system screen. Generally, a device driver is also installed that prevents rebooting to deactivate the log-off system. Other security measures that may be included in automatic log-off products are features that prevent users from changing the screen saver and that allow an authorized person to set local password options in case the user is not connected to the network. Failed log-in attempts may be recorded and reported on, along with statistics on user log-ins, elapsed time, and user identification.

Each user of a health care information system must be assigned a unique identifier. This identifier is a combination of characters and numbers assigned and maintained by the security system. It is used to track individual user activity. This identifier is commonly called the *user ID* or *log-on ID*. It is the *public*, or known, portion of most user log-on procedures. For example, many organizations will assign a log-on identifier that is the same as the user's e-mail address or a combination of the user's last and first name. It is generally fairly easy to identify a user by his or her log-on. John Doe's log-on identifier might be "doej," for example. Because of the public nature of the log-in, additional safeguards, beyond the log-on ID, are needed.

Entity authentication can be implemented in a number of different ways in a health care information system. The most common entity authentication method is a *password system*. Other mechanisms include *personal identification numbers* (PINs), *biometric identification systems, telephone callback systems*, and *tokens*. These implementation methods can be used alone or in combination with other systems. Security experts often encourage *layered* security systems that use more than one security mechanism.

As one security expert has stated, "A series of overlapping solutions works much more effectively, even when you know the solutions are individually fallible. If you line up three security controls that are each 60 percent effective, together they're something like 90 percent effective against a given attack" (Briney, 2000).

Walsh (2003) recommends a system that uses a *two-factor* authentication. He identifies these three methods for authentication, and any two of them used together would constitute a two-factor system:

- Something you know, such as a password or personal identification number (PIN)
- Something you have, such as an ATM card, token, or swipe card
- Something you are, such as a biometric fingerprint, voice scan, or iris or retinal scan [Walsh, 2003].

Password Systems The most common way to control access to a health care information system (or any other computer system for that matter) is through a combination of the user ID and a password or PIN. User IDs and passwords for a system are maintained either as a part of the access control list for the network or local operating system or in a special database. The list or database is then searched for a match before the user is allowed to access the system requested. Although the user ID is not secret, the password or PIN is. Passwords are generally stored in an encrypted form for which no decryption is available (White, 2001; Oz, 2006).

Although password and PIN systems are the most common forms of entity authentication, they also provide the weakest form of security. A *password* is defined by Whatis?.com (2002) as an "unspaced sequence of characters used to determine that a computer user requesting access to a computer system is really that particular user." Typically, a password is made up of four to sixteen characters. One of the biggest problems with passwords is that users may share them or publicly display them. Users will often write down passwords they cannot remember. They may even tape or post the password on the computer workstation. Health care organizations must take steps to prevent this type of password misuse. Clear policies on the use and maintenance of passwords, education for employees, and meaningful sanctions for policy violators are essential.

Another common problem with passwords is that when they are simple enough to remember, they may be simple enough for someone else to guess. Passwords are encrypted, but there are software programs available, called *password crackers*, that can be used to identify an unknown or forgotten password. Unfortunately, unauthorized persons seeking to gain access to computer systems can also use these applications (White, 2001; Whatis?.com, 2002). Health care organizations should establish enforceable, clear guidelines for choosing passwords. The following Perspective offers some suggestions (White, 2001; Whatis?.com, 2002; Reynolds, 2009).

PERSPECTIVE

PASSWORD DOs AND DON'Ts

DON'T

- Pick a password that someone who knows you can easily guess (for example, do not use your Social Security Number, birthday, maiden name, pet's name, child's name, or car name).

- Pick a word that can be found in the dictionary (because cracker programs can rapidly try every word in the dictionary!).

- Pick a word that is currently newsworthy.

- Pick a password that is similar to your previous password.

- Share your password with others.

DO

- Pick a combination of letters and at least one number. Pick a password with at least eight characters, mixing uppercase and lowercase if your password system is case sensitive.

- Pick a word that you can easily remember.

- Change your password often. (Some networks require that you change your password periodically.)

Biometric Identification Systems   Because of the inherent weaknesses of password systems, other identification systems have been developed. Biometric identification systems employ users' biological data, in the form, for example, of a voiceprint, fingerprint, handprint, retinal scan, faceprint, or full body scan. Although some sources (White, 2001) call biometric identification systems the "wave of future," there are indications that the technology is not yet widely used.

Nevertheless, biometrics is likely to play an increasing role in health care information system security. Biometric devices consist of a reader or scanning device, software that converts the scanned information into digital form, and a database that stores the biometric data for comparison. IBM, Microsoft, Novell, and other computer companies are currently working on a standard for biometric devices, called BioAPI. This standard will allow software products from different manufacturers to interact with one another (Whatis?.com, 2002).

Telephone Callback Procedures   Telephone callback procedures are another form of entity authentication in use today. Callback is used primarily when employees have access to a health care information system from home. When a modem dials into the system, a special callback application asks for the telephone number from which the call has been placed. If this number is not an authorized number, the callback application will not allow access (Oz, 2004).

Tokens   Tokens are devices, such as key cards, that are inserted into doors or computers. With token authentication systems, identification is based on the user's possession of the token (Eng, 2001). The disadvantage of tokens is that they can be lost, misplaced, or stolen. When tokens are used in combination with a password or PIN, it is essential that the password or PIN not be written on the token or in a location near where the token is stored.

Audit Trails

Webopedia.com (2004a) defines an *audit trail* as "a record showing who has accessed a computer system and what operations he or she has performed during a given period of time. In addition, there are separate audit trail software products that enable network administrators to monitor use of network resources." Audit trails are generated by specialized software, and they have multiple uses in securing information systems. These uses may be categorized as follows (Gopalakrishna, 2000):

- *Individual accountability.* When employees' or other individuals' actions are tracked with an audit trail these individuals become accountable for their actions, which can be a strong deterrent to violating acceptable policies and procedures.

- *Reconstructing electronic events.* Audit trails can also be used to reconstruct how and when a computer or application was used. This can be quite useful when there is a suspected security breach, whether internal or external.

- *Problem monitoring.* Some types of auditing software can detect problems such as disk failures, overutilization of system resources, and network outages as they occur.

- *Intrusion detection.* When there are attempts to gain unauthorized access to a system, an audit system can detect them.

Data Encryption

Data encryption is used to ensure that data transferred from one location on a network to another are secure from anyone eavesdropping or seeking to intercept them. This becomes particularly important when sensitive data, such as health information, are transmitted over public networks such as the Internet or across wireless networks. Secure data are data that cannot be intercepted, copied, modified, or deleted either while in transit or stored, such as on a disk or tape.

   Cryptography is the study of encryption and decryption techniques. It is a complicated science with a vast number of associated techniques. Only the basic concepts and some current authentication technologies will be discussed in this chapter. Public Key Infrastructure, Pretty Good Privacy, wired equivalent privacy (WEP), and WiFi protected access (WPA) are forms of encryption being used in health care organizations today. (WEP and WPA apply specifically to wireless networks and will be discussed later in this chapter.) These protocols are used to authenticate the senders and receivers of messages transmitted over public networks, such as the Internet or wireless networks.

Some basic terms associated with encryption are plaintext, encryption algorithm, ciphertext, and key. *Plaintext* refers to data before any encryption has taken place. In other words, the original datum or message is recorded in the computer system as plaintext. An *encryption algorithm* is a computer program that converts plaintext into an enciphered form. The *ciphertext* is the data after the encryption algorithm has been applied. The *key* in an encryption and decryption procedure is unique data that are needed both to create the ciphertext and to decrypt the ciphertext back to the original message. Figure 10.1 is a simple diagram of the components of an encryption and decryption system (White, 2001).

The earliest encryption systems used a single, private key. In other words, the same key (or code) was used to generate the ciphertext and to decrypt it. The problems with the single, private (secret) key systems were that both the sender and receiver had to have the key and that this key had to be protected from interception or tampering as well.

Public Key Infrastructure   *Public key cryptography* addresses the basic problems of single, private key systems. In a public key system, there are two keys, a *private key* and a *public key*. Basically, in this two-key system, data encrypted with the public key can be decrypted only by the private key, and data encrypted by the private key can be decrypted only by the public key. With public key cryptography, encrypted data become very difficult to break (White, 2001). The following is a simplified illustration of how public key cryptography works.

A health care clinic in a major city needs to send patient information to the main hospital across town. First, the hospital sends a public key to the clinic and it keeps the corresponding private key in a secure location. The clinic uses the public key to encrypt

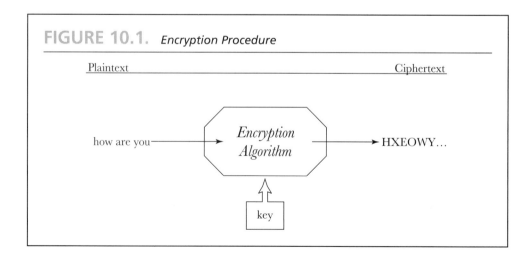

FIGURE 10.1. *Encryption Procedure*

the data before sending it over to the hospital. Now, only the hospital can decode the data, because it has sole possession of the corresponding private key.

Public key cryptography today is a component of Public Key Infrastructure (PKI), an entire system designed to make the use of public key cryptography practical. PKI is a combination of encryption techniques, software, and services. A health care organization can adopt an in-house PKI model or contract with an application service provider (ASP) to host and manage a PKI system for it. One potential use of PKI in health care is sending secure e-mail. To send a secure e-mail in the PKI environment, the sender retrieves the recipient's public key from a directory in his or her organization. After obtaining the public key, the sender encrypts the e-mail message (by selecting the "encrypt" button, for example) and sends the encrypted message. When the e-mail arrives at the recipient's computer, the recipient's private key will automatically decrypt the message (Etheridge, 2001).

There are other potential uses for PKI technology in health care, such as ensuring secure access to Web-based health records or other health care information systems. One example is that Marconi Medical Systems, which makes a picture archiving and communication system (PACS), is integrating PKI into its Web-based products to allow remote access through a standard Web browser. PKI is also being used by an on-line prescription service (Etheridge, 2001). As wonderful as PKI sounds, it has some problems. It is expensive, and many of the systems are proprietary and will not interact with other systems. However, with the HIPAA standards demanding a higher level of security for on-line health care transactions, the use of PKI technology in health care is likely to increase.

Pretty Good Privacy   In the early 1990s, software engineer Phillip Zimmermann created open source encryption software that he called Pretty Good Privacy (PGP). PGP has the specific purpose of allowing the average person to create and send secure e-mail and data files. PGP uses public key cryptography and digital signatures. In order to use PGP, both the sending and the receiving workstations must have the same PGP software. Originally, PGP was available via the Internet. A freeware version is available to individuals in the United States from the PGP Corporation (www.pgp.com), and PGP can also be purchased for commercial use (White, 2001).

Firewall Protection

A *firewall* is "a system or combination of systems that supports an access control policy between two networks" (White, 2001). The term *firewall* may be used to describe software that protects computing resources or to describe a combination of software, hardware, and policies that protects these resources (Oz, 2004; Whatis?.com, 2002). The most common place to find a firewall is between the health care organization's internal network and the Internet. This firewall prevents users who are accessing the health care network via the Internet from using certain portions of that network and also prevents internal users from accessing various portions of the Internet (Oz, 2004; Whatis?.com, 2002).

The basic types of firewalls are (1) packet filter, or network level, and (2) proxy servers, or application level. The *packet filter* firewall is essentially a router that has been programmed to filter out some types of data and to allow other types to pass through. The early versions of these firewalls were fairly easy to fool. As routers have become more sophisticated, the protection offered by this type of firewall has increased. The *proxy server* is a more complex firewall device. The proxy server firewall is software that runs on a computer that acts as the gatekeeper to an organization's network. Any external transaction enters the organization's network through the proxy server. The request for information is actually "stopped" at the proxy server, where a proxy application is created. This proxy is what goes into the organization's network to retrieve the requested information (White, 2001).

As important as firewalls are to the overall security of health care information systems, they cannot protect a system from all types of attacks. Many viruses, for example, can hide inside documents that will not be stopped by a firewall.

Virus Checking

Computer *viruses* come in many different varieties. The common types may be classified as (Whatis?.com, 2002)

- *File infectors*, which attach to program files so that when a program is loaded the virus is also loaded
- *System or boot-record infectors*, which infect system areas of diskettes or hard disks
- *Macro viruses*, which infect Microsoft Word applications, inserting unwanted words or phrases

A *worm* is a special type of computer virus that stores and then replicates itself. Worms usually transfer from computer to computer via e-mail. A *Trojan horse* is a destructive piece of programming code that hides in another piece of programming code that looks harmless, such as a macro or e-mail message (White, 2001).

Fortunately, there are effective antivirus software packages on the market today. These programs have three main features: signature-based scanning, terminate-resident monitoring, and multilevel generic scanning.

Signature-based scanning works by recognizing the unique pattern, or signature, of a virus. As new viruses appear, the antivirus program developers catalogue their signatures. The signature scanning feature of the antivirus software then scans applications, messages, and files as they are downloaded or opened, searching for matches to the signatures in the catalogue. Some types of viruses are designed to avoid detection by the signature scanning feature. *Terminate-and-stay-resident* antivirus software runs in the background while an application runs in the foreground. It is useful for finding hard-to-detect viruses such as stealth viruses and polymorphic viruses. A third feature of most antivirus packages is *multilevel generic scanning*. This type of virus checking employs "expert" analysis techniques to catch viruses the other two features might miss (White, 2001).

Virus checking is an important component of a health information security program. As discussed earlier, virus attacks are very common and can cause extensive damage and loss of productivity. Antivirus software is effective as long as the virus catalogue is updated frequently. Most antivirus software packages can be set to automatically scan the user's computer system periodically to detect and clean any viruses found.

SECURITY IN A WIRELESS ENVIRONMENT

As discussed in earlier chapters, wireless technologies are changing the way health care information systems operate. These technologies cover a wide range of capabilities. Wireless LAN (WLAN) devices allow users to move laptops easily from place to place within the health care organization. Bluetooth technologies allow data synchronization and application sharing across a variety of devices, such as keyboards, printers, and other peripheral devices. Handheld devices allow remote users to synchronize personnel data and to access health care organizations' network services, such as calendars, e-mail, and Internet access. These technologies offer flexibility and new capabilities to health care providers and the individuals that support them (Karygiannis & Owens, 2002). However, the adoption of wireless technologies has been relatively rapid, creating concerns about the level of security they offer in an environment like the health care organization. According to a white paper written by Fluke Networks (2003, p. 1), the issues with wireless security are "exactly the same as with wired security. The problem with wireless is that it's difficult to limit the transmission media to just the areas that we control, or just the hosts we want on our network."

There are specific threats and vulnerabilities to be considered for wireless networks and handheld devices, including the following (Karygiannis & Owens, 2002):

- Malicious entities may gain unauthorized access to a health care organization's computer network through wireless connections, bypassing firewall protections.
- Sensitive information that is not encrypted (or has been encrypted with poor techniques) and is transmitted between two wireless devices may be intercepted and disclosed.
- Denial-of-service attacks may be directed at wireless connections or devices.
- Sensitive data may be corrupted during improper synchronization.
- Handheld devices are easily stolen and can reveal sensitive information.
- Internal attacks may be possible via ad hoc transmissions.
- Unauthorized users may obtain access to the wireless network through piggybacking or war driving. Users who *piggyback* simply gain access through an unsecured wireless internet connection. *War driving* involves unauthorized users driving city streets with an antenna and a wireless computer looking for an Internet connection.

There are currently two cryptographic techniques for the wireless environment, WEP (Wired Equivalent Privacy), and the newer, more secure WPA (Wi-Fi Protected Access). Karygiannis and Owens (2002) note these security problems associated with WEP:

- Security features in vendor products are frequently not enabled.
- Cryptographic keys are short.

- Cryptographic keys are shared.

- Cryptographic keys are not updated automatically.

- There is no user authentication—only device authentication.

In response to these and other security problems with WEP, the new WPA protocol was created by the WiFi Alliance, an industry trade group.

Health care organizations that use wireless technologies should pay close attention to risk analysis for these technologies and make safeguards a part of ongoing risk management. As with other networks and information systems, the organization must know where the threats and vulnerabilities are. Securing the handheld devices and laptop computers commonly associated with a wireless network also poses challenges for the health care organization. Clear policies, and appropriate sanctions for those violating the policies, should be established to govern the downloading of patient-specific information onto personal devices such as these. In addition to the standard inventory control mechanisms and assigning responsibility for portable computers, health care organizations may want to provide their employees with accessories that may minimize theft: for example (Hughes, 2000):

- Cases that do not appear to contain computers.

- Cables with locks that hook onto tables; once this cable is removed from the computer, an unauthorized person cannot turn the computer on.

- Alarms and software that "instruct" the computer to call and "report" its location.

REMOTE ACCESS SECURITY

Health care organizations, like many other modern organizations, allow personnel to work from home. This *remote access* creates additional security issues. In fact there have been a number of security incidents related to the remote use of laptops and other portable devices that store ePHI. In response to these incidents and the potential risk of HIPAA violations due to remote access, CMS issued a HIPAA security guidance document in late December of 2006. The following tables (10.1, 10.2, and 10.3), taken from this HIPAA security guidance document, list potential risks in accessing, storing, and transmitting ePHI when using portable devices in remote locations and describe the management strategies recommended to mitigate these risks.

SUMMARY

Health information is created, maintained, and stored using computer technology. The use of this technology creates new issues in protecting patients' rights to privacy and confidentiality, and demands that health care organizations develop comprehensive information security programs. The publication of the final HIPAA Security Rule in 2003 underscores the importance of securing health information and the need for comprehensive security programs. The standards and specifications of the HIPAA rule can serve as a framework for health care

TABLE 10.1. CMS Recommendations for Accessing ePHI Remotely

Risks	Possible Risk Management Strategies
Log-on/password information is lost or stolen resulting in potential unauthorized or improper access to or inappropriate viewing or modification of EPHI.	Implement two-factor authentication for granting remote access to systems that contain EPHI. This process requires factors beyond general usernames and passwords to gain access to systems (e.g., requiring users to answer a security question such as "Favorite Pet's Name"); Implement a technical process for creating unique usernames and performing authentication when granting remote access to a workforce member. This may be done using Remote Authentication Dial-In User Service (RADIUS) or other similar tools.
Employees access EPHI when not authorized to do so while working offsite	Develop and employ proper clearance procedures and verify training of workforce members prior to granting remote access; Establish remote access roles specific to applications and business requirements. Different remote users may require different levels of access based on job function. Ensure that the issue of unauthorized access of EPHI is appropriately addressed in the required sanction policy.
Home or other offsite workstations left unattended risking improper access to EPHI.	Establish appropriate procedures for session termination (time-out) on inactive portable or remote devices. Covered entities can work with vendors to deliver systems or applications with appropriate defaults.
Contamination of systems by a virus introduced from an infected external device used to gain remote access to systems that contain EPHI.	Install personal firewall software on all laptops that store or access EPHI or connect to networks on which EPHI is accessible; Install, use and regularly update virus-protection software on all portable or remote devices that access EPHI.

Source: CMS Security Guidance, 12/28/2006.

organizations as they design their individual security programs.

Information security programs need to be designed to address internal and external threats to health care information systems, whether those threats are intentional or unintentional. Health information security programs should address administrative, physical, and technical safeguards. This chapter not only outlined the HIPAA security requirements but also provided a discussion of many of the common security measures that can be employed to minimize potential risks to health information.

TABLE 10.2. CMS Recommendations for Storing ePHI on Portable Devices

Risks	Possible Risk Management Strategies
Laptop or other portable device is lost or stolen resulting in potential unauthorized/improper access to or modification of EPHI housed or accessible through the device.	Identify the types of hardware and electronic media that must be tracked, such as hard drives, magnetic tapes or disks, optical disks or digital memory cards, and security equipment and develop inventory control systems;
	Implement process for maintaining a record of the movements of, and person(s) responsible for, or permitted to use hardware and electronic media containing EPHI;
	Require use of lock-down or other locking mechanisms for unattended laptops;
	Password protect files;
	Password protect all portable or remote devices that store EPHI;
	Require that all portable or remote devices that store EPHI employ encryption technologies of the appropriate strength;
	Develop processes to ensure appropriate security updates are deployed to portable devices such as Smart Phones and PDAs;
	Consider the use of biometrics, such as fingerprint readers, on portable devices.
Use of external device to access corporate data resulting in the loss of operationally critical EPHI on the remote device.	Develop processes to ensure backup of all EPHI entered into remote systems;
	Deploy policy to encrypt backup and archival media; ensure that policies direct the use of encryption technologies of the appropriate strength.
Loss or theft of EPHI left on devices after inappropriate disposal by the organization.	Establish EPHI deletion policies and media disposal procedures. At a minimum this involves complete deletion, via specialized deletion tools, of all disks and backup media prior to disposal. For systems at the end of their operational lifecycle, physical destruction may be appropriate.
Data is left on an external device (accidentally or intentionally), such as in a library or hotel business center.	Prohibit or prevent download of EPHI onto remote systems or devices without an operational justification;
	Ensure workforce is appropriately trained on policies that require users to search for and delete any files intentionally or unintentionally saved to an external device;
	Minimize use of browser-cached data in web based applications which manage EPHI, particularly those accessed remotely.
Contamination of systems by a virus introduced from a portable storage device.	Install virus-protection software on all portable or remote devices that store EPHI.

Source: CMS Security Guidance, 12/28/2006.

TABLE 10.3. CMS Recommendations for Transmitting ePHI from Remote Locations

Risks	Possible Risk Management Strategies
Data intercepted or modified during transmission.	Prohibit transmission of EPHI via open networks, such as the Internet, where appropriate;
	Prohibit the use of offsite devices or wireless access points (e.g. hotel workstations) for non-secure access to email.
	Use more secure connections for email via SSL and the use of message-level standards such as S/MIME, SET, PEM, PGP etc.;
	Implement and mandate appropriately strong encryption solutions for transmission of EPHI (e.g. SSL, HTTPS etc.).
	SSL should be a minimum requirement for all Internet-facing systems which manage EPHI in any form, including corporate web-mail systems.
Contamination of systems by a virus introduced from an external device used to transmit EPHI.	Install virus-protection software on portable devices that can be used to transmit EPHI.

Source: CMS Security Guidance, 12/28/2006.

KEY TERMS

Access Control
Administrative safeguards
Assigned security responsibilities
Audit trails
Chief security officer
Covered entity (CE)
Data encryption
Entity authentication
Firewall protection
HIPAA security rule
Media controls
Password
Personal identification number (PIN)

Physical access controls
Physical safeguards
Pretty good privacy (PGP)
Public key infrastructure (PKI)
Remote access
Risk analysis
Systems security evaluation
Technical safeguards
Tokens
Virus checking
WiFi protected access (WPA)
Wired equivalent privacy (WEP)
Wireless LAN (WLAN)

LEARNING ACTIVITIES

1. Do an Internet or library search for recent articles discussing the HIPAA Security Rule. From your research, write a short paper discussing the impact of these

security regulations on health care organizations. How have these regulations changed the way organizations view security? Do you think the regulations are too stringent? Not stringent enough? Just right? Explain your rationale.

2. Interview a chief security officer at a hospital or other health care facility. What are the major job responsibilities of this individual? To whom does he or she report within the organization? What are the biggest challenges of the job?

3. Contact a physician's office or clinic, and ask if the organization has a security plan. Discuss the process that staff undertook to complete the plan, or develop an outline of a plan for them.

SENIOR MANAGEMENT IT CHALLENGES

CHAPTER

ORGANIZING INFORMATION TECHNOLOGY SERVICES

LEARNING OBJECTIVES

- To be able to describe the roles, responsibilities, and major functions of the IT department or organization.

- To be able to discuss the role and responsibility of the chief information officer (CIO), chief medical informatics officer (CMIO), chief security officer (CSO), chief technology officer (CTO), and other key IT staff.

- To be able to describe the different ways IT services might be organized and governed within a health care organization.

- To be able to identify key attributes of highly effective IT organizations.

- To be able to develop a plan for evaluating the effectiveness of the IT function within an organization.

By now you should have an understanding of health care data, the various clinical and administrative applications that are used to manage those data, and the processes of selecting, acquiring, and implementing health care information systems. You should also have a basic understanding of the core technologies that are common to many health care applications, and you can appreciate some of what it takes to ensure that information systems are reliable and secure.

In many health care organizations an information technology (IT) function employs staff who are involved in these and other IT-related activities—everything from customizing a software application to setting up and maintaining a wireless network to performing system backups. In a solo physician practice, this responsibility may lie with the office manager or lead physician. In a large hospital setting, this responsibility may lie with the IT department in conjunction with the medical staff, the administration, and the major departmental units—for example, admissions, finance, radiology, and nursing.

Some health care organizations outsource a portion or all of their IT services; however, they are still responsible for ensuring that those services are of high quality and support the IT needs of the organization. This responsibility cannot be delegated entirely to an outside vendor or information technology firm. Health care executives must manage information technology resources just as they do human, financial, and other facility resources.

This chapter provides an overview of the various functions and responsibilities that one would typically find in the IT department of a large health care organization. We describe the different groups or units that are typically seen in an IT department. We review a typical organizational structure for IT and discuss the variations that are often seen in that structure and the reasons for them. This chapter also presents an overview of the senior IT management roles and the roles with which health care executives will often work in the course of projects and IT initiatives. IT outsourcing, in which the health care organization asks an outside vendor to run IT, is reviewed. Finally, we examine approaches to evaluating the efficiency and effectiveness of the IT department.

INFORMATION TECHNOLOGY FUNCTIONS

The IT department has been an integral part of most hospitals or health care systems since the early days of mainframe computing. If the health care facility was relatively large and complex and used a fair amount of information technology, one would find IT staff "behind the scenes" developing or enhancing applications, building system interfaces, maintaining databases, managing networks, performing system backups, and carrying out a host of other IT support activities. Today the IT department is becoming increasingly important, not only in hospitals but in all health care organizations that use IT to manage clinical and administrative data and processes.

Throughout this chapter we refer to the IT department usually found in a large community hospital or health care system. We chose this setting because it is typically the most complex and IT intensive. Moreover, many of the principles that apply to managing IT resources in a hospital setting also apply in other types of health care facilities, such as an ambulatory care clinic or rural community health center. The breadth and scope of the services provided may differ considerably, however, depending on the extent to which IT is used in the organization.

IT Department Responsibilities

The IT department has several responsibilities:

- Ensuring that an IT plan and strategy have been developed for the organization and that the plan and strategy are kept current as the organization evolves; these activities are discussed in Chapter Twelve.

- Working with the organization to acquire or develop and implement needed new applications; these processes were discussed in Chapters Six and Seven.

- Providing day-to-day support for users: for example, fixing broken personal computers, responding to questions about application use, training new users, and applying vendor-supplied upgrades to existing applications.

- Managing the IT infrastructure: for example, performing backups of databases, installing network connections for new organizational locations, monitoring system performance, and securing the infrastructure from virus attacks.

- Examining the role and relevance of emerging information technologies.

Core Functions

To fulfill their responsibilities, all IT departments have four core functions. Depending on the size of the IT group and the diversity of applications and responsibilities, a function may require several subsidiary departments or subgroups.

Operations and Technical Support The *operations and technical support function* manages the IT infrastructure—for example, the servers, networks, operating systems, database management systems, and workstations. This function installs new technology, applies upgrades, troubleshoots and repairs the infrastructure, performs "housekeeping" tasks such as backups, and responds to user problems, such as a printer that is not working.

This function may have several IT subgroups:

- Data center management: manages the equipment in the organization's computer center.

- Network engineers: manage the organization's network technologies.

- Server engineers: oversee the installation of new servers, and perform such tasks as managing server space utilization.

- Database managers: add new databases, support database query tools, and respond to database problems such as file corruptions.

- Security: ensure that virus protection software is current, physical access to the computer room is constrained, disaster recovery plans are current, and processes are in place to manage application and system passwords.

■ Help desk: provide support to users who call in with problems such as broken office equipment, trouble with operating an application, a forgotten password, or uncertainty about how to perform a specific task on the computer.

■ Deployments: install new workstations and printers, move workstations when groups move to new buildings, and the like.

■ Training: train organization staff on new applications and office software, such as presentation development applications.

Applications Management The *applications management* group manages the processes of acquiring new application systems, developing new application systems, implementing these new systems, providing ongoing enhancement of applications, troubleshooting application problems, and working with application suppliers to resolve these problems.

This function may have several IT groups:

■ Groups that focus on major classes of applications: for example, a financial systems group and a clinical systems group.

■ Groups dedicated to specific applications (this is most likely in large organizations): for example, a group to support the applications in the clinical laboratory or in radiology.

■ An applications development group (this is found in organizations that perform a significant amount of internal development).

■ Groups that focus on specific types of internal development: for example, a Web development group.

Specialized Groups Health care organizations may develop groups that have very specialized functions, depending on the type of organization or the organization's approach to IT. For example:

■ Groups that support the needs of the research community in academic medical centers

■ Process redesign groups in organizations that engage in a significant degree of process reengineering during application implementation

■ Decision-support groups that help users and management perform analyses and create reports from corporate databases: for example, quality-of-care reports or financial performance reports

In addition, the chief information officer (CIO), who is the most senior IT executive, is often responsible for managing the organization's telecommunications function—the staff who manage the phone system, overhead paging system, and nurse call systems. Depending on the organization's structure and the skill and interests of the CIO, one occasionally finds these other organizational functions reporting to the CIO:

■ The health information management or medical records department

■ The function that handles the organization's overall strategic plan development

■ The marketing department

IT Administration Depending on the size of the IT department, one may find groups that focus on supporting IT administrative activities. These groups may perform such tasks as

- Overseeing the development of the IT strategic plan

- Managing contracts with vendors

- Developing and monitoring the IT budget

- Providing human resource support for the IT staff

- Providing support for the management of IT projects: for example, developing project status reports or providing project management training

- Managing the space occupied by an IT department or group

A typical organizational structure for an IT department in a large hospital is shown in Figure 11.1.

IT Senior Leadership Roles

Within the overall IT group, several positions and roles are typically present. These roles range from senior leadership—for example, the chief information officer—to staff who do the day in, day out work of implementing application systems—for example, systems analysts. In the following sections we will describe several senior-level IT positions, including the

- Chief information officer (CIO)

- Chief technology officer (CTO)

- Chief security officer (CSO)

- Chief medical informatics officer (CMIO)

This is not an exhaustive list of all possible senior-level positions, but the discussion provides an overview of typical roles and functions.

The Chief Information Officer Many midsize and large health care organizations employ a *chief information officer* (CIO). The CIO not only manages the IT department but is also seen as the executive who can successfully lead the organization in its efforts to apply IT to advance its strategies.

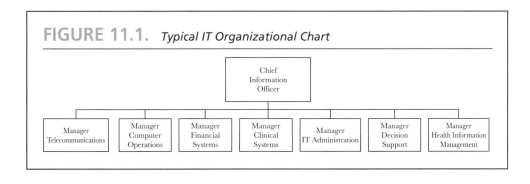

FIGURE 11.1. *Typical IT Organizational Chart*

The role of the CIO in health care and other industries has been the subject of research and debate over the years (Glaser & Williams, 2007). Studies conducted by College of Healthcare Information Management Executives (CHIME) (1998, 2008) have chronicled the evolution of the health care CIO. This evolution has involved debates on CIO reporting relationships, salaries, and titles and the role of the CIO in an organization's strategic planning. Through extensive research, CHIME has identified seven key attributes, or competencies, exhibited by high-performing CIOs (CHIME, 2008). CHIME provides intensive "boot camp" training sessions for its CIO members, to aid in their professional development of these competencies.

1. *Sets vision and strategy.* Collaborates well with senior leaders to set organization vision and strategy and to determine how technology can best serve the organization.

2. *Integrates information technology for business success.* Applies knowledge of the organization's systems, structures and functions to determine how best to advance the performance of the business with technology.

3. *Makes change happen.* Is able to lead the organization in making the processes changes necessary to fully capitalize on IT investments.

4. *Builds technological confidence.* Helps the business assess the value of IT investments and the steps needed to achieve that value.

5. *Partners with customers.* Interacts with internal and external customers to ensure continuous customer satisfaction.

6. *Ensures information technology talent.* Creates a work environment and community that draws, develops and retains top IT talent.

7. *Builds networks and community.* Develops and maintains professional networks with internal and external sources and effectively leverages those networks to further the effective use of IT [CHIME, 2008].

Earlier work by Earl and Feeney (1995) found that CIOs from a wide range of industries who "added value" to their respective organizations had many of these same characteristics. Earl and Feeney found that the value-added CIOs

- Obsessively and continuously focus on business imperatives so that they focus the IT direction correctly.

- Have a track record of delivery that causes IT performance problems to drop off management's agenda.

- Interpret for the rest of the leadership the meaning and nature of the IT success stories of other organizations.

- Establish and maintain good working relationships with the members of the organization's leadership.

▪ Establish and communicate the IT performance record.

▪ Concentrate the IT development efforts on those areas of the organization where the most leverage is to be gained.

▪ Work with the organization's leadership to develop a shared vision of the roles and contributions of IT.

▪ Make important general contributions to business thinking and operations.

Earl and Feeney (1995) also found that the value-added CIO, as a person, has integrity, is goal directed, is experienced with IT, and is a good consultant and communicator. Those organizations that have such a CIO tend to describe IT as critical to the organization, find that IT thinking is embedded in business thinking, note that IT initiatives are well focused, and speak highly of IT performance.

Organizational excellence in IT doesn't just happen. It is managed and led. If the health care organization decides that the effective application of IT is a major element of its strategies and plans, it will need a very good CIO. Failure to hire and retain such talent will severely hinder the organization's aspirations.

Whom the CIO should report to has been a topic of industry debate and an issue inside organizations as well. CIOs will often argue that they should report to the chief executive officer (CEO). This argument is not wrong nor is it necessarily right. The CIO does need access to the CEO and clearly should be a member of the executive committee and actively involved in strategy discussions. However, the CIO needs a boss who is a good mentor, provides appropriate political support, and is genuinely interested in the application of IT. Chief financial officers (CFOs) and chief operating officers (COOs) can be terrific in these regards. In general about one-third of all health care provider CIOs report to the CEO, one-third report to the CFO, and one-third report to the COO.

The Chief Technology Officer   The *chief technology officer* (CTO) has several responsibilities. The CTO must guide the definition and implementation of the organization's technical architecture. This role includes defining technology standards (for example, defining the operating systems and network technologies the organization will support), ensuring that the technical infrastructure is current (for example, that major vendor releases and upgrades have been applied), and ensuring that all the technologies fit. The CTO's role in ensuring fit is similar to an architect's role in ensuring that the materials used to construct a house come together in a way that results in the desired house.

The CTO is also responsible for tracking emerging technologies, identifying the ones that might provide value to the organization, assessing them, and when appropriate, working with the rest of the IT department and the organization to implement these technologies. For example, the CTO may be asked to investigate the possible usefulness of the new biometric security technologies. The CTO role is not often found in smaller organizations but is increasingly common in larger ones. In smaller organizations, the CIO also wears the CTO hat.

The Chief Security Officer   As discussed in Chapter Ten, the *chief security officer* (CSO) is a relatively new position that has emerged as a result of the growing threats to information security and the health care organization's need to comply with HIPAA security regulations. The primary role and functions of the CSO are to ensure that the health care organization has an effective information security plan, that appropriate technical and administrative procedures are in place to ensure that information systems are secure and safe from tampering or misuse, and that appropriate disaster recovery procedures exist.

The Chief Medical Informatics Officer   Like the CSO, the *chief medical informatics officer* (CMIO) is a relatively new position. The CMIO position emerged as a result of the growing interest in adopting clinical information systems and the need for physician leadership in this area. The CMIO is usually a physician, and this role may be filled through a part-time commitment by a member of the organization's medical staff.

Examples of the types of responsibilities a CMIO might assume include

- Leading clinical information system initiatives such as electronic medical record (EMR) implementations
- Serving as physician advocate for computerized provider order entry (CPOE)
- Engaging physicians and other health care professionals in the development and use of the EMR system
- Leading the clinical informatics steering committee or other designated group that serves as the central governance forum for establishing the organization's clinical IT priorities
- Keeping a pulse on national efforts to develop EHR systems, and assuming a leadership role in areas where the national effort and the organization's agenda are synergistic
- Being highly responsive to user needs, such as training, to ensure widespread use and acceptance of clinical systems

Like the CIO and CTO, the role of the CMIO is emerging. Leviss, Kremsdorf, and Mohaideen (2006) conducted structured interview with five CMIOs at health systems that used health information technology widely. The aim of the study was to identify individual skills and organizational structures that helped the CMIO to be effective. Leviss and his colleagues offer the following recommendations to hospital and health system leaders:

- The CMIO should be
  - credible as a good clinician and not be viewed as a "techie doctor" who is only knowledgeable about computers,
  - an effective communicator across services and disciplines,

- an effective consensus builder,
- knowledgeable of hospital operations.
- The hospital CEO and executive leadership must be engaged in the projects involving the CMIO.
- The CMIO should become a senior member of the physician executive leadership team.
  - If the health system organization is large, the CMIO should have budget and operational authority as necessary to support clinical information system initiatives.
- Continuous professional development should be provided to the CMIO. [Leviss et al., 2006]

The CIO, CTO, CSO, and CMIO all play important roles in helping to ensure that information systems acquired and implemented are consistent with the strategic goals of the health care organization, are well accepted and effectively used, and are adequately maintained and secured. Sample job descriptions for the CIO and the CMIO positions are displayed in Exhibits 11.1 and 11.2.

IT Staff Roles

The IT leadership team cannot carry out the organization's IT agenda unilaterally. The department's work relies heavily on highly trained, qualified professional and technical staff to perform a host of IT-related functions. Here are brief descriptions of some key professionals who work in IT:

- The systems analyst
- The programmer
- The database administrator
- The network administrator
- The telecommunications specialist
- Other IT staff

The Systems Analyst   The role of the *systems analyst* will vary considerably depending on the analyst's background and the needs of the organization. Some analysts have a strong computer programming background, whereas others have a business orientation or come from clinical disciplines, such as nursing, pharmacy, or laboratory sciences. In fact, due to the increased interest in the adoption of clinical information systems, systems analysts with clinical backgrounds in nursing, pharmacy, laboratory science, and the like (often referred to as *clinical systems analysts*) are in high demand. Most

EXHIBIT 11.1. *Sample CIO Job Description*

<<XX>> HEALTH CARE SYSTEM, INC.
JOB DESCRIPTION

POSITION TITLE: Chief Information Officer (CIO)
DEPARTMENT: Information Systems & Telecommunications
POSITION REPORTS TO: Chief Financial Officer (CFO)

POSITION SUPERVISES: Information Systems Department, Telecommunications Department

POSITION REQUIREMENTS:
Master of Science Degree in Information Systems or other related field. Five to ten years progressive management experience in Information Systems required. Experience with a multi-unit/integrated health care system preferred. Demonstrated successful leadership in planning, developing, and implementing management information processes, mechanisms, and systems is required. Excellent communication skills, leadership skills, negotiation skills, and motivational abilities are a must.

POSITION SUMMARY:
Responsible for <<XX>> Health Care System's Information Systems Division. This division includes Information Management, Health Information Management and Telecommunications for our multi-location/integrated health care system operating 24 hours a day, 365 days a year. This job description is congruent with the human and community development philosophy of the <<XX>>. The philosophy emphasizes responsibility for human life and the dignity and worth of every person. It also promotes the creation of caring communities in which the needs of those serving and being served are met. It is expected employees will perform their jobs in accordance with the philosophy.

ESSENTIAL FUNCTIONS:

1. Knows, understands, incorporates, and demonstrates the <<XX>> Health Care System Mission, Visions, Values, and Management Philosophy in leadership behaviors, practices, and decisions.

2. Monitors the health care delivery environment in order to anticipate any impact on information systems and communications networks to ensure appropriate utilization of information technology.

3. Examines new systems and develops strategies directed toward increased productivity by improving the work environment through systems and people consistent with the Mission, Vision, Values, and Management Philosophy of the <<XX>> system.

4. Establishes system-wide information management/technology standards and strategies for achieving integration and interoperability of information systems, technology architecture, and selection of software applications.

5. Maintains responsibility for the information system operations including the development and management of operating and capital budgets, policies, human resource utilization, mission effectiveness, and the overall performance of information technology within <<XX>> Health Care System.

6. Develops long-range plans and associated capital and expense budgets and monitors the achievement of these plans in order to ensure the successful performance of the organization.

7. Develops information system plans and programs to improve organization effectiveness and efficiency, ensuring that the information needs of <<XX>> Health Care System information technology staff are met.

8. Creates a seamless process to gather information regarding operational, human resources, financial, and clinical outcomes.

9. Maintains internal and external relationships with all system users and vendors.

10. Responsible for the installation of all new information systems and telecommunication systems for <<XX>> Health Care System.

11. Is a member of the Executive Team providing leadership to <<XX>> Health Care System.

12. Maintains the integrity and security of <<XX>> Health Care System's information systems, complying with all regulatory agencies and statutes.

13. Provides for professional growth and career opportunities for the Information System division staff.

OTHER FUNCTIONS:

1. All other duties as assigned.

_____

APPROVED BY:

_____
DEPARTMENT HEAD   **DATE**

_____
PRESIDENT'S COUNCIL MEMBER   **DATE**

_____
HUMAN RESOURCES DEPARTMENT   **DATE**

REVISION DATES: _____

FOR HUMAN RESOURCES DEPT. USE ONLY: _____ **EXEMPT** _____ **NONEXEMPT**

systems analysts work closely with managers and end users in identifying information system needs and problems, evaluating workflow, and determining strategies for optimizing the use and effectiveness of particular systems. They may specify the inputs to be accessed by a system, design the processing steps, and format the output to meet users' needs.

When an organization decides to implement a new information system, systems analysts are often called upon to determine what computer hardware and software will be needed. They prepare specifications, flowcharts, and process diagrams for computer programmers to follow. They work with programmers to *debug*, or eliminate, errors in the system. Systems analysts may also conduct extensive testing of systems, diagnose problems, recommend solutions, and determine whether program requirements have

EXHIBIT 11.2.   *Sample CMIO Job Description*

JOB DESCRIPTION FOR CHIEF MEDICAL INFORMATION OFFICER

BACKGROUND

The position of Chief Medical Information Officer is a newly created position and reports to the Senior Vice President Information Services, CIO. This individual will lead the development and implementation of automated support for clinicians and clinical analysts through researching, recommending, and facilitating major and advanced clinical information system initiatives for the health care system.

In this role, the incumbent will provide reviews of medical informatics experiences and approaches, develop technical and application implementation strategies, manage implementation of advanced clinical information systems, assist in the development of strategic plans for clinical information systems, and provide project management for co-development relationships with the vendor community.

Information technology at THE HOSPITAL is becoming highly user driven. Governed by the Quality Council, a Clinical Informatics Steering Committee and subcommittees reporting to the Clinical Informatics Steering Committee will be formed to provide a user forum for input, coordination, and integration of information technology with THE HOSPITAL. The Director of Medical Informatics will chair, lead, and support the Clinical Informatics Steering Committee.

The following are ongoing responsibilities of the CHIEF MEDICAL INFORMATION OFFICER:

> Lead the implementation of a computerized patient record (CPR) system for the health care system (hospitals, clinics, physicians offices, ancillary and therapy units). This system should embody an information model focused on the diagnosis, treatment, and process data that will be required in future treatment and preventive care.

> Engage providers with varying roles including independent and employed physicians and clinicians, medical records professionals, and clinical analysts to contribute to the development and use of the CPR and analysis tools.

> Lead and support the Clinical Informatics Steering Committee which serves as the principal user governance forum to determine organizational priorities in this area.

> Stay attuned to the national effort to develop comprehensive, functional, and uniform medical records, and take an active role in areas where the national effort and health care system can mutually benefit.

> Be highly responsive to users' needs, including training, to ensure widespread acceptance and provider use of the clinical systems.

The following are expected accomplishments of the Chief Medical Information Officer for the first 12 to 24 months.

> Gain a thorough understanding of the personality and culture of the organization and community; evaluate and refine the strategic information plan as it relates to clinical informatics.

Develop empathy and understanding of physician needs; build relationships with physicians to gain the support of physician leadership.

Together with a team leader evaluate the skills of the current clinical informatics team, identify needs and build a strong team by enhancing team members' skill base, motivating them and fostering a collaborative approach that values their contribution.

Design a model of the clinical database(s) to support the enterprise-wide CPR. The database(s) should support individual patient care and clinical studies across the full continuum of care.

Guided by the Quality Council, determine an approach and plan for the development and implementation of clinical systems that are components of a computerized patient record. The CPR will be designed to support clinicians in the care of patients throughout the network.

Select the products and vendors for the components of the initial phase of CPR implementation. Be on schedule, according to plan, with the implementations.

Implement physician network services, the transfer of clinical information between network sites, and the presentation of that information on a physician workstation.

The following are the desired credentials, skills, and personality characteristics of the ideal candidate (not listed in priority order):

The successful candidate will have the following profile:

A licensed physician with recent medical practice experience, graduate degree in medical informatics, and one year of work experience in medical informatics. In lieu of graduate training in medical informatics, a minimum of three years work experience in medical informatics systems will be required.

A personable individual with excellent interpersonal and communication skills who can handle a diversity of personalities and interact effectively with people at all levels of the organization.

A strong leader with a mature sense of priorities and solid practical experience to implement the vision for the organization.

An individual who is politically savvy, has a high tolerance for ambiguity, and can work successfully in a matrix management model.

A systems thinker with strong organizational skills who can pull all the pieces together and understand how to deliver ideals.

A strong manager who is adaptable and has a strong collaborative management style.

(Continued)

EXHIBIT 11.2. *(Continued)*

A creative thinker with high energy and enthusiasm.

A team player and consensus builder who promotes the concept of people working together versus individual performance.

A contemporary clinician who understands major trends in health care and managed care and has extensive knowledge of currently available point-of-care products and medical informatics development.

An individual with strong self-confidence who is assertive without being arrogant or ostentatious and who possesses confidence in heavy physician interaction.

---

been met. They may also prepare cost-benefit and return-on-investment analyses to help management decide whether implementing a proposed system will deliver the desired value.

The Programmer   In some organizations the systems analyst and the computer *programmer* fulfill similar roles, particularly if the analyst has a strong programming background. However, many systems analysts do not have such experience, yet they work closely with programmers.

Programmers write, test, and maintain the programs that computers must follow to perform their functions. They also conceive, design, and test logical structures for solving problems with computers. Many technical innovations in programming—advanced computing technologies and sophisticated new languages and programming tools—have redefined the role of programmers and elevated much of the programming work done today (Department of Labor, Bureau of Labor Statistics, 2008).

Programmers are often grouped into two broad types—applications programmers and systems programmers. *Applications programmers* write programs to handle specific user tasks, such as a program to track inventory within an organization. They may also revise existing packaged software or customize generic applications such as integration technologies. *Systems programmers* write programs to maintain and control infrastructure software, such as operating systems, networked systems, and database systems. They are able to change the sets of instructions that determine how the network, workstations, and central processing units within a system handle the various jobs they have been given and how they communicate with peripheral equipment such as other workstations, printers, and disk drives.

The Database Administrator   *Database administrators* work with database management systems software and determine ways to organize and store data. They identify user requirements, set up computer databases, and test and coordinate modifications to these systems. An organization's database administrator ensures the performance of the database systems, understands the platform on which the databases run, and adds new users to the systems. Because they may also design and implement system security, database administrators often plan and coordinate security measures. With the volume of sensitive data growing rapidly, data integrity, backup systems, and database security have become increasingly important aspects of the job for database administrators (Department of Labor, Bureau of Labor Statistics, 2008).

The Network Administrator   As discussed in Part Three of this book, it is essential that the organization has an adequate network or network infrastructure to support all its clinical and administrative applications and also its general applications (such as e-mail, intranets, and the like). Networks come in many variations, so *network administrators* are needed to design, test, and evaluate systems such as local area networks (LANs), wide area networks (WANs), the Internet, intranets, and other data communications systems. Networks can range from a connection between two offices in the same building to globally distributed connectivity to voice-mail and e-mail systems across a host of different health care organizations. Network administrators perform network modeling, analysis, and planning; they may also research related products and make hardware and software recommendations.

The Telecommunications Specialist   Working closely with the network administrator is the *telecommunications specialist*. These specialists manage the organization's telephone systems: for example, the central phone system, cellular telephone infrastructure, and nurse call systems. They often manage the communication network to be used by the organization in the event of a disaster. Because of the progressive convergence of voice networks and data networks, they may design voice and data communication systems, supervise the installation of those systems, and provide maintenance and other services to staff throughout the organization after the system is installed.

Other IT Staff   The growth of the Internet and the expansion of the World Wide Web have generated a variety of occupations related to the design, development, and maintenance of Web sites and their servers. For example, *Web masters* are responsible for all technical aspects of a Web site, including performance issues such as speed of access, and for approving the site content. *Web developers* are responsible for day-to-day site design and creation. Often health care organizations contract with an outside IT company to provide Internet development functions such as those performed by a Web developer.

   The distinctions between the roles and functions of IT staff may seem a bit murky in practice. In one organization the systems analyst might do computer programming, advise on network specifications, and assist in database development. In another organization the systems analyst might have a clinical focus and work primarily with the end users in a particular unit, such as a laboratory, identifying needs, addressing problems, and providing ongoing training and support.

The specific qualifications, roles, and functions of the various IT staff members are generally determined by the pattern of IT development and use within the organization. For example, in a large academic medical center, the IT staff may be actively involved in designing in-house applications, and therefore the organization may employ teams of IT staff to work with faculty and clinicians in developing customized IT tools. This same level of IT expertise would be rare in an organization that relies primarily on IT applications purchased from the health care IT vendor community.

Furthermore, an organization might have an in-house IT services department, yet outsource a number of IT functions, having them performed by staff outside the organization.

Staff Attributes

In addition to ensuring that it has the appropriate IT functions and IT roles (and that the individuals filling these roles are competent), the health care organization must ensure that the IT staff have certain attributes. These attributes are unlikely to arise spontaneously; they must often be managed into existence. An assessment of the IT function (as discussed later in this chapter) can highlight problems in this area and then lead to management steps designed to improve staff attributes.

High-performing IT staff have several general characteristics:

- *They execute well.* They deliver applications, infrastructure, and services that reflect a sound understanding of organizational needs. These deliverables occur on time and on budget, so that those involved in a project give the project team high marks for professional comportment.
- *They are good consultants.* They advise organizational members on the best approach to the application of IT given the problem or opportunity. They advise when IT may be inappropriate or the least important component of the solution. This advice ranges from help desk support to systems analyses to new technology recommendations to advice on the suitability of IT for furthering an aspect of organizational strategy.
- *They provide world-class support.* Information systems require daily care and feeding and problem identification and correction. This support needs to be exceptionally efficient and effective.
- *They stay current in their field of expertise.* They keep up to date on new techniques and technologies that may improve the ability of the organization to apply IT effectively.

Recruitment and Retention of IT Staff

In addition to ensuring that IT staff possess desired attributes, senior leadership may become involved in discussions centered on the attraction and retention of IT staff. Although the IT job market ebbs and flows, the market for talented and experienced IT staff is likely to be competitive for some time (Committee on Workforce Needs in

Information Technology, 2001). In fact, a recent study by Hersh and Wright (2008) estimates that there are approximately 108,000 IT professionals in health care in the United States. As the country moves to higher levels of health information technology adoption, over 40,000 additional IT professionals will be needed. The latest leadership survey conducted by the Healthcare Information and Management Systems Society (HIMSS) among CIOs suggests that organizations are already feeling the shortage. Approximately two-thirds of CIO participants predicted that the number of FTEs in the IT departments at their organizations will increase within the year. The increases are expected to be modest and the most pressing needs are in the areas of clinical application support, network/architecture support and systems integration (HIMSS, 2008a).

Recruitment and retention strategies involve making choices about what work factors and management practices will be changed and how they will be changed in order to improve the organization's ability to recruit and retain. Management may need to determine whether the focus will be on salaries or career development or physical surroundings or some combination of these factors.

For example, the IT managers at Partners HealthCare were asked to identify the factors that make an organization a great place to work and then to rate the Partners IT group on those factors, using letter grades. The factors identified by the managers included

- Salary and benefits
- Physical quality of the work setting, for example, well-maintained surroundings
- Caliber of IT management
- Amount of interesting work
- Importance of the organization's mission
- Opportunities for career growth
- Adequacy of communication about topics ranging from strategy to project status

The managers' grades for Partners IT on these factors are presented in Table 11.1. Using these scores, Partners IT leadership decided to focus on

- Establishing more thorough and better-defined career paths and development programs for all staff
- Improving training opportunities, ranging from brown bag lunches with invited speakers to technical training to supervisory training to leadership training
- Reviewing work environment factors such as parking, free amenities (such as soda), and office furniture
- Improving communication through mechanisms such as sending a monthly e-mail from the CIO, videotaping staff meetings so they could be accessed through streaming media, and having regular dinners and lunches hosted by the CIO and deputy CIO

Taking steps such as these is important. Fundamentally, people work at organizations where the work is challenging and meaningful. They work at places where they

TABLE 11.1. **Managers' Grades for Work Factors**

	A	B	C	D	F
Compensation and benefits	1	14	12	3	
Work environment	4	17	4	3	2
Good management	6	13	8	3	
Interesting work	12	2			
Mission	17	12	1		
Career growth	4	19	5	2	
Communication		8	15	2	5
Status of organization	17	10	3		
TOTAL	61	95	48	13	7

like their coworkers and respect their leadership. They work at places where they are proud of the organization, its mission, and its successes.

ORGANIZING IT STAFF AND SERVICES

Now that we have introduced the various roles and functions found in the health care IT arena, we will examine how these roles and functions can be organized. Essentially, four factors influence the structure of the IT department:

- Definition and formation of major IT units
- Degree of IT centralization or decentralization
- Core IT competencies
- Departmental attributes

Definition and Formation of Major IT Units

There is no single right way to organize IT, and a department may iterate various organizational approaches in an effort to find the one that works best for it. (No approach is free of limitations.) There are several overall approaches to structuring formal departments, and an organization may employ several approaches simultaneously.

First, many IT departments organize their staff according to major job function or service areas. For example, a department might have a communications unit that sets up and manages local area networks and access to wide area networks, a research and development unit that keeps abreast of technology advances and experiments with new products, and a data administration unit that designs and maintains the organization's databases, data warehouses, and data management applications. Under this structure, staff members working in these various areas typically have both specialized and common skills, which they then apply to a wide range of systems or applications throughout the organization.

Second, the IT staff and services may be organized along product lines. That is, IT staff might work as project teams to develop, implement, maintain, and support a particular application or suite of applications. For example, there might be an applications unit comprising five to six major project teams. One team might support the administrative and billing systems, a second might support human and facility resources, and a third might cover clinical areas such as the laboratory, pharmacy, radiology, or nursing. Each team might combine IT staff and end users from the respective area. For example, a CPOE project team might include a systems analyst, a network administrator, a database manager, and key representatives from the clinical areas of medicine, nursing, laboratory, and pharmacy. This approach enables team members to work together closely, gain extensive knowledge about a particular application or suite of applications, and engage in holistic problem solving. In fact the IT staff on the team may be physically located near the user department.

Third, the IT staff may be organized according to critical organizational processes. For example, there may be an IT team that manages and provides IT services to support the patient revenue cycle or patient access or medical services. This arrangement would enable the IT staff to understand all the information systems issues associated with a cross-organization process and develop a comprehensive understanding of critical organizational processes. This approach recognizes that patient care is based not on processes defined by organizational silos, for example, the laboratory or admitting, but rather on processes that cut across silos. Despite the conceptual appeal of this approach, it is not common. Its rarity is due largely to the fact that most organizations are organized by departments and not cross-organization processes: for example, it is rare to see a vice president of patient access. In general it is not intelligent to have IT organized in a way that is radically different from the approach used by the organization overall.

Fourth, the IT department may support a health care organization that is an integrated delivery system (IDS); it has multiple subsidiaries and divisions and may span a wide geography. The form of the IT department in an IDS is invariably matrixed. Kilbridge et al. (1998), in a study of IT organization in integrated delivery systems, found three dimensions that defined this matrix. The *functional* dimension was devoted to IDS-wide infrastructure, such as a communications network and enterprise master person index, and the support of IDS-wide consolidated functions, such as finance. The *geographical* dimension was devoted to supporting distinct geographical sites or logically separate provider sites, such as one of the IDS's community hospitals. The *cross-continuum, process-oriented* dimension might support acute care in general or a *carve-out*, such as oncology services. Figure 11.2 depicts a two-dimensional structure based on function and geography. Figure 11.3 shows a two-dimensional structure based on function and process.

These four approaches are by no means the only way that one might approach organizing IT staff. The CIO, in conjunction with the organization's executive team, should consider a wide range of options for organizing IT staff and resources. As part of this process the executive team should seek input from key constituents, examine

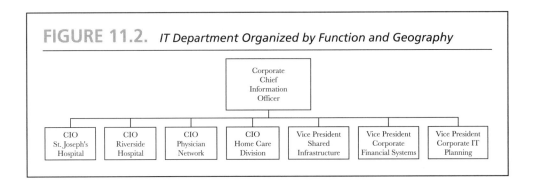

FIGURE 11.2.   *IT Department Organized by Function and Geography*

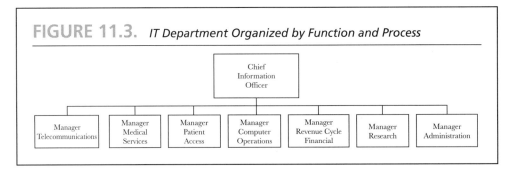

FIGURE 11.3.   *IT Department Organized by Function and Process*

the culture of the organization and the IT department, assess the long-term goals of the organization, and ultimately employ a structure that facilitates IT staff efficiency and effectiveness. In determining the structure of the IT organization, the team may ask these strategic questions: Which approaches will be used? Do the IT groupings represent well-circumscribed clusters of like expertise or common goals? Is the resulting set of departments comprehensive in scope?

Degree of IT Centralization or Decentralization

A critical factor in determining the structure for the IT department is the degree of centralization of organizational decision making. A health care organization might be a highly structured, vertical hierarchy where decisions are made by a few senior leaders. Conversely, an organization might delegate authority to the departmental level, or to the hospital level in an integrated delivery system, resulting in decentralized decision making.

There is no right level of centralization. Centralized organizations can be as effective as decentralized organizations. There are trade-offs. For example, centralized organizations are more likely to be able to effect uniformity of operations and to be more rational in their allocation of capital dollars, whereas decentralized organizations are more likely to be innovative. Moreover, an organization can be centralized in some areas, such as the process for developing the budget, and decentralized in other areas, such as developing marketing plans.

Ideally, the management and structure of IT will parallel that of the executive team's management philosophy; centralized management tends to want centralized control over IT, whereas decentralized management is more likely to be comfortable with IT that can be locally responsive.

One approach is not necessarily better than the other; they both have advantages and trade-offs. Some of the advantages to centralizing IT services are (Oz, 2006)

- *Enforcement of hardware and software standards.* In a centralized structure the organization typically develops software and hardware standards, which can lead to cost savings, facilitate the exchange of data among systems, make installations easier, and promote sharing of applications.

- *Efficient administration of resources.* Centralizing the administration of contracts and licenses and inventories of hardware and software can lead to greater efficiency.

- *Better staffing.* Because it results in a pool of IT staff from which to choose, the centralized approach may be able to identify and assign the most appropriate individuals to a particular project.

- *Easier training.* In a centralized department, staff can specialize in certain areas (hardware, software, networks) and do not need to be jacks of all trades.

- *Effective planning of shared systems.* A centralized IT services unit typically sees the big picture and can facilitate the deployment of systems that are to be used by all units of a health care system or across organizational boundaries.

- *Easier strategic IT planning.* A strategic IT plan should be well aligned with the overall strategic plan of the organization. This alignment may be easier when IT management is centralized.

- *Tighter control by senior management.* A centralized approach to managing IT services permits senior management to maintain tighter control of the IT budget and resources.

Despite the advantages of a more centralized approach to managing IT services, many health care organizations have moved in recent years to a relatively decentralized structure. Some of the advantages to a decentralized structure are (Oz, 2006)

- *Better fit of IT to business needs.* The individual IT units are familiar with their business unit's or department's needs and can develop or select systems that fit those needs more closely.

- *Quick response time.* The individual IT units are typically better equipped to respond promptly to requests or can arrange IT projects to fit the priorities of their business unit or department.

- *Encouragement of end-user development of applications.* In a decentralized IT services structure, end users are often encouraged to develop their own small applications to increase productivity.

- *Innovative use of information systems.* Given that IT staff are closer in proximity to users and know their needs, the decentralized structure may have a better chance of implementing innovative systems.

Most IT services in a health care organization are not fully centralized or decentralized but a combination of the two. For example, training and support for applications may be decentralized, with other IT functions such as application development, network support, and database management being managed centrally. The size, complexity, and culture of the health care organization might also determine the degree to which IT services should be managed centrally. For example, in an ambulatory care clinic with three sites that are fairly autonomous, it may be appropriate to divide IT services into three functional units, each dedicated to a specific clinic. In a larger, more complex organization, such as an integrated delivery network (with multiple hospitals, outpatient clinics, and physician practices), it may be appropriate to form a centralized IT services unit that is responsible for specific IT areas such as systems planning and integration, network administration, and telecommunications, with all other functions being managed at the individual facility level.

Core IT Competencies

Organizations should identify a small number of areas that constitute core IT capabilities and competencies. These are areas where getting an A+ from the "customers" matters. For example, an organization focused on transforming its care processes would want to ensure A+ competency in this area and would perhaps settle for B− competency in its supply chain operations. An organization dedicated to being very efficient would want A+ competency in areas such as supplier management and productivity improvement and would perhaps settle for a B− in delivering superb customer service.

This definition of core competencies has a bearing on the form of the IT organization. If A+ competency is desired in care transformation, the IT department should be organized into functions that specialize in supporting care transformation: for example, a clinical information systems implementation group and a care reengineering group.

Partners HealthCare, for example, defined three areas of core capabilities: base support and services, care improvement, and technical infrastructure.

Base Support and Services   The category of core capabilities at Partners HealthCare included two subcategories:

- Frontline support: for example, PC problem resolution
- Project management skills

The choice of these areas of emphasis resulted in many management actions and steps: for example, the selection of criteria to be used during annual performance reviews. The emphasis on frontline support also led to the creation of an IT function responsible for all frontline support activities, including the help desk, workstation deployments, training, and user account management. The emphasis on project management led to the creation of a project management office to assist in monitoring the status of all projects and a *project center of excellence* to offer training on project management and established project management standards.

Care Improvement Central to the Partners agenda was the application of IT to improve the process of care. One consequence was to establish, as a core IT capability, the set of skills and people necessary to innovatively apply IT to medical care improvement. An applied medical informatics function was established to oversee a research and development agenda. Staff skilled in clinical information systems application development were hired. A group of experienced clinical information system implementers was established. An IT unit of health services researchers was formed to analyze deficiencies in care processes, identify IT solutions that would reduce or eliminate these deficiencies, and assess the impact of clinical information systems on care improvement. Organizational units possessing unique technical and clinical knowledge in radiology imaging systems and telemedicine were also created.

Technical Infrastructure Recognizing the critical role played by having a well-conceived, well-executed, and well-supported technical architecture, infrastructure architecture and design continued to serve as a core competency. A technology strategy function was created, and the role of chief technology officer was created. Significant attention was paid to ensuring that extremely talented architectural and engineering staff were hired along with staff with terrific support skills.

Departmental Attributes

IT departments, like people, have characteristics or attributes. They may be agile or ossified. They may be risk tolerant or risk averse. These characteristics can be stated, and strategies to achieve desired characteristics can be defined and implemented. To illustrate, this section will briefly discuss two characteristics—agility and innovativeness—and discuss how they might affect the organization of IT functions. These two characteristics are representative and are generally viewed as desirable.

There are many steps that an organization can take to increase its overall agility and also that of the IT department (Glaser, 2008a). For example, it is likely to try to *chunk* its initiatives so that there are multiple points at which a project can be reasonably stopped and yet still deliver value. Thus the rollout of a computerized medical record might call for implementation at ten clinics per year but could be stopped temporarily at four clinics and still deliver value to those four. Chunking allows an organization and its departments to quickly shift emphasis from one project to another.

An agile IT department will have the ability to form and disband teams quickly (perhaps every three months) as staff move from project to project. This requires that organizational structures and reporting relationships be flexible so staff can move rapidly between projects. It also means that during a project, the project manager is (temporarily anyway) the boss of the project team members. The team members might report to someone else according to the organizational chart, but their real boss at this time is the project manager. Because team members might move rapidly from project to project, they might have several bosses during the course of a year. And a person might be the boss on one project and the subordinate on another project. Agile organizations and departments are organized less around functions and more around projects. The IT structure must accommodate continuous project team formation, and project managers must have significant authority.

An organization or department that wants to be innovative might take steps such as implementing reward systems that encourage new ideas and successful implementation of innovative applications, and also punishment systems that are loath to discipline those involved in experiments that failed (Glaser, 2008b). The innovative IT department might create dedicated research and development groups. It might form teams composed of IT staff and vendor staff in an effort to cross-fertilize each group of staff with the ideas of the other. It might also permit staff to take sabbaticals or accept internships with other departments in the organization in an effort to expand IT members' awareness of organizational operations, cultures, and issues.

IN-HOUSE VERSUS OUTSOURCED IT

For the past two decades, health care organizations have generally provided IT services in-house. By *in-house* we mean that the organization hired its own IT staff and formed its own IT department. In recent years, however, health care organizations have shown a growing interest in outsourcing part or all of their IT services. Outsourcing IT means that an organization asks a third party to provide the IT staff and be responsible for the management of IT.

The reasons for outsourcing IT functions are varied. Some health care organizations may simply not have staff with the skills, time, or resources needed to take on new IT projects or provide sufficient IT service. Others may choose to outsource certain IT functions, such as help desk services or Web-site development, so that internal IT staff can focus their time on implementing or supporting applications central to the organization's strategic goals. Still other organizations contract with an application service provider (ASP) to run system applications, manage the data, and provide technical support. Outsourcing IT may enable organizations to better control costs. Because a contract is typically established for a defined scope of work to be done over a specific period of time, the IT function becomes a line item that can be more effectively budgeted over time. This does not mean, however, that outsourcing IT services is necessarily more cost effective than providing IT services in-house. At times, new organizational leadership finds an IT function that is in disastrous condition. After years of mismanagement, applications may function poorly, the infrastructure may be unstable, and the IT staff may be demoralized. An outsourcing company may be brought in as a form of rescue mission.

A number of factors come into play and should be considered when evaluating whether outsourcing part or all of IT services is in the best interest of the organization. The questions asked should include the following:

- Does our organization have IT staff with the knowledge and skills needed to provide necessary services? Effectively manage projects? Adequately support current applications and infrastructure?

- How easy or difficult is it to recruit and retain qualified IT staff?

- What are our organization's major IT priorities? How equipped is our organization to address these priorities? Do we have the right mix of skills, time, and resources?

■   What benefits might be realized from outsourcing this IT function? What are the risks? Do the benefits outweigh the risks?

■   What parts, if any, of the IT department does it make the most sense to outsource?

■   If we opt to outsource IT services, whom do we want to do business with? How will we monitor and evaluate IT performance and service? What provisions will we make in the contract with the outsourcing company to ensure timeliness and quality of service? How will the terms of the contract be monitored?

It is important to evaluate the cost and effectiveness of the IT function and services, whether they are performed by in-house staff or outsourced. There are pros and cons to each approach, and the organization must make its decision based upon its strategy goals and priorities. There is no silver bullet or one solution for all.

EVALUATING IT EFFECTIVENESS

Whether IT services are provided by in-house staff or are outsourced, it is important to evaluate IT performance. Is the function efficient? Does it deliver good service? Is it on top of new developments in its field? Does the function have a strong management team?

At times, health care executives become worried about the performance of an IT function. Other organizations have IT functions that seem to accomplish more or spend less. Management and physicians frequently express dissatisfaction with IT; nothing is getting done, it costs too much, or it takes too long to get a new application implemented. Many factors may result in user dissatisfaction: poor expectation setting, unclear priorities, limited funding, or inadequate IT leadership. An assessment of IT services can help management understand the nature of the problems and identify opportunities for improvement.

One desirable approach to assessing IT services is to use outside consultants. Consultants can bring a level of objectivity to the assessment process that is difficult to achieve internally. They can also share their experiences from having worked with a variety of different health care organizations and having observed different ways of handling some of the same issues or problems.

Whether the assessment is done by internal staff or by consultants, several key areas should be addressed:

■   Governance

■   Budget development and resource allocation

■   System acquisition

■   System implementation

■   IT service levels

Governance

How effective is the governance structure? To what degree are IT strategies well aligned with the organization's overall strategic goals? Is the CIO actively involved in strategy discussions? Does senior leadership discuss IT agenda items on a regular basis? We will discuss governance in Chapter Thirteen.

Budget Development and Resource Allocation

The IT budget is often compared to the IT budgets of comparable health care organizations. The question behind a budget benchmark is, Are we spending too much or too little on IT? Budget benchmarks are expressed in terms of the IT operating budget as a percentage of the overall organization's operating budget and the IT capital budget as a percentage of the organization's total capital budget. On average, hospitals spend 2.7 percent of their operating budget and 15 percent of their capital budget on IT (Gartner, 2007).

These budget benchmarks are useful and in some sense required because most boards of directors expect to see them. Management has to be careful in interpreting the results, however. These percentages do not necessarily reflect the quality of IT services or the extent and size of the organization's application base or infrastructure. Hence one can find a poorly performing IT group that has implemented little having the same percentage of the organization's budgetary resources as a world-class IT group that has implemented a stunning array of applications.

Spending a high percentage of the operating budget—for example, 4.5 percent—does not per se mean that the organization is spending too much and should reduce its IT budget. The organization may have decided to ramp up its IT investments in order to achieve certain strategic objectives. A low percentage—for example, 1 percent—does not per se mean that underinvestment is occurring and the IT budget should be significantly increased. The organization may be very efficient, or it may have decided that given its strategies its investments should be made elsewhere.

We will discuss the IT budget and resource allocation in Chapter Thirteen.

System Acquisition

How effective are system acquisitions? How long did they take? What process was used to select the systems? We discussed system acquisition in Chapter Six.

System Implementation

Are new applications delivered on time, within budget, and according to specification? Do the participants in the implementation speak fondly of the professionalism of the IT staff or do they view IT staff as forms of demonic creatures? We discussed system implementation in Chapter Seven.

IT Service Levels

IT staff deliver service every day: for example, they manage system performance, respond to help desk calls, and manage projects. The quality of these services can be measured. An assessment of the IT function invariably reviews these measures and the management processes in place to monitor and improve IT services. IT users in the organization are interested in measures such as these:

- *Infrastructure.* Are the information systems reliable, that is, do they rarely "go down"? Are response times fast?

- *Day-to-day support.* Does the help desk quickly, patiently, and effectively resolve my problems? If I ask for a new workstation, does it arrive in a reasonable period of time?

- *Consultation.* Are the IT folks good at helping me think through my IT needs? Are they realistic in helping me to understand what the technology will and will not do?

An organization faces a challenge in defining what level of IT service it would like and also how much it is willing to pay for IT services. All of us would love to have systems analysts with world-class consulting skills, but we may not be able to afford their salaries. Similarly, all of us would love to have systems that never go down and are as fast as greased lightning, but we might not be willing to pay the cost of engineering very, very high reliability and blazing speed. The IT service conversation attempts to establish formal and measurable levels of service and the cost of providing that service. The organization seeks an informed conversation about the desirability and the cost of improving the service or the possibility of degrading the service in an effort to reduce costs.

In general it can be very difficult to measure the quality and consequences of consultative services. This makes it difficult to understand whether it is worth investing to improve the service other than at the service extremes. For example, it can be clear that you need to fire a very ineffective systems analyst and that you need to treat your all-star analyst very well. But it may not be clear whether paying $10,000 extra for an IT staff member is worth it or not.

Formal, measurable service levels can be established for many infrastructure attributes and day-to-day support. Moreover, industry benchmarks exist for these measures. Infrastructure service metrics may include

- *Reliability:* for example, the percentage of time that systems have unscheduled downtime

- *Response time:* for example, how quickly an application moves from one screen to the next

- *Resiliency:* for example, how quickly a system can recover after it goes down

- *Software bugs:* for example, the number of bugs detected in an application per line of program code or hour of use

Day-to-day support service metrics may include

- The percentage of help desk calls that are resolved within twenty-four hours

- The percentage of help desk calls that are not resolved after five days

- The percentage of help desk calls that are repeat calls: that is, the problem was not resolved the first time

- The time that elapses between ordering a workstation and its installation

It is important that the management team define the desired level of IT service. For example, is the goal to achieve an uptime of 99.99 percent, or does the organization want to have 90 percent of help desk calls closed within twenty-four hours? If the service levels are deemed to be inadequate, a discussion can be held with IT managers to identify the costs of achieving a higher level of service. Additional staff may be needed at the help desk, or the organization may need to develop a redundant network to improve resiliency. Conversely, if the organization needs to reduce IT costs, the management team may need to examine the service consequences of reducing the number of help desk staff.

The assessment of the IT function requires examining areas that range from strategy development to service levels. And the assessment can use a variety of data collection techniques. Exhibit 11.3 is a sample survey used by an IT services department to assess user satisfaction.

Answers to these questions provide an indication, clearly rough, of how well the IT function is being run and, to a degree, of whether the aggregate IT investment is providing value. All these questions come from common sense, management beliefs about what is involved in running an organization well, and tests of IT domain knowledge.

PERSPECTIVE

ASSESSING THE IT FUNCTION

Glaser (2006) proposes a series of questions that can be used to assess the IT function. These questions cover the areas of infrastructure and application performance, execution and strategic alignment.

Infrastructure and application performance

External and internal auditors' reports on IT controls and management. Do these reports note material problems with significant downtime, failure to perform adequate management of the data center, and adequacy of security controls?

IT infrastructure management processes. Does IT track downtime and what steps have been taken to reduce it? Are they current with vendor releases? How does IT manage virus protection? When the infrastructure has problems what are the procedures for responding?

Execution

Achieving desired application outcomes. Picking three recent implementations, what were the objectives? To what degree were the objectives achieved? If the organization fell short in achieving objectives, why did this happen?

(Continued on page 311)

EXHIBIT 11.3. *Sample User Satisfaction Survey*

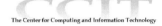

The Center for Computing and Information Technology

CUSTOMER SERVICE SURVEY

University Administration and the Center for Computing and Information Technology (CCIT) are reaffirming their commitment to continuous improvement of their services by asking for your feedback on CCIT's quality of service to you. The questions are intended to give us input on the department's strengths and weaknesses and get a feel as to what you, our customers, would like to see. Please be frank and candid in your answers. Only with your help can we improve the services CCIT provides to you! If you would prefer, you can complete this survey on-line at http://www.musc.edu/ccit/.

Thank you in advance for your participation!

Please, tell us about yourself . . .

You are: (circle one)   Faculty   Staff   Information Technology Corrdinator   Student   Resident   Temp

If "staff" or "temp," where do you work?

College   Ambulatory Care/ Medical Center/UMA   Finance and Administration   University Support (for example, Enrollment Services, Library)

Does your department have a computer support resource (for example, ITC)?   Yes   No   Don't Know

Which CCIT-supported systems do you use? (circle all used routinely)

General

Audix (voice mail)   CentreVu (CMS)   Internet services   PPP server   Telephone

Information References

Auget   *Catalyst*   "Tips"   CCIT web page   Keane newsletter   *PacketXpress*

Educational/Research Systems

American Fundware   CDMIS   Faculty Profile System   Grants Accounting   GCG, Sybil   Homeroom

MUSCLS   Netscape Calendar   Ovid   SPSS (UNIX)   Usenet News   WWW Server

Clinical Systems

AeroMed	ANSOS	AutoTrack	Burn Unit MR	Cerner Pathology	Coding (3M)	
DeMedici	Downtime MPI	DS Plus	EPS	ESI/Nova	GI Trac/ GI Image	
HARP	IDXRad	Infection Control	Keane / PatcomPlus	LANVision	Med Staff
MediLinks	MediScribe	Meduline/Centramax	MRS / Tumor Reg.	MSMeds/Megasource	MSDS
MUSCHealth.com	MUSE	NucMed Pharmacy	Oacis / Passport	Odyssey	Oversite
PACS	PAID	QS1 OP Pharmacy	RenalStar	SMS	Summit
SurgiServer	Trendstar	Velos	VingMed/EchoPac		

Administrative and Financial Systems

Colleague/Datatel   Effort Reporting   HeRMIT   Parking Svcs   SmartStream   STAR/Kronos

Workstation Support (circle your configuration)

ClinLAN   Macintosh   Win 95/'98/NT/2000   Linux / UNIX   FinLAN / Metaframe / Citrix

(Continued)

EXHIBIT 11.3. (Continued)

Now, what do you think about us . . .

Help Desk Staff	Very satisfied	Somewhat satisfied	Neutral	Somewhat dissatisfied	Very dissatisfied
1. Requests are clearly understood	5	4	3	2	1
2. Troubleshooting skills are adequate	5	4	3	2	1
3. If not able to resolve, are able to identify right resource	5	4	3	2	1
4. Professional, friendly, diplomatic	5	4	3	2	1
5. Understands needs and priorities	5	4	3	2	1
6. Treats you with respect and consideration	5	4	3	2	1

Systems Support Staff					
1. Responsive to problems/requests	5	4	3	2	1
2. Professional, friendly, diplomatic	5	4	3	2	1
3. Understands needs and priorities	5	4	3	2	1
4. Treats you with respect and consideration	5	4	3	2	1
5. Communicates well	5	4	3	2	1
6. Quality of work is high	5	4	3	2	1
7. Positive attitude	5	4	3	2	1
8. Plans/manages projects well	5	4	3	2	1

Workstation Support Staff					
1. Responsive to problems/requests	5	4	3	2	1
2. Professional, friendly, diplomatic	5	4	3	2	1
3. Understands needs and priorities	5	4	3	2	1
4. Treats you with respect and consideration	5	4	3	2	1
5. Communicates well	5	4	3	2	1
6. Quality of work is high	5	4	3	2	1
7. Positive attitude	5	4	3	2	1
8. Plans/manages projects well	5	4	3	2	1

Do you have additional comments about your experiences with our staff?

Overall, how satisfied are you with CCIT? very satisfied   satisfied   neutral   not satisfied   very dissatisfied

Would you like to be interviewed? For "yes," please note your name and MUSC extension:

Thank you again for your time and assistance!

PERSPECTIVE (*Continued from page 308*)

User engagement. Do implemented systems improve the operation of key departments? Was the training good? Were the IT group and the vendor responsive to issues and problems?

Managing the implementation. Were clear project charters developed? Are sound project management techniques used? Do most projects get done on time and on budget?

Frontline support. Does the IT organization measure its service? Has the IT organization established service goals? Was the organization's management involved in setting those goals?

Departmental IT liaisons. Who are the IT liaisons to major user departments and do they do a good job? Do the liaisons keep the department up to date on IT plans? Are liaisons considered to be members of department's team?

Alignment of the IT Agenda with the Organization's Agenda

IT linkage to organizational strategy. Can the major elements of the organization's strategy be mapped to the IT initiatives needed to support the strategic plan? Is there a regular senior leadership discussion of the IT agenda and does the leadership take responsibility for making decisions about which IT initiatives to fund?

Governance. What processes and committees are used to set priorities? Is the process for setting the IT budget well understood, efficient, sufficiently rigorous and perceived as fair? Is there a well-accepted approach for acquiring new applications?

Source: Glaser, 2006, p. 104.

PERSPECTIVE

MANAGING CORE IT PROCESSES

Agarwal and Sambamurthy have identified eight core IT processes that must be managed well for an IT department to be effective:

1. *Human capital management* involves the development of IT staff skills and the attraction and retention of IT talent.

2. *Platform management* is a series of activities that designs the IT architecture and constructs and manages the resulting infrastructure.

(*Continued*)

PERSPECTIVE (*Continued*)

3.   *Relationship management* centers on developing and maintaining relationships between the IT function and the rest of the organization and on partnerships with IT vendors.

4.   *Strategic planning* links the IT agenda and plans to the organization's strategy and plans.

5.   *Financial management* encompasses a wide range of management processes—developing the IT budget, defining the business case for IT investments, and benchmarking IT costs.

6.   *Value innovation* involves identifying new ways for IT to improve business operations and ensuring that IT investments deliver value.

7.   *Solutions delivery* includes the selection, development, and implementation of applications and infrastructure.

8.   *Services provisioning* centers on the day-to-day support of applications and infrastructure: for example, the help desk, workstation deployments, and user training.

Source: Agarwal & Sambamurthy, 2002, p. 43.

SUMMARY

It is critical that health care organizations have access to appropriate IT staff and resources to support their health care information systems and system users. IT staff perform several common functions and have several common roles. In large organizations, the IT department often has a management team comprising the chief information officer, chief technology officer, chief security officer, and chief medical informatics officer, who provide leadership to ensure that the organization fulfills its IT strategies and goals. Having a CIO with strong leadership skills, vision, and experience is critical to the organization achieving its strategic IT goals. Working with the CIO and IT management team, one will often find a team of professional and technical staff including systems analysts, computer programmers, network administrators, database administrators, and Web designers and support personnel. Each brings a unique set of knowledge and skills to support the IT operations of the health care organization.

The organizational structure of the IT department is influenced by several factors: definition of major units, level of centralization, core IT competencies, and desired attributes of the IT department.

IT services may be provided by in-house staff or outsourced to an outside vendor or company. Many factors come into play in deciding if and when to outsource all or part of the IT services. Availability of staff, time constraints, financial resources, and the executive management team's view of IT may determine the appropriateness of outsourcing.

Whether IT services are provided in-house or outsourced, it is important for the management team to assess the efficiency and effectiveness of IT services. The governance structure, how the IT resources are allocated, the track record of system acquisitions and system implementations, and user satisfaction with current IT service levels are some of the key elements that should be examined in any assessment. Consultants may be employed to conduct the assessment and offer the organization an outsider's objective view.

KEY TERMS

Applications manager
Chief information officer (CIO)
Chief medical informatics officer (CMIO)
Chief security officer (CSO)
Chief technology officer (CTO)
Clinical systems analyst
Database administrator
Governance
IT centralization

IT decentralization
IT functions
Network administrator
Outsourced IT
Programmer
Systems analyst
Telecommunications specialist
Web developer
Web master

LEARNING ACTIVITIES

1. Visit an IT department in a health care facility in your community, and interview the CIO or department director. Examine the IT department's organizational structure. What functions or services does the IT department provide? How centralized are IT services within the organization? Does the organization employ a CMIO, CSO, or CTO? If so, what are each person's job qualifications and responsibilities?

2. Find an article in the literature that outlines either the advantages or disadvantages, or both, of outsourcing IT. Discuss the findings with your classmates. What have others learned about outsourcing that may be important to your organization?

3. Plan and organize a panel discussion with CIOs from local health care facilities. Find out what some of their greatest challenges are and what a typical day is like for them. To what degree are their organizations facing workforce shortages? In what areas, if any? What strategies do they employ to recruit and retain top-notch staff?

4. Assume that your organization is concerned about employee satisfaction with IT services. How might the organization assess employee satisfaction? What methods and tools might be used? How would you use these methods and tools?

5.   Investigate any one of the following roles, and interview someone working in this type of position. Find out the individual's roles, responsibilities, qualifications, background, experience, and challenges.

- Chief medical informatics officer
- Chief security officer
- Chief technology officer
- Nursing informatics specialist
- Clinical systems analyst
- Biomedical informatics expert

CHAPTER

12

IT ALIGNMENT AND STRATEGIC PLANNING

LEARNING OBJECTIVES

- To be able to understand the importance of an IT strategic plan.
- To review the components of the IT strategic plan.
- To be able to understand the processes for developing an information technology strategy.
- To be able to discuss the challenges of developing an IT strategy.
- To be able to appreciate the ability of information technology to improve organizational competitiveness and performance.

Information technology (IT) investments serve to advance organizational performance. These investments should enable the organization to reduce costs, improve service, enhance the quality of care, and in general, achieve its strategic objectives. The goal of IT alignment and strategic planning is to ensure a strong and clear relationship between IT investment decisions and the health care organization's overall strategies, goals, and objectives. For example, an organization's decision to invest in a new claims adjudication system should be the clear result of a goal of improving the effectiveness of its claims processing process. An organization's decision to implement a computerized provider order entry system should reflect an organizational strategy of improving patient care.

Developing a sound alignment can be very important for one simple reason; if you define the IT agenda incorrectly or even partially correctly, you run the risk that significant organizational resources will be misdirected; the resources will not be put to furthering strategically important areas. This risk has nothing to do with how well you execute the IT direction you choose. Being on time, on budget, and on specification is of little value to the organization if it is doing the wrong thing!

The IT alignment and strategic-planning process has several broad objectives:

■ Ensure that IT plans and activities are well linked to the plans and activities of the organization. This means that the IT needs of each aspect of organizational strategy are clear, and the overall portfolio of IT plans and activities can be mapped to organizational strategies and operational needs.

■ Ensure that the alignment is comprehensive. In other words:

Each aspect of strategy has been addressed from an IT perspective, recognizing that not all aspects have an IT component and not all IT components will be funded.

The non-IT organizational initiatives have been addressed, such as any process reengineering needed to ensure maximum leverage of the IT initiative.

The organization has not missed a strategic IT opportunity: for example, one that might result from new technologies.

■ Develop a tactical plan that details approved project descriptions, timetables, budgets, staffing plans, and plan risk factors.

■ Create a communication tool that can inform the organization of the IT initiatives that will be undertaken and those that will not.

■ Establish a political process that helps to ensure that the IT plan has sufficient organizational support.

At the end of the alignment and strategic-planning process an organization should have an outline that at a high level resembles Table 12.1. With this outline the leadership can see the IT investments needed to advance each of the organization's strategies. For example, the goal of improving the quality of patient care may lead the organization

TABLE 12.1. **IT Support of Organizational Goals**

Goal	IS Initiatives
Research and education	Research patient data registry Genetics and genomics platform Grants management
Patient care: Quality improvement	Quality measurement databases Order entry Electronic medical record
Patient care: Sharing data across the system	Enterprise master person index Clinical data repository Common infrastructure
Patient care: Nonacute services	Nursing documentation Transition of care
Financial stability	Revenue system enhancements PeopleSoft Cost accounting

to invest in databases to measure and report quality, computerized provider order entry (CPOE), and an electronic medical record (EMR) system.

Despite the simplicity implied by Table 12.1, the development of well-aligned IT strategies has been notoriously difficult for many years, and there appears to be no reason to expect that crafting this alignment will become significantly easier over time.

This chapter discusses the challenges of and approaches to IT alignment and strategic planning. We will address

- An overview of strategy
- The areas requiring IT strategy
- The vectors for arriving at IT strategy
- The IT asset and governing concepts
- A normative approach to developing IT alignment and strategy
- The challenges of IT strategy and alignment
- Information technology as a competitive advantage

OVERVIEW OF STRATEGY

The strategy of an organization has two major components (Henderson & Venkatraman, 1993): formulation and implementation.

Formulation

Formulation of strategy involves making decisions about the mission and goals of the organization and the activities and initiatives it will undertake to achieve that mission and those goals. Formulation may involve, for example, determining that

- Our mission is to provide high-quality medical care.
- We have a goal of reducing the cost of care while preserving the quality of that care.
- One of our greatest leverage points lies in reducing inappropriate and unnecessary care.
- To achieve this goal we emphasize, for example, reducing the number of inappropriate radiology procedures.
- We will carry out initiatives that enable us to intervene at the time of procedure ordering if we need to suggest a more cost-effective modality.

The organization's members may also recognize other goals directed to achieving the same mission. For each goal they can envision multiple leverage points, and for each leverage point they may see multiple initiatives. An inverted tree that cascades from the mission to a series of initiatives will emerge.

Formulation of initiatives involves understanding competing ideas and choosing between them. In the example just given, leadership could have arrived at a different set of goals and initiatives. It could have decided to improve quality with less emphasis on care costs. It could have decided to focus on reducing the cost per procedure. It could have decided to produce retrospective reports, by provider, of radiology utilization and to use this feedback to manage behavioral change, rather than deciding to intervene at the time of ordering.

IT strategy also needs formulation. For example, in keeping with an IT mission to use technology to support the improvement of the quality of care, an organization may have a goal to integrate clinical application systems. To achieve this goal, it may examine and have to choose between the following ideas:

- Provide a common way to access all systems (single sign-on).
- Interface existing heterogeneous application systems.
- Require that all applications use a common database.
- Implement a common suite of clinical applications from one vendor.

Implementation

Implementation involves making decisions about how the organization structures itself, acquires skills, establishes capabilities, and alters processes in order to achieve the goals and carry out the activities defined during formulation. For example, if organizational leadership has decided to reduce care costs by reducing inappropriate procedure use, it may need to implement

- An organizational unit of providers with health service research training to analyze care practices and identify deficiencies

- A steering committee of clinical leaders to guide these efforts and provide political support

- A CPOE system to provide real-time feedback on order appropriateness

- Data warehouse technologies to support the analyses of utilization

Returning to the clinical applications integration example, an organization may, on the one hand, determine that it needs to acquire interface engine technology, adopt HL7 standards, and form an IT function that manages the technology and interfaces applications. Or, on the other hand, it may decide it needs to engage external consulting assistance for selection of a clinical application suite and that it needs to hire a group to implement the suite.

The implementation component of strategy development is not the development of project plans and budgets. Rather it is the identification of those capabilities, capacities, and competencies that the organization will need if it is to carry out the results of the formulation component of strategy.

AREAS REQUIRING IT STRATEGY

IT strategy is very important in three major areas (which are discussed further in subsequent sections).

First, an IT strategy is important in the development of the *application agenda*, an inventory of desired applications or major improvements to existing applications. Table 12.1 is an example of such an agenda.

Second, the IT strategy shapes initiatives designed to improve the *IT asset*. An organization's IT applications, infrastructure, data, staff and department, and governance make up its IT asset. Initiatives can be designed to add major capabilities to this asset—the ability to access the organization's applications around the globe, for example. Or initiatives might aim to enhance characteristics of the asset—to make the IT organization more agile, for example.

Third, the IT strategy involves concepts that govern the approach to a class of initiatives and applications. The notion of *governing concepts* can be difficult to get your mind around. However, it is essential to do so. Governing concepts define how an organization "thinks about" or "views" many different things. Some governing concepts will concern IT applications or the IT function. For example, does the organization want to be on the cutting edge of IT, or would it prefer to be more conservative, and why? Are Internet technologies viewed as tools that will enable organizational transformation, or are they seen as normal, incremental improvements in technology? Is the EMR system viewed primarily as solving problems associated with the accessibility of the patient record, or is it seen primarily as a means to improve disease management? Is it considered preferable to buy IT systems or build them?

IT STRATEGY VECTORS

In many ways the content of Table 12.1 is deceiving. The table presents a tidy, orderly linkage between the IT agenda and the strategies of the organization. One might assume that this linkage is established through a linear, rational, and straightforward series of steps. But the process of arriving at a series of connections like those in Table 12.1 is complex, iterative, and at times driven by politics and instincts.

There are five major vectors an organization may follow to arrive at an IT strategy. IT strategy may grow out of

1. Organizational strategies
2. Continuous improvement of core processes and information management
3. Examination of the role of new information technologies
4. Assessment of strategic trajectories
5. Fundamental views about competition or the nature of organizations

By *vectors* we mean the perspectives and approaches through which an organization chooses to determine its IT investment decisions. For example, the first vector (derived from organizational strategies) involves answering a question such as this: Given our strategy of improving patient safety, what IT applications will we need? However, the third vector (determined by examining the role of new information technologies) involves answering a question such as this: There is a great deal of discussion about wireless technologies. What types of applications would wireless enable us to perform, and would these applications be important to us? Figure 12.1 illustrates the convergence of these five vectors into a series of iterative leadership discussions and debates. These debates lead to an IT agenda composed of an application inventory, IT asset initiatives, and governing concepts.

Organizational Strategies Vector

The first vector involves deriving the IT agenda directly from the organization's goals and plans. For example, an organization may decide that it intends to become the

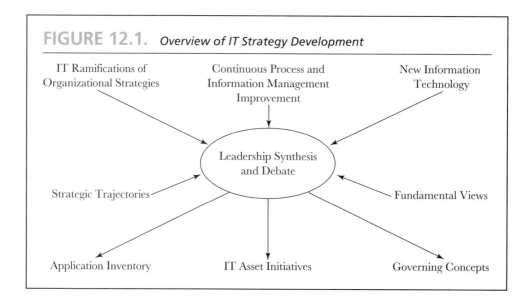

FIGURE 12.1. *Overview of IT Strategy Development*

IT Ramifications of Organizational Strategies

Continuous Process and Information Management Improvement

New Information Technology

Leadership Synthesis and Debate

Strategic Trajectories

Fundamental Views

Application Inventory

IT Asset Initiatives

Governing Concepts

low-cost provider of care. It may decide to achieve this goal through the implementation of disease management programs, the reengineering of inpatient care, and the reduction of unit costs for certain tests and procedures that it believes are inordinately expensive.

The IT strategy development then centers on answering questions such as this one: How do we apply IT to support disease management? The answer might involve Web-based publication of disease management protocols for use by providers, data warehouse technology to assess the conformance of care practice to the protocols, provider documentation systems based on disease guidelines, and CPOE systems that employ the disease guidelines to guide ordering decisions. An organization may choose all or some of these responses and develop various sequences of implementation. Nonetheless, it has developed an answer to the question of how to apply IT in the support of disease management. The IT plan would define the application systems and resources—for example, staff and budgets—needed to support the goals.

Most of the time the linkage between organizational strategy and IT strategy involves developing the IT ramifications of organizational initiatives such as adding or changing services and products, growing market share, or reducing costs. At times, however, an organization may decide that it needs to change or add to its core characteristics or culture. The organization may decide that it needs its staff to be more care quality or service-delivery or bottom-line oriented. It may decide that it needs to decentralize decision making or to recentralize decision making. It may decide to improve its ability to manage knowledge, or it may not. These characteristics, and there are many others, can point to initiatives for IT.

In the cases where characteristics are to be changed, IT strategies must be developed that answer questions like this: What is our basic IT approach to supporting a decentralized decision-making structure? The organization might answer this question by permitting decentralized choices of applications as long as those applications meet certain standards: for example, run on a common infrastructure or support a common database standard. It might answer the question of how IT supports an emphasis on knowledge management by developing an intranet service that provides access to preferred treatment guidelines.

Continuous Improvement Vector

All organizations have a small number of core processes and information management tasks that are essential for the effective and efficient functioning of the organization. For a hospital these processes might include ensuring patient access to care, ordering tests and procedures, and managing the revenue cycle. For a restaurant these processes might include menu design, food preparation, and dining room service. For a managed care organization, information management needs might point to a requirement to understand the costs of care or the degree to which care practices vary by physician.

Using the vector of continuous improvement of core processes and information management to determine IT strategies involves defining the organization's core processes and information management needs. The organization measures the performance of core processes and uses the resulting data to develop plans to improve its performance. The organization defines core information needs, identifies the gap between the current status and its needs, and develops plans to close those gaps. These plans will often point to an IT agenda.

This vector may be a result of a strategy discussion but not always. An organization may make ongoing efforts to improve processes regardless of the specifics of its strategic plan. For example, every year it may set initiatives designed to reduce costs or improve services.

Table 12.2 illustrates a process orientation. It provides an organization with data on the magnitude of some problems that plague the delivery of outpatient care. These problems afflict the processes of referral, results management, and test ordering. The organization may decide to make IT investments in an effort to reduce or eliminate these problems. For example, outpatient CPOE could reduce the prevalence of adverse drug events. Reminders in an EMR system could help the physician remember to order cholesterol tests for patients at high risk of hypercholesterolemia.

When this vector is used, the IT agenda is driven at least in part by a relentless, year in, year out focus on improving core processes and information management needs.

New Information Technology Vector

The third vector involves considering how new IT capabilities may enable a new IT agenda or significantly alter the current agenda. For example, telemedicine capabilities may enable the organization to consider a strategy that it had not previously considered, such as extending the reach of its specialists across the globe, or may alter its approach to achieving an existing strategy, so that, for example, it relies less on specialists visiting regional health centers and more on teleconsultation. Wireless technologies may enable the organization to consider applications that previously were not effective because there was no good way to address the needs of the mobile worker—for example, medication

TABLE 12.2. Summary of Scope of Outpatient Care Problems

For every...	There appear to be...
1,000 patients coming in for outpatient care	14 with life-threatening or serious adverse drug events (ADEs)
1,000 outpatients who are taking a prescription drug	90 who seek medical attention because of drug complications
1,000 prescriptions written	40 that have medical errors
1,000 women with a marginally abnormal mammogram	360 who will not receive appropriate follow-up care
1,000 referrals	250 referring physicians who have not received follow-up information 4 weeks later
1,000 patients who qualify for secondary prevention of high cholesterol	380 who will not have a low-density-lipoprotein cholesterol (LDL-C) measurement recorded within the next 3 years

administration systems can now be used at the bedside rather than requiring the nurse to return to a central work area to document administration.

In this vector the organization examines new applications and new base technologies and tries to answer the question, Does this application or technology enable us to advance our strategies or improve our core processes in new ways? For example, applications that support communication between physician and patient through the Internet might lead the organization to think of new approaches to providing feedback to the chronically ill patient. Holding new technologies up to the spotlight of organizational interest can lead to decisions to invest in a new technology.

An extreme form of this mechanism occurs when a new technology or application suggests that fundamental strategies or even the organization's existence may be called into question or need to undergo significant transformation. Although IT-induced transformation is rare in health care, it is being seen in other industries. The Internet, for example, is transforming and in some case challenging the existence of a range of companies that distribute content. Examples are companies such as bookstores, record and CD stores, publishers, travel agents, and stockbrokers.

Strategic Trajectories Vector

Organizational and IT strategies invariably have a fixed time horizon and fixed scope. These strategies might cover a period of time two to three years into the future. They outline a bounded set of initiatives to be undertaken in that time period. Assessment of strategic trajectories asks the question, What do we think we will be doing after that time horizon and scope? Do we think that we will be doing very different kinds of things, or will we be carrying out initiatives similar to the ones that we are doing now?

For example, an organization might be planning to introduce decision support into its CPOE application. This decision support would point out drug-drug interactions and drug–lab test interactions. Answering the question about trajectories for that decision support might indicate to that patient genetic information will eventually need to be part of the organization's decision-support approach, because genetic makeup can have a significant impact on patient tolerance of a drug. Or an organization might be in the process of implementing electronic data interchange to support the basic payer-provider transactions: for example, eligibility determination and claims submission. Organization leaders expect that this support will significantly improve the efficiency of these transactions. Answering the question about trajectories for systems that link the provider to the payer might indicate that the organization is heading into a time of ever-tighter integration between payer and provider information systems. This integration might become so strong that it should examine the merger of its master patient index with the payer subscriber database in order for both provider and payer to eliminate problems associated with misidentification of patients or subscribers.

The trajectory discussion may be grounded on IT applications, as in the examples just given. It may also be grounded on today's organization, with an effort being made to envision the organization as it would like to be in the future. That vision may point to IT strategy directions and needs. For example, a vision of an organization with exceptional patient service might indicate the need to move toward applications that enable patients to book their own appointments.

The strategic trajectory discussion can be highly speculative. It might be so forward looking and speculative that the organization decides not to act today on that discussion. Yet it can also point to initiatives to be undertaken within the next year to better understand this possible future and to prepare the organization's information systems for it. For example, if the organization believes that its information systems will eventually need to store genetic information, it would be worth understanding whether the new clinical data repository it will be selecting soon will be capable of storing these data.

Fundamental Views Vector

Several IT strategic-planning methodologies are based on fundamental views of the nature of organizations, organizational processes, or competition. Often these views are found first in literature that examines management and strategy issues in general, and then they are adapted for use in IT strategic planning.

The competitive forces model (Porter, 1980) is an example of a fundamental view, and we'll use it to illustrate this vector. The competitive forces model examines forces that shape the competitive environment and hence an industry's (and its member organizations') profitability. Porter (1980) identifies five competitive forces that determine an industry's profitability: the bargaining power of buyers, the bargaining power of suppliers, the threat of new entrants, the threat of substitute products, and the rivalry among existing competitors.

Consider some health care examples of these forces. The competitive strength of a managed care organization is weakened if employers (buyers of insurance) have significant bargaining power. If a hospital has already made a significant commitment to an IT vendor, then it has a difficult time negotiating a reduction in fees because the vendor (the supplier) knows that the hospital is unlikely to deinstall a large number of applications. Community-based primary care physicians may be threatened by the arrival of minute clinics in large stores. A breakthrough in outpatient surgery (a substitute product) could mean that lucrative inpatient surgery volume will diminish. Clearly, a market with several, strong nursing home competitors will lead to smaller margins for all nursing home organizations than will a market with only weak competition.

In order to gain a competitive advantage, companies must devise methods to counter each of these forces. IT can be one of those methods. Conversely, the use of IT by others might threaten an organization's competitive position. For example, the bargaining power of patients (buyers) over providers and payers may be increased by consumer-oriented Web sites that rate provider quality. The barriers that new entrants in some industries must surmount have increased due to the large investments needed to remain on the cutting edge of IT: for example, organizations often join integrated delivery systems because of the capital cost of the information technology viewed as necessary in order to compete. The Internet can reduce the role of traditional channels, such as the referring physician (a buyer of specialty services), by supporting the patient's ability to find and access a specialist. Internet-based health insurance companies, often focusing on supporting a movement to defined contributions, can be viewed as offering a substitute product and thus are a threat to a traditional payer.

IT can also enable the creation of new health care industries and businesses—for example, Internet-based health care consumer content, health insurance products, and providers of second opinions—all of which alter the rivalry force.

Porter's framework could guide the development of IT strategy by encouraging the organization to ask questions such as, How can we apply IT to strengthen our role as a supplier (for example, by providing access to clinical systems to our referring physicians)? or, Can we use IT to develop substitute products (for example, by using telemedicine as a replacement for face-to-face interaction with a specialist)? The process of arriving at an IT strategic plan using the competitive forces framework requires a very different conversation from the conversation that centers on the organization's published strategic plan.

Vector Summary

Developing IT alignment and strategy requires the convergence of five vectors of thinking and discussion, although the fifth vector (IT strategy based on fundamental views about competition and organizations) is not commonly used in health care. These vectors bring multiple orientations to strategy formulation and implementation, and each often results in a different management discussion.

Methodologies have been developed to help guide organizations through the necessary discussions. Organizations commonly use consultants for this purpose; they can provide not only methodologies but also perspectives on new technologies and the IT agenda and the experiences of other health care organizations.

Whether methodologies or consultants are used or not, the development of the IT strategy is not a cookbook exercise. At its core the alignment with organizational strategy is achieved because smart, thoughtful organizational leaders take the time to discuss the IT strategy. On the one hand alignment sounds very simple—smart people talk about it. On the other hand such simplicity means that there is a significant amount of art to this process. In general the accountability for developing an aligned IT agenda should rest with the CIO.

THE IT ASSET AND GOVERNING CONCEPTS

The discussion of vectors and alignment up to this point has focused generally on the development of an application agenda as the outcome. In other words, the completion of the IT strategy discussion is an inventory of systems, such as the EMR system, customer relationship management system, and clinical laboratory system, that are needed to further overall organizational strategies. However, the application inventory is a component of the larger idea of the IT asset. And in addition to the IT asset, the IT strategy conversation must address governing concepts. These areas are discussed in the following sections.

The IT Asset

The *IT asset* is composed of those IT resources that the organization has or can obtain and that are applied to further the goals, plans, and initiatives of the organization. The IT strategy discussion identifies specific changes or enhancements to the composition of the asset—for example, the implementation of a new application—and general properties of the asset that must exist—for example, high reliability of the infrastructure. The IT asset has five components: applications, infrastructure, data, IT staff, and IT governance.

Applications   *Applications* are the systems that users interact with: for example, scheduling, billing, and electronic medical record systems. In addition to developing an inventory of applications, the organization may need to develop strategies regarding properties of the overall portfolio of applications.

For example, if the organization is an integrated delivery system, decisions will need to be made about the degree to which applications should be the same across the organization. E-mail systems ought to be the same, but is there a strategic reason to have the same clinical laboratory system across all hospitals? Should an organization buy or build its applications? Building applications is risky and often requires skills that most health care organizations do not possess. However, internally developed applications can be less expensive and can be tailored to an organization's needs.

Strategic thinking may center on the form and rigor of the justification process for new applications. Formal return on investment analyses may be emphasized so that all application decisions will emphasize cost reduction or revenue gain. Or the organization may decide to have a decision process that takes a more holistic approach to acquisition decisions, so that factors such as improving quality of care must also be considered.

In general, strategy discussions surrounding the application asset as a whole focus on a few key areas:

- *Sourcing.* What are the sources for our applications? And what criteria determine the source to be used for an application? In other words, should we buy or build applications? If we buy, should we get all applications from the same vendor or will we use a small number of approved vendors?

- *Application uniformity.* If we are a large organization with many subsidiaries or locations, to what degree should our applications be the same at all locations? If some have to be the same but some can be different, how do we decide where we allow autonomy? This discussion often involves a trade-off between local autonomy and the central desire for efficiency and consistency.

- *Application acquisition.* What processes and steps should we use when we acquire applications? Should we subject all acquisitions to rigorous analyses? Should we use a request for proposal for all application acquisitions? This discussion is generally an assessment of the extent to which the IT acquisition process should follow the degree of rigor applied to non-IT acquisitions (of diagnostic equipment, for example).

Infrastructure   *Infrastructure* needs may arise from the strategic-planning process. An organization desiring to extend its IT systems to community physicians will need to ensure that it can deliver low-cost and secure network connections. Organizations placing significant emphasis on clinical information systems must ensure very high reliability of their infrastructure; computerized provider order entry systems cannot go down.

In addition to initiatives designed to add specific components to the infrastructure— for example, new software to monitor network utilization—architecture strategies will focus on the addition or enhancement of broad infrastructure capabilities and characteristics.

Capabilities are defined by completing this sentence: "We want our applications to be able to . . ." Organizations might complete that sentence with phrases such as "be accessed from home," "have logic that guides clinical decision making," or "share a pool of consistently defined data."

Characteristics refer to broad properties of the infrastructure, such as reliability, agility, supportability, integrability, and potency. An organization may be heading into the implementation of mission-critical systems and hence must ensure very high degrees of reliability in its applications and infrastructure. The organization may believe that it is in the middle of a large amount of environmental uncertainty and hence must place a premium on agility. The asset plans in these cases involve discussions and analyses that are intended to answer the questions: What steps do we need to take to significantly improve the reliability of our systems? or, If we need to change course quickly, how do we ensure an agile IT response?

Data *Data* and *information* were discussed in Chapters One and Two and *data management* in Chapter Eight. Strategies surrounding data may center on the degree of data standardization across the organization, accountability for data quality and stewardship, and determination of database management and analyses technologies.

Data strategy conversations may originate with questions such as, We need to better understand the costs of our care. How do we improve the linkage between our clinical data and our financial data? or, We have to develop a much quicker response to outbreaks of epidemics. How do we link into the city's emergency rooms and quickly get data on chief complaints?

In general, strategies surrounding data focus on acquiring new types of data, defining the meaning of data, determining the organizational function responsible for maintaining that meaning, integrating existing sets of data, and obtaining technologies used to manage, analyze, and report data.

IT Staff *IT staff* are the analysts, programmers, and computer operators who, day in and day out, manage and advance information systems in an organization. IT staff were discussed in Chapter Eleven. Alignment discussions may highlight the need to add IT staff with specific skills, such as Web developers and clinical information system implementation staff. Organizations may decide that they need to explore outsourcing the IT function in an effort to improve IT performance or obtain difficult-to-find skills. The service orientation of the IT group may need to be improved.

In general the IT staff strategies focus on the acquisition of new skills, the organization of the IT staff, the sourcing of the IT staff, and the characteristics of the IT department—is it, for example, innovative, service oriented, and efficient?

IT Governance   *IT governance* is the organizational mechanisms by which IT priorities are set, IT policies and procedures are developed, and IT management responsibility distributed. IT governance will be discussed in Chapter Thirteen.

In addition to creating an application inventory, the IT strategy can lead to asset strategies and plans. Strategies may be developed that alter the asset, as a response to questions such as these:

- What is our approach to ensuring that it will become easier to integrate applications?

- What is our approach to attracting and retaining superb IT talent?

- How do we improve our prioritization of IT initiatives?

- Which data should be consistently defined across the organization, and how do we develop those definitions?

In general, significant changes to the IT asset are defined during the alignment discussion as a result of answering two questions:

- Does our IT strategy suggest that we should make major changes to any portion of our IT asset?

- Are there areas of our IT asset that require significant improvements in performance?

Governing Concepts

At times, classes of technology, applications, and IT management techniques (which we will refer to collectively as *technologies* in this section) appear to have the potential to make a significant impact on the health care industry and its organizations and on the way those organizations implement and apply information systems. Examples today include Web 2.0, service-oriented architectures, knowledge management, and electronic medical record systems.

It may not be clear initially how particular technologies could further organizational strategies or what their impact could be on the IT asset. As organizations adopt or explore the adoption of technologies, they develop concepts that guide how they think about these technologies, which in turn has great influence over whether and how they will adopt a technology and how they will evaluate its success. For example, there are several ways to think about the various technologies that compose Web 2.0:

- A powerful means for communities of patients to learn from each other but not something that the hospital can influence

- Something that teenagers and people who are bored do

- A mechanism that the hospital can use (by sponsoring sites and guiding conversations) to leverage its support of patients with chronic diseases

- A way to keep track of what people are saying about an organization

All these concepts are correct in that all can be effective. However, once an organization chooses a concept or concepts it tends to think about the technology in that way, often to the exclusion of other ways to think about it. Moreover the organization's concept may be wrong or only half-potent. For example, if an organization views cell phones as a consumer but not an organizational technology, it will miss an extraordinary set of other opportunities for these technologies.

Governing concepts have a considerable impact on all aspects of our lives, and their ramifications are significant. For example:

- One can view the Bible as literal, allegorical, or something that one doesn't think about at all.

- One can view the role of the federal government as being to protect shores and individual freedoms or to compensate for and overcome injustice and deficiencies in the free market.

- One can view an individual's destiny as being heavily influenced by his or her environment and genes, largely determined by the choices he or she makes in life, or preordained by larger forces in the universe.

- One can view the goal of a college education as being preparing for a job, garnering knowledge of one's society and civilization, or attending a prolonged party.

There is no one formula or cookbook for arriving at governing concepts. The strategic-planning vectors discussed earlier in this chapter represent different governing concepts. This chapter will not attempt to present a methodology for concept development. Concepts emerge from complex and not well understood phenomena involving insight, discussions among members of the organization's leadership, examinations of the strategic efforts of others, the organization's successes and failures (and the reasons it assigns for success and failure), and organizational values and history that form the basis for judging views. The basis for concept formation is a small number of questions. These questions are often easy to state. For example:

- What is it about the EMR that makes it important to us?

- Should we view electronic prescribing (the electronic linkage of a provider's medication ordering with the pharmacy benefits manager's eligibility determination function with the retail pharmacy's fulfillment function) as a competitive advantage, or should we view it as a regional utility? If we view it as the former, we should proceed unilaterally. If we view it is as the latter, we should put together a regional collaborative to develop it.

- When we say that we want to integrate our systems, what does integration mean to us? Common data? Common interface? Common application logic?

- Should IT be a tightly controlled resource, or should we encourage multiple instances of IT innovation? What would cause us to choose one approach over the other?

Developing thoughtful and insightful answers to questions such as these is difficult. Nonetheless, forming such concepts is critical.

A minority of the elements that make up the IT strategy will require the discussion about governing concepts. The IT strategy may be clear and not helped by high-altitude conceptual discussions. If the organization needs a new patient accounting system, it may not gain any ground by examining the conceptual nature of patient accounting systems. That said, it is not easy to know where conceptual discussions might be helpful. In general these discussions may have merit for those elements of the IT strategy that are deemed to be particularly critical, that possess a high degree of uncertainty because they are new to the industry and hence real experience is limited, or that require a very large investment.

A NORMATIVE APPROACH TO IT STRATEGY

You may now be asking yourself, How do I bring all of this together? In other words, is there a suggested approach that an organization can take to develop its IT strategy that takes into account these various vectors? And by the way, what does an IT strategic plan look like?

Across health care organizations the approaches taken to developing, documenting, and managing an IT strategy are quite varied. Some organizations have well-developed, formal approaches that rely on the deliberations of multiple committees and leadership retreats. Other organizations have remarkably informal processes—a small number of medical staff and administrative leaders meet, in informal conversations, to define the organization's IT strategy. In some cases the strategy is developed during a specific time in the year, often preceding the development of the annual budget. In other organizations IT strategic planning goes on all the time, permeating a wide range of formal and informal discussions.

There is no right way to develop an IT strategy and to ensure alignment. However, the process for developing IT strategy should be similar in approach and nature to the process used for overall strategic planning. If the organization's core approach to strategy development is informal, so should be its approach to IT strategy development.

Recognizing this variability, a normative approach to the development of IT strategy can be offered.

Strategy Discussion Linkage

Organizational strategy is generally discussed in senior leadership meetings. These meetings may be focused specifically on strategy or strategy may be a regular agenda item. These meetings may be supplemented with retreats centered on strategy development and with task forces and committees that are asked to develop recommendations for specific aspects of the strategy: for example, a committee of clinical leadership might be asked to develop recommendations for improving patient safety.

Regardless of their form, the organization's CIO should be present at such meetings or kept informed of the discussion and its conclusions. If task forces and committees supplement strategy development, an IT manager should be asked to be a member. The CIO (or the IT member of a task force) should be expected to develop an assessment of the IT ramifications of strategic options and to identify areas where IT can enable new approaches to strategy. The CIO will not be the only member of the leadership team who will perform this role. CFOs, for example, will frequently identify the IT ramifications of plans to improve claims processing. However, the CIO should be held accountable for ensuring that the linkage does occur.

As strategy discussions proceed, the CIO must be able to summarize and critique the IT agenda that should be put in place to carry out the various aspects of the strategy. Two examples follow. The first displays an IT agenda that might emerge from a strategy designed to improve the patient service experience in outpatient clinics. The second displays a health plan IT agenda that could result from a strategy designed to improve patient access to health information and self-service administrative tasks.

PERSPECTIVE

SAMPLE IT AGENDA FOR A STRATEGY TO IMPROVE PATIENT SCHEDULING SERVICE

Strategic Goal

Improve service to outpatients.

Problem

- Patients have to call many locations to schedule a series of appointments and services.
- The quality of the response at these locations is highly variable.
- Locations inconsistently capture necessary registration and insurance information.
- Some locations are over capacity and others are underutilized.

IT Solution

- Common scheduling system for all locations.
- A call center for "one-stop" access to all outpatient services.
- Development of master schedules for common service groups: for example, preoperative testing.
- Integration of scheduling system with electronic data interchange connection to payers for eligibility determination, referral authorization, and copay information.
- Patient support material—for example, maps and instructions—to be mailed to patient.

PERSPECTIVE

SAMPLE IT AGENDA FOR A STRATEGY TO IMPROVE HEALTH INFORMATION ACCESS AND SELF-SERVICE FOR PATIENTS

Strategic Goals

- Improve service to subscribers.
- Reduce costs.

Problem

- Subscribers have difficulty finding high-quality health information.
- The costs of performing routine administrative transactions—for example, changes of address and responses to benefits questions—is increasing.
- Subscriber perceptions are that the quality of service in performing these transactions is low.

IT Solution

- A plan portal that provides subscribers with

    Health information content from high-quality sources

    Access to chronic disease services and discussion groups

    Self-service functions to perform routine administrative transactions

    Access to benefit information

    The ability to ask questions

    Plan ratings of provider quality

- A plan-sponsored provider portal that enables subscribers to

    Conduct routine transactions with their provider: for example, request appointments or renew prescriptions.

    Have electronic visits with their provider for certain conditions: for example, back pain.

    Ask care questions of their provider.

IT Liaisons

All major departments and functions—for example, finance, nursing, and medical staff administration—should have a senior IT staff person who serves as the function's point of contact. As these functions examine ways to improve their processes—for example, lower their costs and improve their services—the IT staff person can work with them to identify IT activities necessary to carry out their endeavors. This identification often emerges with recommendations to implement new applications that advance the performance of a function, such as a medication administration record application to improve the nursing workflow. Here is an example of output from a nursing leadership discussion on improving patient safety through the use of a nursing documentation system.

PERSPECTIVE

SAMPLE OF RECOMMENDATIONS FOR IT NURSING DOCUMENTATION SUPPORT TO IMPROVE PATIENT SAFETY

Problem Statement

- Both the admitting physician(s) and nurse document medication history in their admission notes.
- Points of failure have been noted:

    Incompleteness due to time or recall constraints, lack of knowledge, or lack of clear documentation requirements

    Incorrectness due to errors in memory, transcription between documents, and illegibility

    Multiple inconsistent records due to failure to resolve conflicting accounts by different caregivers

- Most of the clinical information required to support appropriate clinician decision making is obtained during the history-taking process.

Technology Interventions and Goals

- A core set of clinical data should be made available to the clinician at the point of decision making:

    Demographics

(Continued)

PERSPECTIVE (*Continued*)

> Principle diagnoses and other medical conditions
>
> Drug allergies
>
> Current and previous relevant medications
>
> Laboratory and radiology reports
>
> ▪ Required information should be gathered only once:
>
>> Multidisciplinary system of structured, templated documentation
>>
>> Clinical decision support rules, associated with specific disciplines, to guide gathering
>>
>> Workflow that supports the mobile caregiver with integrated wireless access to clinical information
>
> ▪ Needed applications could be implemented in phases:
>
>> Nursing admission assessment
>>
>> Multidisciplinary admission assessment
>>
>> Planning and progress
>>
>> Nursing discharge plan
>>
>> Multidisciplinary discharge plan

New Technology Review

The CIO should be asked to discuss, as part of the strategy discussion or in a periodic presentation in senior leadership forums, new technologies and their possible contributions to the organization's goals and plans. These presentations may lead to suggestions that the organization form a task force to closely examine a technology. For example, a multidisciplinary task force could be formed to examine the role of wireless technology in nursing care, materials management, and service provision to referring physicians. Table 12.3 provides an example of a review of the potential contribution of wireless technology; various potential uses of wireless technology are assessed according to their expected ability to increase revenue, reduce costs, improve care quality, and improve patient service.

Synthesis

The CIO should be asked to synthesize, or summarize, the conclusions of these discussions. This synthesis will invariably be needed during the development of the annual

TABLE 12.3. **Potential Value Proposition for Wireless Technology**

Function	Value			
	Revenue	Cost Savings	Care Quality	Service
Medical information or textbooks	L	L	M	L
Lab test orders	M	L	L	L
Medication orders	H	M	H	M
Results retrieval	L	M	M	L
Patient charting	M	L	M	L
Charge capture	H	M	L	M
Supply management	L	H	L	L

Note: H = High, M = Medium, L = Low.

budget. And the synthesis will be a necessary component of the documentation and presentation of the organization's strategic plan. Table 12.4 presents an example of such a synthesis.

The organization should expect that the process of synthesis will require debate and discussion: for example, trade-offs will need to be reviewed, priorities set, and

TABLE 12.4. **Sample Synthesis of IT Strategic Planning**

Strategic Challenge	IT Agenda
Capacity and growth management	Emergency Department tracking Inpatient electronic bed board Ambulatory clinic patient tracking
Quality and safety	Inpatient order entry Anticoagulation therapy unit Online discharge summaries Medication administration record
Performance improvement	Registration system overhaul Anatomic pathology Pharmacy Order communication Transfusion and donor services
Budget management and external reviews	Disaster recovery Joint Commission preparation Privacy policy review

the organization's willingness to implement embryonic technologies determined. This synthesis and prioritization process can occur in the course of leadership meetings, through the work of a committee charged to develop an initial set of recommendations, and during discussions internal to the IT management team.

An example of an approach to prioritizing recommendations is to give each member of the committee "$100" to be distributed across the recommendations. The amount a member gives to each recommendation reflects his or her sense of its importance. For example, a member could give one recommendation $90 and another $10 or give five recommendations $20 each. In the former case the committee member believes that only two recommendations are important and the first one is nine times more important than the second. In the latter case the member believes that five recommendations are of equal importance. The distributed dollars are summed across the members, with a ranking of recommendations emerging.

For an example of the scoring of proposed IT initiatives, see Figure 12.2. It lists categories of organizational goals—for example, improve service and invest in people—along with goals within the categories. The leadership of the organization, through a series of meetings and presentations, has underscored the contribution of the IT initiative to the strategic goals of the organization. The contribution to each goal may be critical (*must do*), *high, moderate,* or *none*. These scores are based on data but nonetheless are fundamentally judgment calls. The scoring and prioritization will result in a set of initiatives deemed to be the most important. The IT staff will then construct preliminary budgets, staff needs, and timelines for these projects.

Figure 12.3 provides an overview of the timeline for these initiatives and the cost of each. Management will discuss various timeline scenarios, considering project interdependence and ensuring that the IT department and the organization are not overwhelmed by too many initiatives to complete all at once. The organization will use the budget estimates to determine how much IT it can afford. Often there is not enough money to pay for all the desired IT initiatives, and some initiatives with high and moderate scores will be deferred or eliminated as projects. The final plan, including timelines and budgets, will become the basis for assessing progress throughout the year.

Overall, a core role of the organization's chief information officer is to work with the rest of the leadership team to develop the process that leads to alignment and strategic linkage.

Once all is said and done, the alignment process should produce these results:

■ An inventory of the IT initiatives that will be undertaken. These initiatives may include new applications, major enhancements to the infrastructure, and projects designed to improve the IT asset.

■ A diagram or chart that illustrates the linkage between the initiatives and the organization's strategy and goals.

■ An overview of the timeline and the major interdependencies between initiatives.

■ A high-level analysis of the budget needed to carry out these initiatives.

■ An assessment of any material risks to carrying out the IT agenda, and a review of the strategies needed to reduce those risks.

FIGURE 12.2.   IT Initiative Priorities

Color Key: **High** | **Moderate** | **Must Do**

	Service		People		Financial		Growth		Quality and Safety		Infra-structure	Overall Priority
	Enhances Patient Care	Strengthens Community Outreach	Strengthens Physician Integration	Strengthens Employee Support	Enhances Operational Efficiency	Minimizes Investment Level	Invests in Current Scalable Technology	Supports Growth with Strong ROI	Addresses Significant System Deficiency	Addresses Compliance Issues (Must Do)	Mandatory Technology Building Block	
Clinical applications												
1. Physician order entry	✓		✓		✓				✓	✓		Start now
2. Patient care documentation	✓				✓				✓	✓		Plan it
3. Clinical data repository			✓		✓		✓		✓			Start now
4. Computerized medical record	✓		✓		✓							Delay it
5. PACS (phase I)					✓				✓			Start now
6. Expand physician practice mgmt.			✓		✓	✓	✓					Plan it
7. Departmental systems												Ongoing
Data integration												
8. Integration engine							✓		✓		✓	Plan it
Administrative and financial systems												
9. General financials					✓		✓					Plan it
10. Materials management				✓	✓		✓					Plan it
11. Scheduling application		✓		✓	✓				✓			Plan it
12. Decision-support system					✓	✓			✓			Start now
Emerging technologies												
13. Wireless LAN & WAN			✓		✓		✓	✓				Plan it
14. Voice recognition			✓		✓		✓					Start now
Infrastructure												
15. Server consolidations/upgrades											✓	Plan it
16. Network upgrades											✓	Ongoing
17. Security: SSO, HIPAA, policies					✓				✓	✓	✓	Plan it
Governance												
18. Project/change mgmt. office				✓	✓	✓					✓	Start now
19. U.S. governance (steering, business liaisons, SLAs)				✓	✓	✓						Ongoing

Note: SSO = Single Sign On; SLA = Service Level Agreement.

FIGURE 12.3. Plan Timelines and Budget

Hospital It Migration Path	Priority	Funded	FY2002 Capital (in $1000) Actual	FY2003 Capital Expense (in $1000) Low	High	FY2004 Capital Expense (in $1000) Low	High	FY2005 Capital Expense (in $1000) Low	High	Annual Recurring Operate
Clinical Applications										
1. Physician order entry	Start now	Funded	$ 200		$ 1,800					$ 270
2. Patient care documentation	Plan it			$ 333	$ 467	$ 167	$ 233			$ 70
3. Clinical data repository	Start now				$ 25					$ 4
4. Computerized medical record	Delay it					$ 50	$ 125	$ 150	$ 375	
5. PACS (phase I)	Start now			$ 500	$ 500	$ 50	$ 150			$ 75
6. Expand physician practice management	Plan it									
7. Departmental systems	Ongoing			$ 167	$ 333	$ 167	$ 333	$ 167	$ 333	$ 50
Data integration										
8. Integration engine	Plan it			$ 100	$ 200					
Administrative and financial systems										
9. General financials	Plan it					$ 300	$ 500			
10. Materials management	Plan it					$ 200	$ 333	$ 100	$ 167	
11. Scheduling application	Plan it					$ 75	$ 150	$ 225	$ 450	
12. Decision-support system	Start now	$ 100		$ 50						$ 8
Emerging technologies										
13. Wireless LAN & WAN	Plan it					$ 167	$ 667	$ 83	$ 333	$ 75
14. Voice recognition	Start now	Pending		$ 100	$ 300					$ 45
Infrastructure										
15. Server consolidations or upgrades	Plan it			$ 250	$ 500					$ 75
16. Network upgrades	Ongoing	Funded	$ 100	$ 33	$ 133	$ 33	$ 133	$ 33	$ 133	$ 20
17. Security: SSO, HIPAA, policies	Plan it			$ 33	$ 67	$ 17	$ 33			$ 10
Governance										
18. Project or change management office	Start now	Funded		$ 10	$ 20					$ 3
19. U.S. governance (steering, business liaisons, SLAs)	Ongoing	N/A		N/A	N/A	N/A	N/A	N/A	N/A	N/A

Timeline / FTE Staffing (FY02 Q4 through FY2005 Q4) is shown in the right-hand columns of the figure with approximate project timelines and FTE staffing numbers indicated per quarter.

Note: "Annual Recurring" is the ongoing operating cost of the system. Approximate project timelines are shown in the right-hand columns. Numbers below the timeline headings indicate the number of IT staff (0.5 and so forth) needed to implement each project.

It is important to recognize the amount and level of discussion, compromise, and negotiation that go into the strategic alignment process. Inventories, linkages, timelines, and analyses that are produced without going through the preceding thoughtful process will be of little real benefit.

IT STRATEGY AND ALIGNMENT CHALLENGES

Creating IT strategy and alignment is a complicated organizational process. The following sections present a series of observations about that process.

Persistent Problems with Alignment

Despite the apparent simplicity of the normative process we have described and the many examinations of the topic by academics and consultants, achieving IT alignment has been a top concern of senior organizational leadership for several decades. A survey of CIOs from across industries found improving IT alignment with business objectives to be the number one IT management priority for 2007 and 2008 (Alter, 2007). There are several reasons for the persistent difficulty of achieving alignment (Bensaou & Earl, 1998):

- Business strategies are often not clear or are volatile.
- IT opportunities are poorly understood.
- The organization is unable to resolve the different priorities of different parts of the organization.

Weill and Broadbent (1998) note that effective IT alignment requires that organizational leaders clearly understand and strategically and tactically well integrate (1) the organization's strategic context (its strategies and market position), (2) the organization's environment, (3) the IT strategy, and (4) the IT portfolio (including the current applications, technologies, and staff skills). Understanding and integrating these four continuously evolving and complex areas is exceptionally difficult.

At least two more factors that make alignment difficult can be added to this list:

- The organization finds that it has not achieved the gains, apparently achieved by others, that it has heard or read about, nor have the promises of the vendors of the technologies materialized.
- Often the value of IT, particularly in terms of infrastructure, is difficult to quantify, and the value proposition is fuzzy and uncertain.

In both these cases the organization is unsure whether the IT investment will lead to the desired strategic gain or value. This is not strictly an alignment problem. However, alignment does assume that the organization believes that it has a reasonable ability to achieve desired IT gains. We will discuss the IT value challenge in Chapter Fifteen.

Limitations of Alignment

As we shall also see in Chapter Thirteen, although alignment is important it will not guarantee effective application of IT. Planning methodologies and effective use of vectors cannot, by themselves, overcome weaknesses in other factors that can significantly diminish the likelihood that IT investments will lead to improved organizational performance. These weaknesses include poor relationships between IT staff and the rest of the organization, inadequate technical infrastructure, and ill-conceived IT governance mechanisms. IT strategy also cannot overcome unclear overall strategies and cannot necessarily compensate for material competitive weaknesses.

If one has mediocre painting skills, a class on painting technique will make one a better painter but will not turn one into Picasso. Similarly, superb alignment techniques will not turn an organization limited in its ability to implement IT effectively into one brilliant at IT use. Perhaps this reason, more than any other, is why the alignment issue persists as a top-ranked IT issue. Organizations are searching for IT excellence in the wrong place; it cannot be delivered purely by alignment prowess.

Alignment at Maturity

Organizations that have a history of IT excellence appear to evolve to a state where their alignment process is *methodology-less*. A study by Earl (1993) of organizations in the United Kingdom with a history of IT excellence found that their IT planning processes had several characteristics:

IT planning was not a separate process. IT planning and the strategic discussion of IT occurred as an integral part of each organization's strategic-planning processes and management discussions. In these organizations, management did not think of separating out an IT discussion during the course of strategy development any more than it would run separate finance or human resource planning processes. IT planning was an unseverable, intertwined component of the normal management conversation. This would suggest not forming a separate IT steering committee. (IT steering committees will be discussed in Chapter Thirteen.)

IT planning had neither a beginning nor an end. In many organizations, IT planning processes start in a particular month every year and are completed within a more or less set period. In the studied organizations the IT planning and strategy conversation went on all the time. This does not mean that an organization doesn't have to have a temporally demarked, annual budget process. Rather it means that IT planning is a continuous process reflecting the continuous change in the environment and in organizational plans and strategies.

IT planning involved shared decision making and shared learning between IT and the organization. IT leadership informed organizational leadership of the potential contribution of new technologies and the constraints of current technologies. Organizational leadership ensured that IT leadership understood the business plans and strategies and their constraints. The IT budget and annual tactical plan resulted from shared analyses of IT opportunities and a set of IT priorities.

The IT plan emphasized themes. A provider organization may have themes of improving care quality, reducing costs, and improving patient service. During the course of any given year, IT will have initiatives that are intended to advance the organization along these themes. The mixture of initiatives will change from year to year, but the themes endure over the course of many years. Because themes endure year after year, organizations develop competence around them. Organizations become, for example, progressively better at managing costs and improving patient service. This growing prowess extends into IT. Organizations become more skilled at understanding which IT opportunities hold the most promise and at managing the implementation of these applications. And the IT staff become more skilled at knowing how to apply IT to support such themes as improving care quality and at helping leadership assess the value of new technologies and applications.

IT Strategy Is Not Always Necessary

There are many times in IT activities when the goal, or the core approach to achieving the goal, is not particularly strategic, and strategy formulation and implementation are not needed. Replacing an inpatient pharmacy system, enhancing help desk support, and upgrading the network, although requiring well-executed projects, do not always require leadership to engage in conversations about organizational goals or to take a strategic look at organizational capabilities and skills. Such discussions would produce little substantive change in the organization's understanding of what it has to do and how it should go about doing it.

There are many times when there is little likelihood that the way an organization achieves a goal will create a distinct competitive advantage. For example, an organization may decide that it needs to provide wireless access to patients and visitors but it does not expect that that support, or its implementation, will be so superior to a competitor's patient wireless access that an advantage accrues to the organization.

Much of what IT does is not strategic nor does it require strategic thinking. Many IT projects do not require hard looks at organizational mission, thoughtful discussions of fundamental approaches to achieving organizational goals, or significant changes in the IT asset.

IT Alignment and Strategy Summary

The development of IT alignment and strategic linkage is a complex undertaking. Five vectors, each complex, must converge. Organizational strategy is often volatile and uncertain and will invariably be developed in multiple forums, making it difficult to have a static, comprehensive picture of the strategy. The ability of IT to support a strategy can be unclear and the trade-offs between IT options can be difficult to assess. The complexity of this undertaking is manifest in the frequent citing of IT alignment in surveys of major organizational issues and problems. There are no simple answers to this problem. At the end of the day, good alignment requires talented leaders (including the CIO) who have effective debates and discussions regarding strategies and who have very good instincts and understandings about the organization's strategy and the potential contribution of IT.

It appears that organizations that are mature in their IT use have evolved these IT alignment processes to the point where they are no longer distinguishable as separate processes. This observation should not be construed as advice to cease using planning approaches or disband effective IT steering committees. Such an evolution, to the degree that it is normative, may occur naturally, just as kids will eventually grow up (at least most of them will).

IT AS A COMPETITIVE ADVANTAGE

Competitive strategy involves identifying goals in ways that are materially superior to the ways that a competitor has defined them (formulation). It also involves developing ways to achieve those goals and capabilities that are materially superior to the methods and capabilities of a competitor (implementation) (Lipton, 1996). For example, an organization and its chief competitor may both decide to create a network of primary care providers. However, the first organization might believe that it can move faster and use less capital than its competition does if it contracts with existing providers rather than buy their practices. Or an organization and its competition may both have a mission to delivery high-quality care, but the competitor may have decided to focus on selected carve-outs or *focused factories* (Herzlinger, 1997) whereas the first organization may be attempting to create a full-spectrum care delivery capacity.

Competitive strategy should attempt to define superiority that can be sustained. For example, an organization may believe that if it moves quickly, it can capture a large network of primary care providers and limit the ability of the competition to create its own network. Being *first to market* can provide a sustainable advantage, although no advantage is sustainable for long periods of time. Similarly, an organization with access to large amounts of capital can have an advantage over an organization that does not. Wealth can provide a sustainable advantage.

As organizations examine strategies and capabilities, an entirely reasonable question is, Can the application of information technology provide a competitive advantage to an organization? Over the last two decades, across a wide range of industries, answers to this question have been explored and developed, most recently through the lens of the Internet (see, for example, Porter, 2001). Perhaps, as a result of continued evolution of the technology and continued transformation of industries and economies, answers to such questions will always be explored.

These explorations have examined uses of IT that are now legendary; the American Airlines SABRE system for travel reservations, the American Hospital Supply ASAP system for hospital supply ordering, the Federal Express suite of applications for tracking packages, and the Amazon.com approach to Internet-based retailing. In these cases and others an organization was able to achieve an advantage over its competitors through the thoughtful application of IT. Consider these brief overviews of the competitive use of IT by Harrah's Entertainment, Enterprise Rent-a-Car, and Con-Way Transportation Services.

CASE STUDY

Con-Way Transportation Services A subsidiary of California-based CNF Inc., Con-Way Transportation Services, Inc., is a $2 billion transportation and services company that provides time-definite and day-definite freight delivery services and logistics for commercial and industrial businesses. A leader in less-than-truckload (LTL) shipping, Con-Way boasts more next-day delivery combinations than any other LTL carrier, and 99 percent on-time reliability in next-day services.

The key to Con-Way's success was the development and implementation of an automated line-haul system. Born out of what was thought to be a logistically and financially impossible task, the system optimizes personnel, equipment, and individual routes for the nighttime movement and timely relay of freight shipments in the United States and Canada. Built around Con-Way's successful core business model and designed using historical performance, human intuitive skills and experience, and selected iterative processes including linear programming, the system transformed a tedious, expensive, and time-consuming manual process into an efficient, automated process that completely routes over 95 percent of each day's shipments in about seven minutes.

The automated line-haul system has given Con-Way several competitive advantages in the industry, some of which were not even foreseen:

- *Dispatch personnel management.* Originally, dispatcher positions were difficult to fill, and new dispatchers had a long learning curve, sometimes as long as eighteen months. The procedures and business rules the dispatchers followed were undocumented, making the company uncomfortably dependent on the knowledge in the dispatchers' heads. The automated system completes the dispatchers' jobs faster and more consistently, letting dispatchers use their time to troubleshoot problems that could jeopardize on-time delivery. Con-Way has been able to reduce its dispatch personnel by three people (through attrition) and can keep the group small as it adds business.

- *Customer benefits.* Con-Way was able to extend its cutoff time for customers requesting overnight shipments. This allows customers to submit orders right up until the end of the business day, which gives Con-Way a competitive advantage because businesses don't want to arrange their activities around shippers' schedules. Additionally, the new system, in coordination with the work of dispatch personnel in troubleshooting problems such as bad weather and road closures, has attained a 99 percent on-time delivery rate.

- *Efficiency.* The line-haul automation system has seen efficiency improvements of 1 percent to 3 percent over the results achieved with manual route planning. Although a modest improvement by industry standards, the incremental effect has resulted in savings of $4 million to $5 million annually from paying fewer drivers, moving trucks fewer miles, packing more freight per trailer, and reducing damage from rehandling freight.

Con-Way plans to expand its automated system into other business units, including Con-Way Western Express and Con-Way Southern Express, and is expecting to generate additional operational savings and customer conveniences.

Source: Adapted from Pastore, 2003.

CASE STUDY

Harrah's Entertainment   A leader in the gaming industry, Harrah's Entertainment operates twenty-six casinos in thirteen states under the brand names of Harrah's, Rio, Harvey's, and Showboat. As one of the most recognized names in an overwhelmingly competitive industry, Harrah's is focused on building loyalty and value for its customers, shareholders, employees, business partners, and communities by being the most service-oriented, technology-driven, geographically diversified company in gaming.

In an industry where it is hard for one casino to differentiate itself from another, Harrah's has made the important decision to put its dollars into building customer loyalty rather than high-priced themed casinos. It is Harrah's belief that customer demand is stimulated by a company knowing its customers, not building an attractive spectacle. To do this, Harrah's invested $30 million into WINet (Winner's Information Network) to advance its customer relationship management (CRM) strategy through its Total Rewards Program.

Before the advent of WINet, each Harrah's casino operated independently of the others, with each having its own rewards program—just like every other casino in the country. Each of the casinos had its own information systems that tracked customer data, but none of them were linked or shared information with each other. Harrah's felt it could gain a competitive advantage in the gaming industry by capitalizing on player loyalty. To that end, WINet was developed to standardize and connect the information systems throughout all its casinos, tracking and sharing information about customers and their gaming preferences and practices.

Through WINet, players who were part of Harrah's Total Rewards Program could use their player's card at any of Harrah's casinos throughout the country. In return, Harrah's was able to capture information about its players to use in direct marketing, promotions, contests, customer service, and predictive modeling. Additionally, Harrah's was able to save over $20 million per year on its overall costs and increase same-store sales growth. The number of customers playing at more than one Harrah's casino increased by 72 percent, and cross-market revenues increased from $113 million to $250 million.

Harrah's strategic use of information technology has made other industry players take notice. Harrah's is taking steps to solidify its competitive advantage by patenting the innovative technology that has given it the edge to become a leader in the cut-throat gaming industry.

Source: Adapted from Levinson, 2001.

CASE STUDY

Enterprise Rent-a-Car   A leader in the car and truck rental industry, Enterprise Rent-a-Car has more than 530,000 cars in its fleet in over 5,000 locations in five countries. With over 50,000 employees, Enterprise has annual revenues over $6 billion. Enterprise is focused on providing excellent customer service, as one of its core values, by listening and acting on customer feedback.

Enterprise has been able to remain the leading rental car company in part through its innovative use of information technology to improve customer service and enhance the efficiency of core processes. Ninety-five percent of Enterprise's business comes through local rentals, of which a significant number are replacement rentals, paid for by insurance companies on behalf of drivers whose cars have been in accidents and need to be repaired. In order to make this process efficient and customer friendly, Enterprise developed an Internet-based system called ARMS (Automated Rental Management System) that allows Enterprise and its customers to streamline and automate a once-tedious, time- and resource-consuming process.

The concept of ARMS is simple, but its effect on the car rental industry has been staggering. The insurance company, the repair shop, and the Enterprise rental center are brought together through the Enterprise-supported ARMS Internet site. The insurance company logs into the Web site to search for and make a reservation for its policyholder, the driver whose car needs to be repaired. The driver simply picks up and uses the rental car while his or her car is at a repair shop. Meanwhile, the repair shop updates the status of that car daily until the repair is complete. The repair shop then sends a message to ARMS, which sends a message to the insurance company, who calls the driver with the information that the car is ready. The driver returns the rental car and is driven to the repair shop to pick up his or her own car. Meanwhile, a bill is generated and sent to the insurance company for payment.

Having invested $28 million to develop and implement ARMS, which has an annual maintenance cost of $7.5 million, Enterprise processes more than $1 billion in transactions through the system, which is used by twenty-two of the nation's twenty-five biggest insurance companies (and by over 150 insurance companies in all), more than doubling its business with certain companies since the advent of ARMS. Moreover, insurance companies are doing more business with Enterprise because the insurance industry saves between $36 million and $107 million annually due to shorter rental times (due to eliminating phone calls to Enterprise and repair shops and to eliminating time-consuming paperwork), and shorter repair times (because mechanics don't have to continuously field phone calls from the insurance company).

Source: Adapted from Berkman, 2002.

Improving competitive position is a critical element of all strategy discussions. The question to be answered is, What have these experiences taught us about the role of IT as a competitive weapon?

Core Sources of Advantage

The experiences just described and similar experiences among other organizations have led to a series of observations and conclusions about the use of IT to provide a competitive advantage.

In most cases, organizations seeking a competitive advantage through IT, use it to

- Leverage organizational processes.
- Enable rapid and accurate provision of critical data.
- Enable product and service differentiation and occasionally creation.
- Support the alteration of overall organizational form or characteristics.

Leveraging Organizational Processes IT can be applied in the effort to improve organizational processes by making them faster, less error prone, less expensive, more convenient, and available at more times and places. In effect, the *transaction cost* of the process, from the customer's perspective, has been reduced. Examples abound:

- Third-party payer Web sites make the process of enrollment and benefit determination more convenient.

- Accounts receivable applications make accounting processes less expensive and faster.

- EMR systems make the process of accessing information about a patient's prior encounters more efficient.

These examples and countless others have highlighted several process lessons.

IT leverage of processes is most effective when the processes being leveraged are critical, core processes that

- Are used by customers to judge the performance of the organization.
- Define the core business of the organization.

Patients are more likely to judge a provider organization by its ambulatory scheduling processes and billing processes than by its accounts payable and human resource processes. Moreover, certain attributes of these processes and their end products matter more than other attributes. For example, patients may judge appointment availability as more important than the organization's ability to process no-shows.

Making diagnostic and therapeutic decisions is a core provider organizational process; a process that is essential to its core business. It is unlikely that there are a large number of organizational processes that have no bearing on and make no contribution to organizational performance. However, there are processes that are more essential than others to the mission of the organization and its goals. Customers may have limited ability to judge or evaluate these processes. For example, most patients cannot judge how well a provider organization makes diagnostic and therapeutic decisions, despite the growing use and sophistication of quality measures.

Keen 1997 defines the importance of processes along two dimensions. *Worth* is a measure of the difference between the cost of a process and the revenue it generates. *Salience* is a measure of the degree to which a process is critical to the identity of an organization or to its effectiveness. The referral process may have high worth. The ambulatory scheduling process may be a critical contributor to the organization's efforts to be identified as "patient friendly." Medical management may be critical to a payer's effectiveness.

IT can enable an organization to materially alter the nature of its processes. For example, technology can enable processes or business activities to be extended over a wider geography than the immediate service area. Telemedicine enables consultations with patients across the globe. The Internet enables patients in many countries to enroll in clinical trials. IT can give subscribers a self-service option for resolving claims and benefits issues.

Processes can be altered or created in a manner that enables the organization to craft or significantly enhance strategic partnerships with other organizations. A process can be moved from one organization to another, as it is in outsourcing. For example, a hospital and a managed care organization, rather than conducting credentialing separately, could share that responsibility. Providers and materials suppliers have established just-in-time inventory replenishment processes that move the inventory function from the provider to the supplier. These approaches and others are predicated on a strong IT core.

Process reexamination should accompany any effort to apply IT to process improvement. If underlying problems with processes are not remedied, the IT investment can be wasted or diluted. IT applications may result in existing processes continuing to perform poorly only faster. Moreover, it can be harder to fix flawed processes after the application of IT because the IT-supported process now has an additional source of complexity, cost, and ossification to address, the "new computer system." Process reexamination, addressed elsewhere in this book, can range from incremental, although valuable, change to more radical reengineering.

In addition to examining and improving the mechanics of the process that is the target of the information system, the reexamination should question whether the process is defined correctly. Process definitions often incorporate the mechanics of the process into the core definition of the process, inappropriately narrowing the reexamination effort. For example:

- A definition of a process as "obtaining cash from the bank" might lead a reengineering effort to place ATMs only at the bank. Such ATMs might ease the burden of standing in line on a Saturday morning and hence be viewed as an improvement. However, a statement of the process as "obtaining cash" might lead one to consider all the places where people need cash—malls, theaters, and airports. This might result in the placement of ATMs in many and varied locations, leading to a far more powerful improvement in the process. Similarly, a statement of this process as "buying something" might lead one to create debit cards as cash surrogates.

- A definition of a process as "obtaining a referral number" might lead one to construct an EDI link between the managed care application and the systems in the physician's office. A statement of this process as "managing referrals" might lead one to abandon entirely the process of obtaining the referral number.

Rapid and Accurate Provision of Critical Data   Organizations define critical elements of their plans, operations, and environment. These elements must be monitored to ensure that the plan is working, service quality is high, the organization's fiscal situation is sound, and the environment is behaving as anticipated. Clearly, data are required to perform such monitoring.

IT can improve a competitive position by providing such data. Examples abound:

- Gathering data during registration about the patient's referring physician can help a hospital understand whether its outreach activities and market share growth strategies are working.

- Obtaining data about why subscribers do not reenroll in a health insurance plan aids the plan in identifying major service deficiencies.

- Bar-code scanners at supermarkets and department stores tell product suppliers which products are being purchased. This knowledge can ensure that valuable shelf space is filled with the optimal mix of products. This knowledge can also improve inventory management and manufacturing capacity utilization. Bar-code data in combination with other data about the customer, obtained when the customer presents a store card to obtain discounts, enables the store and the product manufacturer to understand the demographics of their customers, leading to more focused advertising.

- Provider order entry systems that request the reason or clinical indication for a procedure being ordered not only assist receiving department staff to understand what they are supposed to do but also assist quality assurance and utilization review efforts to understand the dynamics of procedure utilization.

These and other instances of data use have generated several lessons.

Rapid *and* accurate *are relative terms.* Data about product movement should be gathered and analyzed in as close to real time as possible because one can change things such as shelf space use almost instantly. Analysis of physician referral patterns need not be done in real time because the organization is unlikely to be able to effect a change in patterns instantly. Complete accuracy about the cost of performing laboratory tests may not be necessary because it can be clear from allocations whether a cost structure is too high or is reasonable. High accuracy in linking providers and the medications they order may be critical in order to get provider acceptance of any utilization analyses.

The rapid and accurate gathering of data may be the most significant and important source of a competitive advantage. Having good data about utilization may be more important than efficient ordering processes. Having good data about referring physicians may be more important than an error-free registration process. Knowing the demographics of the customers who consume your snack food, what else they buy when they buy your product, and where and when they buy may be far more important than well-run inventory management. Knowing who your passengers are, their fare tolerance, what time of year they fly, and their destinations may be more important than managing full utilization of the aircraft.

The role of data should not imply that well-run processes are irrelevant. People prefer to obtain services from organizations with well-run processes. Often a well-run, efficient, and convenient process may be necessary to get high-quality data. But in some cases the process is subordinate to the need for the data. There are many examples of the competitive use of IT that show an organization, accepting that its rivals will mimic process gains, focusing on the uses of the data. For example, systems to support the making of an airline reservation evolved into the use of the reservation data to develop frequent flyer programs, establish mileage programs linked to credit cards, and engage in fare wars. Those organizations that developed the reservation systems sold the use of them to their competitors, recognizing that exclusive use of the system itself did not provide a sustainable process advantage.

Product and Service Differentiation   IT can be used to differentiate and customize products and services. Again, examples abound:

- Financial planners may offer prospective customers Web sites that help an individual assess the savings needed to achieve financial goals such as funding college for children or having a certain income at retirement. Customers discover, after running the software, that they will be insolvent within a week after retirement. Fortunately, the financial planner is there to work with the customer to ensure that such a gloomy outcome does not occur.

- Health care providers establish Web sites with news and information about health, classes to reduce health risk, new research, and basic triage algorithms. Such information is an effort to differentiate the provider's care from that of others.

- Supermarkets send information to customers about upcoming sales. This information is often based on knowledge of prior customer purchases. Hence a family that has purchased diapers and baby food will be seen as a household with young children. Information about sales on infant products and products directed to young parents will be sent to that household and not to households where a steady pattern of purchasing hot dogs, snack food, and beer indicates a single male. The supermarket is attempting to differentiate its service by helping the household plan its purchases around store specials.

Customization and differentiation often rely on data. Effective *customization* presumes that an organization knows something about the customer. *Differentiation* assumes that it knows something about the customer's criteria for evaluating its kind of organization so that it can differentiate its processes, products, and services in a way deemed to have value.

Customization and differentiation often center on organizational processes. Existing processes can be made unique. New processes can be created. For example, financial services firms enable clients to move their money between money market, stock, and bond accounts by creating new processes that enable such asset movements.

IT has enabled the development of new products and services and the formation of new companies and industries. For several years around the turn of the millennium, new Internet-based services and companies seemed to be spawned (and to die) daily. Companies that provide comparative analyses of health care claims and utilization data owe their existence to IT. Capitation as a scheme for financing and managing risk would be extraordinarily difficult without information technology. Several academic medical centers now provide international telemedicine consultations, although it is arguable whether that is an extension of existing service or a new business.

Change in Organizational Form or Characteristics   IT can be used to improve or change certain organizational attributes or characteristics. Such attributes or characteristics might involve service quality orientation, communication, decision making, and collaboration. Consider these examples of using IT to encourage change:

- Most business and medical schools require students to perform their assignments using tools on the school's network. This emphasis is intended to accomplish several objectives, one of which is to enhance the student's comfort and skill with the technology for professional purposes.

- Organizations have implemented various types of Web 2.0 technologies in an effort to foster collaboration.

- Senior management teams have implemented quality measurement systems in an effort to encourage other managers to be more data driven and focused on key quality parameters—in other words, "to think quality."

The value of such efforts or their impact is often unclear because the organization is changing deep but largely intangible attributes. For example, becoming more data driven can be a profound change, but it is difficult to measure the value of being data driven or to know if an organization has progressed 50 percent or 80 percent of the way toward that desired change. These characteristics tend to be difficult to measure at anything other than a very crude level.

Often a change in organizational characteristics is inadvertent or an unintended consequence of an IT implementation. Electronic mail has been implemented to improve communication, but it has also had the effect of speeding up decision making and altering power structures. Staff will use e-mail to seek information from other staff whom they would feel uncomfortable approaching face to face, for example, to schedule a meeting with the chief of medicine.

Advantage Sustainability

It is difficult to sustain an IT-enabled or IT-centric advantage. Competitors, noting the advantage, are quick to attempt to copy the application, lure away the original developers, or obtain a version of the application from a vendor who has seen a market opportunity in the success of the original developers. And a sufficient number of these competitors will be successful. Often their success may be less expensive and faster to achieve than the first organization's success was because they learn from the mistakes of the leader. A provider organization that offers Web access to patient results to its referring physicians finds that its competitors will also provide such capabilities. A managed care organization that provides consumer health information and benefits management capabilities to its subscribers finds that its competitors are quite capable of doing the same.

The result can be a sort of IT arms race, a race that provides no advantage for long, a race that you have to run often because customers come to think of the new system as a basic service. No one today would bank at a financial institution that did not offer ATM service.

Knowing that today's IT advantage is tomorrow's core capability possessed by all industry participants, the organization has several strategies that it can adopt:

Attempt to out hustle the competition by aggressive and focused introduction of a series of enhancements to a core system that enables that system to evolve faster than the competition can and to hold a lead.

Freeze the system by ceasing major investments in it and relegating it to the role of a core production system where efficiency and reliability of operation, rather than the possession of superior capabilities, become the objectives. In this case the organization may turn its sights to new systems that attempt to create an advantage in other ways.

Change the basis of competition by using the technology to make the competitive strengths of rivals no longer competitive. Amazon.com attempts to decrease the value of an asset possessed by other retail booksellers, a nationwide network of stores. This network could have been a barrier to entry for Amazon.com; it is expensive to build hundreds of stores. Instead, Amazon.com attempts to make such a network irrelevant and possibly a liability because the network is expensive to maintain.

There are ways that an advantage can be sustained over a prolonged period of time. A single application cannot by itself result in a prolonged sustained advantage. However, an advantage can be sustained for longer than a brief period of time by

- Leveraging other significant organizational strengths
- Leveraging a well-developed, strong IT asset

Leveraging Other Strengths   Organizations can have strengths that are difficult for their competitors to duplicate (Cecil & Goldstein, 1990). Such strengths may include market share, access to capital, brand-name recognition, and proprietary know-how. IT can be used to reinforce or extend such strengths, as in the following examples.

A large integrated delivery system (IDS) and a large retail pharmacy chain, both with significant market shares in a region, may decide to link the IDS's ambulatory care medication order entry system to the pharmacy's dispensing and medication management system. The IDS's system learns from the pharmacy's system whether the entered medication order was filled, which improves the IDS's medical management programs. The IDS is also able to provide a service to its patients because it can now route a prescription to a pharmacy near a patient's home. The pharmacy is able to channel customers to its stores where it believes that as they pick up medications, they will also make other purchases.

The IDS and the retail pharmacy chain find each other attractive because of their respective shares of the market. The IDS is able to ensure significant geographical coverage for patients who need to fill prescriptions. The pharmacy chain is able to ensure a large volume of customers visiting its stores. Neither party might find another party with less market share as attractive as a partner. For both organizations, this partnership leverages an existing strength of market share.

A well-known academic medical center may be able to leverage its brand name and cohort of foreign-born physicians who trained at the medical center to establish a telemedicine-based international consultation service. It may also be able to leverage its brand name to improve the attractiveness of its consumer-oriented health information Web site. Consumers, confused and worried about the quality of information on the Internet, may take comfort in knowing that information is being generated by a respected source.

These advantages do not result purely from an application system or inherently from process improvement, data gathering, or service differentiation or customization. They result from capitalizing upon some core, difficult-to-replicate strength of the organization, through the application of IT.

Although an organization may have difficult-to-replicate strengths, it should be mindful that IT might also be used to undermine those strengths (Christensen, 2001). For example, most integrated delivery systems have a strength of economies of scope, in other words, they offer a full range of medical services and amortize fixed costs, such as clinical laboratory costs, over this range. When economies of scope exist, the incremental cost of the next medical service is small. Conversely, the incremental savings that result from eliminating a service are small.

If this country moves toward defined contributions as a means of offering health insurance, the employee or patient may be able to select his or her own network of providers, using a Web-based application and bypassing the network defined by the IDS. The employee might select cardiology services from one provider and oncology services from another provider. This *cherry picking* enabled by information technology reduces the advantages of economies of scope. The IDS's revenue from its services that are not picked becomes small, but costs have not been reduced proportionally. The IDS will face competition from organizations that focus on one service line, such as oncology. Compared to the IDS, these focused service providers may also be able to obtain fixed-cost services at less cost. For example, they may obtain testing as a service, supported by IT, from a laboratory service provider.

Leveraging the IT Asset   For most of the health care industry, the technology and applications being implemented today are available to all industry participants, including competitors. Any provider organization can acquire and implement systems from Eclipsys, Cerner, GE, HBOC, or Siemens. Similarly, why would one payer believe that its claims adjudication system can provide an advantage if its competitor can buy the same system (particularly if the organization has no other advantage—for example, market share—that it is able to leverage with that system)?

An advantage can be obtained if one or both of two things happen. First, one organization might do a more thoughtful and effective job than its competitors do of understanding and then effecting the changes in processes or data gathering associated with the system to be implemented. The application does not provide an advantage, but the way that it is implemented does. We all see the difference that execution makes every day in all facets of our lives. It is the difference between a great restaurant and a mediocre one or a terrific movie and a terrible one. In neither case is the idea—for example, "let's make meals and sell them"—or the fact that one executes on the idea—"we've hired a cook and purchased silverware"—the advantage. It is the manner of execution that distinguishes.

Second, one organization might be consistently able to outrun the other. If an organization is able to develop means to implement programs and processes faster or cheaper, it may be able to outrun its competition, even if its implementations, one for one, are of no higher quality than its competitors'. Perhaps over a certain period of time one organization implements four applications whereas the other implements three. Or perhaps for a given amount of capital one organization implements five applications whereas the other implements three.

In general, organizations may be able to sustain an IT-based or IT-supported competitive advantage because they have an established and exceptionally strong IT asset:

for example, talented IT staff, strong relationships between that staff and the organization, and an agile technical platform (Ross, Beath, & Goodhue, 1996). This asset may be able to consistently and efficiently deliver high-quality applications that enable the organization to improve its competitive position.

Technology Is a Tool

Information technology can provide a competitive advantage. However, IT has no magic properties. In particular, technology cannot overcome poor strategies, inadequate management, inept execution, or major organizational limitations. For example a system that enables a reduction in nursing staff may not make the salary savings desired if the average nurse's salary is very high or the staff are unionized. Information systems are tools. If the objectives of a building are not well understood, its design flawed, the carpenter unskilled, and certain tools missing, the quality of the hammer and saw used to build it are irrelevant. In those cases where a significant organizational advantage has been realized, superior strategy, a deep understanding of the business, an ability to execute complex transformations of the business and its core processes, and an ability to capitalize upon IT prowess led to the gains. IT was necessary but not sufficient.

PERSPECTIVE

HOW GREAT COMPANIES USE IT

In his seminal book *Good to Great*, Jim Collins identified companies that made and sustained a transition from being a good company to being a great company. His research noted that these companies had several consistent orientations to IT. They

- Avoided IT fads, but were pioneers in the application of carefully selected technologies.

- Became pioneers when the technology showed great promise in leveraging that which they were already good at doing (their core competency) and that which they were passionate about doing well.

- Used IT to accelerate their momentum toward a being great company, but did not use IT to create that momentum. In other words, IT came after the vision had been set and the organization had begun to move toward that vision. IT was not used to create the vision and start the movement.

- Responded to technology change with great thoughtfulness and creativity, driven by a burning desire to turn unrealized potential into results. Mediocre

(Continued)

PERSPECTIVE (*Continued*)

> companies often reacted to technology out of fear, adopting it because they were worried about being left behind.
>
> ■ Achieved dramatically better results with IT than did rival companies using the exact same technology.
>
> ■ Rarely mentioned IT as being critical to their success.
>
> ■ "Crawled, walked and then ran" with new IT even when they were undergoing radical change.
>
> *Source:* Collins, 2001,p. 162.

In a large number of cases in which IT is used as a competitive weapon, the IT system leverages an existing capability (Freedman, 1991). If that capability is weak, IT may not be able to overcome the weakness. Organizations won't use, for example, a supply ordering system if the supplies are inferior in quality, comparatively expensive, and of limited scope. The experiences of Internet-based e-tailers have highlighted the problems created by sloppy inventory management, poor understanding of customer buying behaviors such as returning purchases, and insufficient knowledge of customer price tolerance.

Referring physicians will not find valuable, and probably will not use, a system that gives them access to hospital data if the consulting physicians at the hospital are remiss in getting their consult notes completed on time or at all. High-quality, comprehensive data on care quality diminish in value if the organization has limited ability or skill to improve the practice of care.

Other factors that can limit the utility of the IT tool have been seen (Cash, McFarlan, & McKenney, 1992):

■ Introducing applications too early, with the result that the organization has been unable to overcome not-ready-for-prime-time technology and an unreceptive customer environment.

■ Having an inadequate understanding of buying dynamics across market segments. An academic medical center that hopes its consumer-oriented Web page will lead to increased admissions may not have fully comprehended its own referral process and that 80 percent of referrals to it are made by the patient's physician.

■ Being too far ahead of the customer's comfort level. For example, a large percentage of the public today is uncomfortable with the idea of transmitting individually identifiable health data over the Internet. This discomfort has not been assuaged by the incorporation of advanced security and encryption technologies into these systems.

Finally, the pace of technology evolution is rapid, and new technologies are arriving that enable new ways of supporting processes, gathering data, and differentiating and customizing products and services. In the cases where a significant advantage could be obtained, organizations have been quick to assess new technologies and thoughtful in their application. The incorporation of Radio Frequency ID and the Internet into health care organization activities are examples of effectively leveraging new technologies. This behavior suggests that

- Organizations should have a function that scans for new industry-relevant technologies and engages in evaluating them and experimenting with them.

- To assess new technology well, organizations must develop an understanding of the characteristics of that technology that provide value: for example, what is it about Web 2.0 that might produce a significant improvement in care delivery capabilities? This assessment also involves the development of governing concepts.

- Organizations should be careful not to fall in love with their current technology; they need to be able to ruthlessly jettison technology as its ability to provide a competitive distinction wanes.

Singles and Grand Slams

When one looks back at organizations that have been effective in the strategic application of IT over a reasonably long time, one sees what looks like a series of singles punctuated by an occasional leap, a *grand slam* (McKenney, Copeland, & Mason, 1995). One doesn't see a progression of grand slams or, in the parlance of the industry, *killer applications* (Downes & Mui, 1998). In the course of improving processes, differentiating services, and gathering data, organizations carry out a series of initiatives that improve their performance. The vast majority of these initiatives do not by themselves fundamentally alter the competitive position of the organization, but in the aggregate they make a significant contribution, just as the difference between a great hotel and a mediocre hotel is not solely the presence of clean sheets or hot water but one thousand of such things.

In addition, at various points in time, the organization may have an insight that leads to a major leap in its application of IT to its performance. For example, airlines, having developed their initial travel reservation systems, continued to improve them. At some point they realized that the data gathered by a reservation system had enormous potency and frequent flyer programs resulted. American Hospital Supply, having developed its supply ordering system, continued to improve it. At some point it realized that it was in a materials management partnership with its hospital customers and not strictly in the supply ordering business. No organization has ever delivered a series of killer, or grand slam, applications in rapid succession.

Organizations must develop their IT asset in such a way that they can affect the types of continuous improvement that managers and medical staff will see as possible, day in and day out. For example, in an ideal world an organization would be able to capitalize on the improvements in ambulatory scheduling that a middle manager thinks up and also be able to capitalize on a thousand other good ideas and opportunities. The organization must also develop antennae that sense the possibility of a leap, and the ability to focus that enables it to effect the systems needed to make the leap. Ensuring that these antennae are working is one of the key functions of the chief information officer. The resulting pattern may look like the graph line in Figure 12.4, continuous improvement (singles) in performance using IT, punctuated by periodic leaps, or grand slams.

It is also clear that organizations have a limited ability to see more than one leap at a time. Hence they should be cautious about visions that are too visionary or that have a very long time horizon. Organizations have great difficulty understanding a world that is significantly different from the one they inhabit now or that can be only vaguely understood in the context of the next leap. We might understand frequent flyer programs now. But they were not well understood, nor was their competitive value well understood at the time they were conceived. Moreover, the organizational changes required to support and capitalize upon a leap can take years, five to seven years at times (McKenney et al., 1995).

Competitive Baggage

The pursuit of IT as a source of competitive advantage can create baggage, or a hangover. This baggage can occur in several forms.

Significant investment in capital projects, creating an increase in depreciation and an increase in IT operating budgets, can erode margins. If several competitors are making similar investments, they may all arrive at a position where the customer sees better service or lower prices, but none of the competitors has developed a system that truly differentiates itself, and they all have reduced their margins in the process. ATMs are an example (Lake, 1998). Customers are better off with ATMs, but no bank distinguishes itself by its ATM capabilities. Banks must now carry the cost of operating the ATM system and funding periodic upgrades in ATM technology. The average ATM machine has a net cost of $20,000 to $25,000 after subtracting fees charged to banks and customers for its use. For the health care provider, investment in personal health records may have a similar outcome.

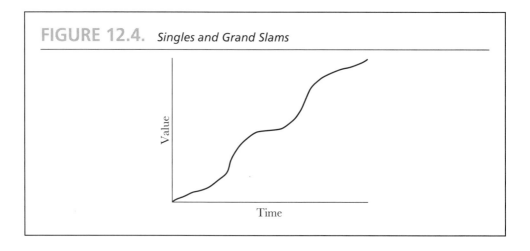

FIGURE 12.4. *Singles and Grand Slams*

Organizations may find themselves in an IT arms race from which prudence has fled, the conversation being replaced by the innate desire to outfeature the competitor. The original thoughtfulness surrounding the use of IT to improve processes of care, expand market share, or reduce costs has been replaced by ego.

Governing concepts that were poorly constructed or that fail to evolve can blind organizations to new opportunities. For example, the belief that personal computers were only for hobbyists and had no major role in a large organization was true in 1978 but had become dead wrong by 1984. The belief that the Internet was a realm of interest solely to hackers, voyeurs, and academics also became wrong very quickly. Organizations often hold to beliefs and concepts long after they should be buried. This is particularly likely to happen when the initial belief led to an IT innovation that was very successful. People and organizations are loath to jettison beliefs that "got them here." Such blindness has put companies out of business (Christensen, 1997).

IT rigidity can result from poor architecture design or poor partnership selection. Many hospitals have seen, belatedly, the consequences of failure to design for application integration as they attempt to integrate systems acquired over years of a best-of-breed strategy. The pursuit of the advantage to each department of implementing the best product on the market failed to consider the infrastructure properties (the ability to integrate applications efficiently) that would be needed to continue to innovate efficiently later.

Organizations that are overly sensitive to the IT market and grasping for an advantage may pursue new technologies and ideas well before the utility of the idea, if any, is known. They do not want to be the only organization not pursuing the latest technology or idea and as a result of this nonpursuit destined for the dustbin of also-rans. However, a very large number of ideas, technologies, and management techniques fail to live up to their initial hype. This does not mean they have no utility, just that their utility has not lived up to their press releases. The desire to achieve a competitive advantage can cause organizations to lose their senses, perspective, and at times, appropriate caution.

Finally, extensive use of IT results in dependency on IT. This dependence can affect many resources, from staff to infrastructure. Investment in technologies leaves organizations dependent on their ability to continue to attract and retain scarce and expensive talent. Failure to plan for this dependency can leave the organization exposed when staff turnover occurs. Similarly, organizations that have become reliant on a computerized medical record, with a corresponding intolerance of downtime, are dependent on having a highly reliable and high-performing technical infrastructure. Pursuit of a competitive advantage needs to plan for the dependencies that will be incurred.

SUMMARY

IT planning has several objectives: the alignment of IT with the strategies, plans, and initiatives of the organization; the development of support for the plan; and the preparation of tactical plans.

IT strategies are developed through five vectors. Each vector is complex, and the integration of the vectors is challenging.

IT planning is a very important organizational process. However, alignment of IT with the organization has been and remains a major challenge. This process is quite difficult. IT planning prowess cannot guarantee organizational excellence in applying IT.

IT can be very effective in supporting an organization's effort to improve its competitive position. This support generally occurs when IT is employed to leverage core organizational processes, support the collection of critical data, customize or differentiate products and services, and transform core characteristics and capabilities.

IT is incapable of providing these advantages by itself. Utility occurs when IT is applied by intelligent and experienced leadership in the pursuit of well-conceived strategies and plans. IT cannot overcome weak leadership, inadequate strategies and plans, or inferior products and services.

Organizations pursuing an IT-supported advantage should be careful of acquiring the baggage that can result: reduced margins with no improvement in competitive position, process ossification, and nonrational pursuit of mirage technologies.

KEY TERMS

Alignment challenges and limitations
Governing concepts
IT alignment
IT Asset

IT as a competitive advantage
IT strategy vectors
Strategy formulation
Strategy implementation

LEARNING ACTIVITIES

1. Describe how an EMR system can advance the strategies of a health care provider organization.

2. Describe how a customer relationship management system can advance the strategies of a payer organization.

3. Pick an example of a new technology, such as personal health records. Discuss how this technology might leverage the strategy of a provider or a payer organization.

4. If a health care organization has a strategy of lowering its costs of care, what types of IT applications might it consider? If the organization has a strategy of improving the quality of its care, what types of IT applications might it consider? Compare the two lists of applications.

CHAPTER

13

IT GOVERNANCE AND MANAGEMENT

LEARNING OBJECTIVES

- To be able to understand the scope and importance of information technology governance.
- To review the IT roles and responsibilities of users, the IT department, and senior management.
- To review the factors that enable sustained excellence in the application of IT.
- To be able to discuss the components of an IT budget and the processes for developing the budget.

In this chapter we discuss an eclectic but important set of information technology (IT) governance and management processes, structures, and issues. Developing, managing, and evolving IT governance and management mechanisms is often a central topic for organizational leadership. In this chapter we will cover the following areas:

- *IT governance.* IT governance is composed of the processes, reporting relationships, roles, and committees that an organization develops to make decisions about IT resources and activities and to manage the execution of those decisions. These decisions involve such issues as setting priorities, determining budgets, defining project management approaches, and addressing IT problems.

- *IT effectiveness.* Over the years several organizations have demonstrated exceptional effectiveness in applying IT; they include American Express, Bank of America, Schwab, and American Airlines. This chapter discusses what the management of these organizations did that led to such effectiveness. It also examines the attributes of IT-savvy senior leadership.

- *IT budget.* Developing the IT budget is a complex exercise. Organizations always have more IT proposals than can be funded. Some proposals are strategically important and others involve routine maintenance of existing infrastructure, making proposal comparison difficult. Although complex and difficult, the effective development of the IT budget is a critical management responsibility.

IT GOVERNANCE

IT governance refers to the principles, processes, and organizational structure that govern the IT resources (Drazen & Straisor, 1995). When solid governance exists, the organization is able to give a coherent answer to the following questions:

- Who sets priorities for IT, and how are those priorities set?

- What organizational structures are needed to support the linkage between IT and the rest of the organization?

- Who is responsible for implementing information system plans, and what principles will guide the implementation process?

- How are IT responsibilities distributed between IT and the rest of the organization and between centralized and decentralized (local) IT groups in an integrated delivery system?

- How are IT budgets developed?

    At its core, governance involves

- Determining the distribution of the responsibility for making decisions, the scope of the decisions that can be made by different organizational functions, and the processes to be used for making decisions

---

Lists quoted from Applegate, Austin, & McFarlan, 2003, McGraw-Hill © 2002, are reproduced with permission of The McGraw-Hill Companies.

- Defining the roles that various organizational members and committees fulfill for IT—for example, which committee should monitor progress in clinical information systems, and what is the role of a department head during the implementation of a new system for his or her department?

- Developing IT-centric organizational processes for making decisions in such key areas as

    IT strategy development

    IT prioritization and budgeting

    IT project management

    IT architecture and infrastructure management

- Defining policies and procedures that govern the use of IT. For example, if a user wants to buy a new network for use in his or her department, what policies and procedures govern that decision?

PERSPECTIVE

THE FOUNDATION OF IT GOVERNANCE

Peter Weill and Jeanne Ross have identified five major areas that form the foundation of IT governance. The organization's governance mechanisms need to create structures and processes for these areas.

- *IT principles:* high-level statements about how IT is used in the business.

- *IT architecture:* an integrated set of technical choices to guide the organization in satisfying business needs. The architecture is a set of policies, procedures, and rules for the use of IT and for evolving IT in a direction that improves IT support for the organization.

- *IT infrastructure strategies:* strategies for the existing technical infrastructure (and IT support staff) that ensure the delivery of reliable, secure, and efficient services.

- *Business application needs:* processes for identifying the needed applications.

- *IT investment and prioritization:* mechanisms for making decisions about project approvals and budgets.

Source: Weill & Ross, 2004, p. 27.

Developing and maintaining an effective and efficient IT governance structure is a complex exercise. Moreover, governance is never static. Continuous refinements may be needed as the organization discovers imperfections in roles, responsibilities, and processes.

Governance Characteristics

Well-developed governance mechanisms have several characteristics.

They are perceived as objective and fair. No organizational decision-making mechanisms are free from politics, and some decisions will be made as part of "side deals." It is exceptionally rare for all managers of an organization to agree with any particular decision. No matter how good an individual is at performing his or her IT governance role, there will be members of the organization who will view that individual as a lower life form. Nonetheless, organizational participants should generally view governance as fair, objective, well reasoned, and having integrity. The ability of governance to govern is highly dependent on the willingness of organizational participants to be governed.

They are efficient and timely. Governance mechanisms should arrive at decisions quickly, and governance processes should be efficient, removing as much bureaucracy as possible.

They make authority clear. Committees and individuals who have decision authority should have a clear understanding of the scope of their authority. Individuals who have IT roles should understand those roles. The organization's management must have a consistent understanding of its approach to IT governance. There will always be occasions where decision rights are murky, roles are confusing, or processes are unnecessarily complex, but these occasions should be few.

They can change as the organization, its environment, and its understanding of technology changes. For example, several organizations spun off portions of their IT groups to create e-commerce departments intended to support the organization's undertakings during the Internet frenzy from 1999 to 2001. This spinning off was an effort to, among other objectives, free e-commerce initiatives from the normal bureaucracy of these organizations' governance structures. This separation was meant to allow the e-commerce groups to operate in "Internet time." These groups have been largely dismantled as a more mature understanding of the role of the Internet developed. Likewise, the potential regional efforts to effect interoperability between clinical information systems will require new governance mechanisms that bring representatives from the partnering organizations together to deal with interorganizational IT issues. Governance mechanisms evolve as IT technology and the organization's use of that technology evolve.

Linkage of Governance to Strategies

Governance structures and the distribution of responsibilities should be heavily influenced by basic strategic objectives. For example, the desire of several provider organizations to be integrated will have ramifications for governance design. In this section we present two examples of governance that is linked to a strategic objective.

Governance to support the integration of the components of an integrated delivery system (IDS) might have these characteristics:

- A central IDS IT committee develops the IT priorities, to maintain the perspective of overall integration and to ensure that initiatives that support integration of the system of care are given a higher priority than those that do not.

- A centralized IT department or group exists, and it has authority over local IT groups.

- IT budgets developed locally are subject to central approval.

- The IT plan specifies the means by which an integrated infrastructure, including integrated applications, will be achieved and the boundaries of that plan: for example, local organizations are free to select from a set of patient care system options but, whatever the selection, the patient care system must interface with the IDS clinical data repository.

- Members of the IDS are constrained in their selection of applications to support ancillary departments, having to choose from those on an "approved" list.

- Certain pieces of data—for example, payer class or patient problems—and certain identifiers—for example, patient identifier and provider identifier—have to use a common dictionary or standard.

- All IDS members must use the same electronic mail system.

This approach is designed to ensure that the applications used by all the organizations within the IDS can be well integrated. The need for this high degree of application integration originates in the IDS's strategy of integrating its care. This approach (referring back to our discussion in Chapter Twelve) represents one of the organization's *governing concepts*, its definition of integration.

Governance to support the ability of the IDS member organizations to be *locally responsive* might have these characteristics:

- A small, central IT group is created to assist in local IT plan development; develop technical, data, and application standards; and perform technical research and development. This group has an advisory and coordination relationship with the local IT organizations.

- Local IT steering committees develop local IT plans according to processes and criteria defined locally. A central IT steering committee with an advisory role reviews these plans to identify and advise on areas of potential redundancy or serious inconsistency.

- IT budgets are developed locally according to overall budget guidelines established centrally—for example, there are rules for capitalizing new systems and selecting the duration to use for depreciation.

- Certain pieces of data are standardized to ensure that the IDS can prepare consolidated financial statements and patient activity counts.

- Local sites are free to, for example, select any e-mail system, but that system must be able to send and receive messages using Internet protocols and the local e-mail system directory must be accessible to other e-mail directories.

This approach reflects a strategy of ensuring that each IDS member has the latitude to respond to local market needs. This approach also reflects a governing concept in the form of a definition of integration. Each of the examples we have just given offers a different definition of integration, and both definitions are correct. As a result of these different definitions, IT governance will be different in these organizations, and both approaches to governance are correct.

IT governance structures and approaches must be designed so that they further organizational goals and strategies. They should not be brought into existence purely to perform some normative task. For example, the thinking that says, "all organizations have IT steering committees with a broad representation of senior leadership and hence so should we," is misguided. If the organization has, for example, an objective of being locally responsive that may mean that no central steering committee should exist or that its powers should be limited.

IT, User, and Senior Management Responsibilities

Effective application of IT involves the thoughtful distribution of IT responsibilities between the IT department, users of applications and IT services, and senior management. In general these responsibilities address decision-making rights and roles. Although different organizations will arrive at different distributions of these responsibilities, and an organization's distribution may change over time, there is a fairly normative distribution (Applegate, Austin, & McFarlan, 2003).

IT Department Responsibilities The IT department should be responsible for the following:

- Developing and managing the long-term architectural plan and ensuring that IT projects conform to that plan.
- Developing a process to establish, maintain and evolve IT standards in several areas:

    Telecommunications protocols and platforms

    Client devices, e.g., workstations and PDAs, and client software configurations

    Server technologies, middleware and database management systems

    Programming languages

    IT documentation procedures, formats and revision policies

    Data definitions (this responsibility is generally shared with the organization function, e.g., finance and health information management, that manages the integrity and meaning of the data)

    IT disaster and recovery plans

    IT security policies and incident response procedures

- Developing procedures that enable the assessment of sourcing options for new initiatives, e.g., build vs. buy new applications or leveraging existing vendor partner offerings versus utilizing a new vendor when making an application purchase

- Maintaining an inventory of installed and planned systems and services and developing plans for the maintenance of systems or the planned obsolescence of applications and platforms
- Managing the professional growth and development of the IT staff
- Establishing communication mechanisms that help the organization understand the IT agenda, challenges and services and new opportunities to apply IT
- Maintaining effective relationships with preferred IT suppliers of products and services [Applegate, Austin, & McFarlan, 2003, p. 56].

The scope and depth of these responsibilities may vary. Some of the responsibilities of the IT group may be delegated to others. For example, some non-IT departments may be permitted to have their own IT staff and manage their own systems. This should be done only with the approval of senior management. And the IT department should be asked to provide oversight of the departmental IT group to ensure that professional standards are maintained and that no activities that compromise the organization's systems are undertaken. For example, the IT department can ensure that virus control procedures and software are effectively applied.

The organization may decide that the IT department should have almost imperial authority in carrying out its responsibilities or that its role should be closer to adviser to senior management. Organizations generally arrive at a level of authority in between imperial and advisory—a level based on experience and recent history.

In general the IT department is responsible for making sure that both individual and organizational information systems are reliable, secure, efficient, current, and supportable. It is also usually responsible for managing the relationship with suppliers of IT products and services and ensuring that the processes that lead to new IT purchases are rigorous.

User Responsibilities IT users (primarily middle managers and supervisors) have several IT-related responsibilities:

- Understanding the scope and quality of IT activities that are supporting their area or function
- Ensuring that the goals of IT initiatives reflect an accurate assessment of the function's needs and challenges and that the estimates of the function's resources (personnel time, funds and management attention) needed by IT initiatives, e.g., to support the implementation of a new system, are realistic

- Developing and reviewing specifications for IT projects and ensuring that ongoing feedback is provided to the IT organization on implementation issues, application enhancements and IT support, e.g., ensuring that the new application has the functionality needed by the user department

- Ensuring that the applications used by a department are functioning properly, e.g., by periodically testing the accuracy of system-generated reports and checking that passwords are deleted when staff leave the organization

- Participating in developing and maintaining the IT agenda and priorities [Applegate, Austin, & McFarlan, 2003, p. 62].

These responsibilities constitute a minimal set. In Chapter Seven, we discussed an additional, and more significant, set of responsibilities during the implementation of new applications.

Senior Management Responsibilities The primary IT responsibilities of the senior leadership are as follows:

- Ensuring that the organization has a comprehensive, thoughtful and flexible IT strategy

- Ensuring an appropriate balance between the perspectives and agendas of the IT organization and the users, e.g., the IT organization may want a new application that has the most advanced technology while the user department wants the application that has been used in the industry for a long time

- Establishing standard processes for budgeting, acquiring, implementing and supporting IT applications and infrastructure

- Ensuring that IT purchases and supplier relationships conform to organizational policies and practices, e.g., contracts with IT vendors need to use standard organizational contract language

- Developing, modifying and enforcing the responsibilities and roles of the IT organization and users

- Ensuring that the IT applications and activities conform to all relevant regulations and required management controls and risk mitigation processes and procedures

- Encouraging the thoughtful review of new IT opportunities and appropriate IT experimentation [Applegate, Austin, & McFarlan, 2003, p. 68].

PERSPECTIVE

PRINCIPLES FOR IT INVESTMENTS AND MANAGEMENT

Charlie Feld and Donna Stoddard have identified three principles for effective IT investments and management. They note that the responsibility for developing and implementing these principles lies with the organization's senior leadership.

1. *A long-term IT renewal plan linked to corporate strategy.* Organizations need IT plans that are focused on achieving the organization's overall strategy and goals. The organization must develop this IT renewal plan and remain focused, often over the course of many years, on its execution.

2. *A simplified, unifying corporate technology platform.* This IT platform must be well architected and be defined and developed from the perspective of the overall organization rather than the accumulation of the perspectives of multiple departments and functions.

3. *A highly functional, performance-oriented IT organization.* The IT organization must be skilled, experienced, organized, goal-directed, responsive, and continuously work on establishing great working relationships with the rest of the organization.

Source: Feld & Stoddard 2004 p. 3.

Although organizations will vary in the ways they distribute decision-making responsibility and roles and the ways in which they implement them, problems may arise when the distribution between groups is markedly skewed (Applegate, Austin, & McFarlan, 2003).

Too much user responsibility can lead to a series of uncoordinated and under-managed user investments in information technology. This occurs when a number of independent user departments make IT decisions that result in a wide range of technologies and vendors, making it difficult to manage and integrate these systems. Users can also underestimate the difficulty of managing IT platforms and make poor technology decisions. This can result in

- An inability to achieve integration between highly heterogeneous systems.

- Insufficient attention to infrastructure, resulting in application instability.

- High IT costs, due to insufficient economies of scale, significant levels of redundant activity, and the cost of supporting a high number of heterogeneous systems.

- A failure to leverage IT opportunities because of user ignorance or fear of IT: for example, users won't invest in needed applications because they are afraid to do so.

■ A lack of, or uneven, rigor applied to the assessment of the value of IT initiatives: for example, insufficient homework may be done and an application selected that has serious functional limitations.

Too much IT responsibility can lead to

■ Too much emphasis on technology, to the detriment of the fit of an application with the user function's need: for example, when a promising application does not completely satisfy the IT department's technical standards, IT will not allow its acquisition.

■ A failure to achieve the value of an application due to user resistance to a solution imposed by IT: "We in the IT department have decided that we know what you need. We don't trust your ability to make an intelligent decision."

■ Too much rigor applied to IT investment decisions; excessive bureaucracy can stifle innovation.

■ A very high proportion of the IT budget devoted to infrastructure, to the detriment of application initiatives, as the IT department seeks to achieve ever greater levels (although perhaps not necessary levels) of reliability, security, and agility.

■ Reduction in business innovation when IT is unwilling to experiment with new technologies that might have stability and supportability problems.

Either extreme can clearly create problems. And no compromise position will make the IT department and the IT users happy with all facets of the outcome. An outcome of "the best answer we can develop but not an answer that satisfies all" is an inevitable result of the leadership discussion of responsibility and role distribution.

Specific Governance Structures

In any organization there may be a plethora of committees and a series of complex reporting relationships and accountabilities, all of which need to operate with a fair degree of harmony in order for governance to be effective. Among them should be five core structures for governing IT:

1. Board responsibility for IT.
2. A senior leadership forum that guides the development of the IT agenda, finalizes the IT budget, develops major IT-centric policies, and addresses any significant IT issue that cannot be resolved elsewhere. This core structure includes subcommittees, designated by the forum, that have specific roles and responsibilities: for example, a privacy committee or a care improvement committee that is charged with overseeing the implementation of a clinical information system.
3. Initiative- and project-specific committees and roles (this structure will be discussed in Chapter Fourteen).
4. IT liaison relationships.
5. A chief information officer (CIO) and other IT staff (described in Chapter Eleven).

The Board The health care organization's board holds the fundamental accountability for the performance of the organization, including the IT function. The board must decide how it will carry out its responsibility with respect to IT.

At a minimum this responsibility involves receiving a periodic update (perhaps annually), at a board meeting, from the CIO about the status of the IT agenda and the issues confronting the effective use of IT. In addition, financial information system controls and IT risk mitigation are often identified and discussed by the board's audit committee, and the IT budget is discussed by the finance committee.

Some organizations create an IT committee of the board. Realizing that the normal board agenda might not always allow sufficient time for discussion of important IT issues and that not all board members have deep experience in IT, the board can appoint a committee of board members who are seasoned IT professionals (IT academics, CIOs of regional organizations, and leaders in the IT industry). The committee, chaired by a trustee, need not be composed entirely of board members. IT professionals who are not on the board may serve as members too. This committee informs the board of its assessments of a wide range of IT challenges and initiatives and makes recommendations about these issues.

The charter for such a committee might charge the committee to

- Review and critique IT application, technical, and organizational strategies.
- Review and critique overall IT tactical plans and budgets.
- Discuss and provide advice on major IT issues and challenges.
- Explore opportunities to leverage vendor partnerships.

Committee meeting agenda items might include

- Assessments of the value of clinical information systems
- Long-term plans for the organization's financial systems
- IT staff recruitment and retention issues
- The annual IT budget

Organizational leaders should not believe, however, that appointing an IT committee gets the board off the hook for having to deal with IT issues. Rather, this committee should be viewed as a way for all board members to continue their efforts to become more knowledgeable and comfortable with the IT conversation.

Senior Leadership Organizational Forum Most health care organizations have a committee called something like the *executive committee*. Composed of the senior leadership of the organization, this committee is the forum in which strategy discussions occur and major decisions regarding operations, budgets, and initiatives are made. It is highly desirable to have the CIO as a member of this committee.

Major IT decisions should be made at the meetings of this committee. These decisions will cover a gamut of topics, such as approving the outcome of a major system selection process, defining changes in direction that may be needed during the course of significant implementations, setting IT budget targets, and ratifying the IT component of the strategic-planning efforts.

This role does not preclude the executive committee from assigning IT-related tasks or discussions to other committees. For example, a medical staff leadership committee may be asked to develop policies regarding physician use of computerized provider order entry. A committee of department heads may be asked to select a new application to support registration and scheduling. A committee of human resource staff may be charged with developing policies regarding organizational staff use of the Internet while at work.

The executive committee, major departments and functions, and several high-level committees will regularly be confronted with IT topics and issues that do not arise from the organization's IT plan and agenda. For example, a board member may ask if the organization should outsource its IT function. Several influential physicians may suggest that the organization assess a new information technology that seems to be getting a lot of hype. The CEO may ask how the organization should (or whether it should) respond to an external event: for example, a new Institute of Medicine report. The organization may need to address new regulations: for example, rules devolving from the Health Insurance Portability and Accountability Act (HIPAA).

When it is not clear which person or committee should address these issues or topics, they could be brought forth during an executive committee meeting for triage. (Alternatively, the CEO, CIO, chief financial officer [CFO], or chief operating officer [COO] may decide where an issue should be handled.) The executive committee can form a task force to examine the issue and develop recommendations, or it can request that an existing forum or function address the issue. For example, a task force of clinicians and IT staff could be asked to examine the ramifications of a new Institute of Medicine report. The organization's compliance department could be charged with developing the organization's response to new regulations.

Some organizations create an IT steering committee and charge this committee with addressing all IT issues and decisions. The use of such committees is uneven in health care organizations. Approximately half have such a committee, and most of these committees are not regarded as functioning effectively.

If an organization has an IT steering committee that works well, it should leave it alone. In general, however, such committees are not a good idea. They tend not to be composed of the most senior leadership, and hence their links to the thinking process of the CEO and the executive committee are not strong. They tend to view IT issues in isolation from the overall issues facing the organization, and few IT issues can be dealt with well in isolation. And committee members often wind up fighting each other over parochial slices of the pie during the IT budget discussion.

IT steering committees are often seen as a senior leadership effort to get "IT problems" off their plate and onto someone else's plate. This is an abdication of responsibility.

IT Liaison Relationships   All major functions and departments of the organization—for example, finance, human resources, member services, medical staff affairs, and nursing—should have an IT liaison. The IT liaison is responsible for

- Developing effective working relationships with the leadership of each major function

- Ensuring that the IT issues and needs of these functions are understood and communicated to the IT department and the executive committee
- Working with function leadership to ensure appropriate IT representation on function task forces and committees that are addressing initiatives that will require IT support
- Ensuring that the organization's IT strategy, plans and policies, and procedures are discussed with function leadership

The IT liaison role is an invaluable one. It ensures that the IT department and the IT strategy receive needed feedback and that function leaders understand the directions and challenges of the IT agenda. It also promotes an effective collaboration between IT and the other functions and departments.

PERSPECTIVE

IMPROVING COORDINATION AND WORKING RELATIONSHIPS

Carol Brown and Vallabh Sambamurthy have identified five mechanisms used by IT groups to improve their coordination and working relationships with the rest of the organization.

1. *Integrators* are individuals who are responsible for linking a particular organization department or function with the IT department. An integrator might be a CIO who is a participant in senior management forums. An integrator might also be an IT person who is responsible for working with the finance department on IT initiatives that are centered on that function; such a person might have a title such as *manager, financial information systems.*

2. *Groups* are committees and task forces that regularly bring IT staff and organization staff together to work collectively on IT issues. These groups could include, for example, the information systems steering committee or a standing joint meeting between IT and nursing to address current IT issues and review the status of ongoing IT initiatives.

3. *Processes* are organizational approaches to management activity such as developing the IT budget, selecting new applications, and implementing new systems. These processes invariably involve both IT and non-IT staff.

4. *Informal relationship building* includes a series of activities such as one-on-one meetings, IT staff presentations at department head meetings, and co-location of IT staff and user staff.

(Continued)

PERSPECTIVE (*Continued*)

> 5. *Human resource practices* include training IT staff on team building, offering user feedback to IT staff during their reviews, and having IT staff spend time in a user area observing work.
>
> *Source:* Brown & Sambamurthy, 1999, p. 68.

Variations The specific governance structures just described are typical in medium-sized and large provider or payer organizations. In other types of health care settings these structures will be different.

A medium-sized physician group might not have a separate board. The physicians and the practice manager might make up both the board and the senior leadership forum. The group might not need a CIO. Instead the practice administrator might manage contracts and relationships with companies that provide practice management systems and support workstations and printers. The practice administrator also might perform all user liaison functions.

A division within a state department of public health would not have a board, but it should have a forum where division leadership can discuss IT issues. IT decisions might be made there or at meetings of the leadership of the overall department. Similarly, the CIO for the department might not have organized IT in a way that results in a division CIO. And the staff of the department CIO might provide user liaison functions for the division.

Despite these variations, effective management of IT still requires

- A senior management forum where major IT decisions are made

- A person responsible for day-to-day management of the IT function and for ensuring that an IT strategy exists

- Mechanisms for ensuring that IT relationships have been established with major organizational functions

In addition, although the structures will vary, the guidance for the respective roles of the IT group, users, and management remains the same. The desirable attributes of the person responsible for IT are unchanged. And the properties of good governance do not change.

PERSPECTIVE

ARCHETYPES OF IT GOVERNANCE DECISION MAKING

Peter Weill and Jeanne Ross have identified six archetypes of IT governance. Each archetype describes an approach to making major IT decisions.

1. *Business monarchy:* a group of business executives, often an executive committee; may include the CIO

2. *IT monarchy:* a group of IT executives or the CIO individually

3. *Feudal:* a committee of business unit leaders or key process owners

4. *Federal:* a committee of senior leadership and business unit leaders; may include IT leadership and senior managers

5. *IT duopoly:* IT executives and one other group: for example, IT leadership and finance leadership

6. *Anarchy:* each individual or business unit on its own

Any one health care organization may have several of these forms of governance but apply them in different areas. For example, a business monarchy may decide IT strategy but an IT monarchy may be used to establish architecture standards. In addition, an IT duopoly may be asked to select and implement a new revenue management system.

Source: Weill & Ross, 2004, p 59.

IT EFFECTIVENESS

Several studies have examined organizations that have been particularly effective in the use of IT. Determining effectiveness is difficult, and these studies have defined organizations that show effectiveness in IT in a variety of ways. Among them are organizations that have developed information systems that defined an industry—as Amazon.com has altered the retail industry, for example—organizations that have a reputation for being effective over decades, and organizations that have demonstrated exceptional IT innovation.

The studies have attempted to identify those organizational factors or attributes that have led to or created the environment in which effectiveness has occurred. In other words, the studies have sought to answer the question, What are the organizational attributes that result in some organizations developing truly remarkable IT prowess?

If an organization understands these attributes and desires to be very effective in its use of IT, then it is in a position to develop strategies and approaches to create or modify its own attributes. For example, one attribute is having strong working relationships between the IT function and the rest of the organization. If an organization finds that its own relationships are weak or dysfunctional, strategies and plans can be created to improve them.

The studies suggest that organizations that aspire to high levels of effectiveness and innovation in their application of IT must take steps to ensure that the core capacity of the organization to achieve such effectiveness is developed. It is a critical IT responsibility of organizational leadership to continuously (year in and year out) identify and effect steps needed to improve overall effectiveness in IT. The development of this capacity is a challenge different from the challenge of identifying specific opportunities to use IT in the course of improving operations or enhancing management decision making. For an analogy, consider running. A runner's training, injury management, and diet are designed to ensure the core capacity to run a marathon. This capacity development is different from developing an approach to running a specific marathon, which must consider the nature of the course, the competing runners, and the weather.

Although having somewhat different conclusions (resulting in part from somewhat different study questions), the studies have much in common regarding capacity development. Four of these studies are summarized in the following sections.

Factors Leading to Visionary IT

The Financial Executives Research Foundation sponsored a study, conducted by Sambamurthy and Zmud (1996), to identify factors that have led to the development of visionary IT applications. Visionary applications are "applications that help managers make decisions, introduce new products and services more quickly and frequently, improve customer relations, and enhance the manufacturing process. Visionary IT applications seek to transform some of a firm's business processes in 'frame breaking' ways. These applications create a variety of benefits to businesses that not only affect their current operations but also provide opportunities for new markets, strategies and relationships" (p. 1).

The study had several findings:

The nature of visionary applications. Visionary applications focused on one or more of these activities: leveraging core business operations, enhancing decision making, improving customer service, or speeding up the delivery of new products and services. These applications were platforms that enabled the business to handle multiple work processes. An example of such a platform in health care is the electronic health record system.

Roles associated with visionary projects. Visionary projects required the participation of four key players. Envisioners conceptualized the initial ideas for a project. Project champions were instrumental in selling an envisioner's idea and its value to senior executives. Executive sponsors acted as champions, with seed funding and political support. IT experts supplied the necessary technical vision and expertise to ensure that the idea would work.

Ways to facilitate investment in visionary IT applications. Several factors facilitated investment in visionary applications:

- A climate existed that offered employees the power, and the support, to undertake visionary applications that often carried significant personal and organizational risk.

- Mechanisms existed for investing continuously in the IT infrastructure.

- Coordinating mechanisms were established to bring together envisioners, project champions, executive sponsors, and IT experts.

- The role of the CIO, in addition to that of envisioner and IT expert, was to ensure that envisioners' proposals furthered the interests of the business, to be an architect and advocate for the corporate IT infrastructure, and to serve as the architect of IT-related coordinating mechanisms.

Rationales for undertaking visionary IT applications. Visionary IT applications were generally defended using one of two distinct rationales: their contribution to critical work processes or their support of a primary strategic driver. In addition to the discussion and analyses that surrounded the selected application, prototypes, best-practice visits to other organizations, and consultants were often used to further organizational understanding of the proposed initiative.

Factors Producing Long-Term IT Competitiveness

Ross, Beath, and Goodhue (1996) examined those factors that enable organizations to achieve long-term competitiveness in the application of IT. This study identified the development and management of three key IT assets as critical to achieving a sustained, IT-based competitive advantage:

The IT human resource asset. The study found that a well-developed, highly competent IT human resource asset was one that "consistently solves business problems and addresses business opportunities through information technology." This asset had three dimensions:

1. IT staff had the technical skills needed to craft and support applications and infrastructures and to understand and appropriately apply new technologies.

2. IT staff had superior working relationships with the end-user community and were effective at furthering their own understanding of the business: its directions, cultures, work processes, and politics.

3. IT staff were responsible, and knew that they were responsible, for solving business problems. This orientation went beyond performing discreet tasks and led IT staff to believe that they "owned" the challenge of solving business problems and had the power to carry out that ownership.

The technology asset. The technology asset consists of "sharable technical platforms and databases." An effective technology asset had two distinguishing characteristics:

1. A well-developed technology architecture

2. Standards that limited the variety of technologies that would be supported

Failure to create a robust architecture can result in applications that are difficult to change, not integrated, expensive to manage, and resistant to scaling (Weill & Broadbent, 1998). These limitations hinder the ability of the organization to advance. IT resources, efforts, and capital can be consumed by the difficulty of managing the current, poorly constructed infrastructure, and applications and relatively modest advances can be too draining.

The relationship asset. When the relationship asset was strong, IT and each business unit's management shared the risk and responsibility for effective application of IT in the organization. A solid relationship asset was present when the business unit was the owner, and was accountable for, all unit IT projects, and top management led the IT priority-setting process.

This study also noted the interrelationships among the assets. IT and user relationships were strengthened by the presence of a strong IT staff. A well-developed, agile infrastructure enabled the IT staff to execute project delivery at high levels and be more effective at solving business problems.

Factors Leading to Industry-Changing Systems

McKenney, Copeland, and Mason (1995) studied those factors that resulted in managerial team success in creating and implementing innovative information systems. They were particularly interested in those examples where the resulting information systems became the dominant design in a particular industry. They studied American Airlines, Bank of America, United States Automobile Association, Baxter Travenol-American Hospital Supply, and Frito-Lay. Their study generated several conclusions:

Management team. IT innovations were led proactively by a management team driven to change its processes through the means of IT. The management team had to play three essential roles:

1. The CEO or other senior executive was both visionary and a good businessperson. He or she had sufficient power and prestige to drive technological innovation.

2. A *technology maestro*, often the CIO, had a remarkable combination of business acumen and technological competence. The CIO had to deliver the system and had to recruit, energize, and lead a superb technical team.

3. The technical team understood how to apply the technology in innovative ways and was capable of developing new business processes that leveraged the technology.

In addition to exceptional competence in each role, in the companies studied there was a rare chemistry between the players of the roles. A change in a role's incumbent often stalled the innovation. This suggests that a great CIO in one setting may not be a great CIO in another setting.

Evolution of the innovation. Innovative systems evolved over time and generally went through several phases of evolution:

■ A business crisis developed: Bank of America, for example, was overwhelmed by the volume of paper transactions—and a search began for an IT solution.

■ IT competence was built as necessary research and development was done for potential IT solutions, particularly the application of emerging technologies.

■ The IT solution was planned and developed.

■ IT was used to restructure the organization and its processes and to lead changes in organizational strategies.

■ The strategy evolved and the systems were refined. Competitors began to emulate the success.

Throughout these phases the capabilities of the technology heavily influenced and constrained the operational changes that were envisioned and implemented. This series of phases occurred over five to seven years, reflecting the magnitude of the organizational change and the time required to experiment with, understand, and implement new information technology at scale. This interval suggests that a CIO (or CEO) average tenure of three years or less risks hindering the organization's ability to make truly innovative, IT-based transformations.

Capitalizing on IT innovation. A particular IT innovation was identified by the organization early in the life of that innovation as being the breakthrough necessary to resolve a business crisis or challenge. Across the cases studied the breakthroughs were the transistor, time-sharing, and cheap mass storage. Today a breakthrough innovation might be the radio frequency ID or the personal health record.

Factors Increasing the Value of IT Investments

Weill and Broadbent (1998) studied firms that "consistently achieve more business value for their information technology investment." This study noted that these organizations were excellent or above average in five characteristics:

Commitment to the strategic and effective application of IT. This commitment was widely known within each organization. Management participated actively in IT strategy discussions, thoughtfully assessed the business contribution of proposed IT investments, and provided seed funding to innovative and experimental IT projects.

Low political turbulence. IT investments often served to integrate processes and groups across the organization. Political conflict can reduce the likelihood and the success of interdisciplinary initiatives. IT investments can require that proposals for one part of the organization be funded at the expense of other parts or of proposed non-IT initiatives. Political turbulence can reduce the likelihood that such "disproportionate" investments will occur.

Satisfied users. When organizational staff had had good experiences with IT projects, they were more likely to view IT as something that could assist their endeavors and less likely to see it as a burden or a function that was anchoring the organization to one spot.

Integrated business information technology planning. Organizations that did a very good job of aligning IT plans and strategies with overall organizational plans and strategies were more effective with IT than those that did not align well.

Experience. Organizations that were experienced in their use and application of the technology, and had had success in those experiences, were more thoughtful and focused in their continued application of IT. They had a better understanding of the technology's capabilities and limitations. Users and their IT colleagues had a better understanding of their respective needs and roles and the most effective ways of working together on initiatives.

Summary of Studies

The studies discussed in the preceding pages suggest that organizations that aspire to effectiveness and innovation in their application of IT must take steps to ensure that their core capacity for IT effectiveness is developed to the point where high levels of progress can be achieved and sustained. The development of this capacity is a challenge different from the task of identifying specific opportunities to use IT in the course of improving core processes or ensuring that the IT agenda is aligned with the organizational agenda.

Although having somewhat different conclusions, the four studies have much in common when they consider capacity development:

Individuals and leadership matter. It is critical that the organization possess talented, skilled, and experienced individuals. These individuals will occupy a variety of roles: CEO, CIO, IT staff, and user middle managers. These individuals must be strong contributors. Although such an observation may seem trite, too often organizations, dazzled by the technology or the glorified experiences of others, embark on technology crusades and substantive investments that they have insufficient talent or leadership to effect well. The studies found that leadership is essential. It is an essential trait of the organization's senior management (or executive sponsors), the CIO, and the project team. Leaders must understand the vision, communicate the vision, be able to recruit and motivate a team, and have the staying power to see the innovation through several years of work with disappointments, setbacks, and political problems along the way.

Relationships are critical. Not only must the individual players be strong, the team must be strong. There are critical senior executive, IT executive, and project team roles that must be filled by highly competent individuals, and great chemistry must exist between the individuals in these distinct roles. Substitutions among team members, even when involving a replacement by an equally strong individual, can diminish the team. This is as true in IT innovation as it is in sports. Political turbulence diminishes the ability to develop a healthy set of relationships among organizational players.

The technology and the technical infrastructure both enable and hinder. New technologies can provide new opportunities for organizations to embark on major transformations of their activities. This implies that the health care CIO must have not only superior business and clinical understanding but also superior understanding of the technology. This does not imply that CIOs must be able to rewrite operating systems as well as the best system programmers, but it does mean that they must have superior understanding of the maturity, capabilities, and possible evolution of various information technologies. Several innovations have occurred because an IT group was able to identify and adopt an emerging technology that could make a significant contribution to addressing a current organizational challenge. The studies also stress the importance of well-developed technical architecture. Great architecture matters. Possessing state-of-the-art technology can be far less important than having a well-architected infrastructure.

The organization must encourage innovation. The organization's (and the IT department's) culture and leadership must encourage innovation and experimentation. This encouragement needs to be practical and goal directed: a real business problem, crisis, or opportunity must exist, and the project must have budgets, political protection, and deliverables.

True innovation takes time. Creating visionary applications or industry-dominant designs or an exceptional IT asset takes time and a lot of work. In the organizations studied by McKenney, Copeland, and Mason 1995, it often took five to seven years for the innovation to fully mature and for the organization to recast itself. Applications and designs will proceed through phases that are as normative as the passage from being a child to being an adult. Innovation, like the maturation of a human being, will see some variations in timing, depth, and success in moving through phases.

Evaluation of IT opportunities must be thoughtful. Visionary and dominant-design IT innovations should be analyzed and studied thoroughly. Nonetheless, organizations engaged in these innovations should also understand that a large amount of vision, management instinct, and "feel" guides the decision to initiate investment and continue investment. The organization that has had more experiences with IT, and more successful experiences, will be more effective in the evaluation (and execution) of IT initiatives.

Processes, data, and differentiation form the basis of an IT innovation. All the innovations studied were launched from management's fundamental understanding of current organizational limitations. Innovations should focus on the core elements discussed in Chapter Twelve as the basis for achieving an IT-based advantage: significant leveraging of processes, expanding and capitalizing on the ability to gather critical data, and achieving a high level of organizational differentiation. Often an organization can pursue all three simultaneously. At other times an organization may evolve from one core element to another as the competition responds or as it sees new leverage points.

Alignment must be mature and strong. The alignment between the IT activities and the business challenges or opportunities must be strong. It should also be mature in the sense that it depends on close working relationships rather than methodologies.

The IT asset is critical. Strong IT staff, well-designed IT governance, well-crafted architecture, and a superb CIO are critical contributors to success. There is substantial overlap between the factors identified in these studies and the components of the IT asset.

PERSPECTIVE

PRINCIPLES FOR HIGH PERFORMANCE

Robert Dvorak, Endre Holen, David Mark, and William Meehan have identified six principles at work in a high-performance IT function:

1. IT is a business-driven line activity and not a technology-driven IT staff function. Non-IT managers are responsible for selecting, implementing, and realizing the benefits of new applications. IT managers are responsible for providing cost-effective infrastructure to enable the applications.

2. IT funding decisions are made on the basis of value. Funding decisions require thorough business cases. IT decisions are based on business judgment and not technology judgment.

3. The IT environment emphasizes simplicity and flexibility. IT standards are centrally determined and enforced. Technology choices are conservative and packaged applications are used wherever possible.

(Continued)

PERSPECTIVE (*Continued*)

4. IT investments have to deliver near-term business results. The 80/20 rule is followed for applications, and projects are monitored relentlessly against milestones.

5. The IT operation engages in year-to-year operation productivity improvements.

6. A business-smart IT function and an IT-smart business organization are created. Senior leadership is involved in and conversant with IT decisions. IT managers spend time developing an understanding of the business.

Source: Dvorak, Holen, Mark, & Meehan, 1997, p. 166.

The Senior Leader in the Information Age

Earl and Feeney (2000) assessed the characteristics and behaviors of senior leaders (in this case CEOs) who were actively engaged and successful in the strategic use of IT. These leaders were convinced that IT could and would change the organization. They placed the IT discussion high on the strategic agenda. They looked to IT to identify opportunities to make significant improvements in organizational performance, rather than viewing the IT agenda as secondary to strategy development. They devoted personal time to understanding how their industry and their organization would evolve as IT evolved. And they encouraged other members of the leadership team to do the same.

Earl and Feeney 2000 observed five management behaviors in these leaders:

1. They studied rather than avoided IT. They devoted time to learning about new technologies and, through discussion and introspection, developed an understanding of the ways in which new technologies might alter organizational strategies and operations.

2. They incorporated IT into their vision of the future of the organization and discussed the role of IT when communicating that vision.

3. They actively engaged in IT architecture discussions and high-level decisions. They took time to evaluate major new IT proposals and their implications. They were visibly supportive of architecture standards. They established funds for the exploration of promising new technologies.

4. They made sure that IT was closely linked to core management processes:

   They integrated the IT discussion tightly into the overall strategy development process. This often involved setting up teams to examine aspects of the strategy and having both IT and business leaders at the table.

   They made sure IT investments were evaluated as one component of the total investment needed by a strategy. The IT investments were not relegated to a separate discussion.

They ensured strong business sponsorship for all IT investments. Business sponsors were accountable for managing the IT initiatives and ensuring the success of the undertaking.

5.   They continually pressured the IT department to improve its efficiency and effectiveness and to be visionary in its thinking.

CEOs and other members of the leadership team have an extraordinary impact on the tone, values, and direction of an organization. Hence their beliefs and daily behaviors have a significant impact on how effectively and strategically information technology is applied within an organization.

IT BUDGET

Developing budgets is one of the most critical management undertakings. The budget process forces management to make choices between initiatives and investments and requires analysis of the scope and impact of any initiative: for example, it answers questions such as, Will this initiative enable us to reduce supply costs by 3 percent?

Developing the IT budget is challenging, for several reasons:

- The IT projects proposed at any one time are eclectic. In addition to the IT initiatives proposed as a result of the alignment and strategic planning process, other initiatives may be put forward by clinical or administrative departments that desire to improve some aspect of their performance. Also on the table may be IT projects designed to improve infrastructure: for example, a proposal to upgrade servers. These initiatives will all be different in character and in the return they offer, making them difficult to compare.

- Dozens, if not hundreds, of IT proposals may be made, making it challenging to fully understand all the requests.

- The aggregate request for capital and operating budgets can be too expensive. It is not unusual for requests to total three to four times more money than the organization can afford. Even if it wanted to fund all of the requests, the organization doesn't have enough money to do so.

And yet the budget process requires that the organization grapple with these complexities and arrive at a budget answer.

Basic Budget Categories

To facilitate the development of the IT budget, the organization should develop some basic categories that organize the budget discussion.

Capital and Operating   The first category distinguishes between capital and operating budgets. Financial management courses are the best place to learn about these two categories. In brief, however, *capital budgets* are the funds associated with purchasing and deploying an asset. Common capital items in IT budgets are hardware and applications. *Operating budgets* are the funds associated with using and maintaining the asset. Common operating items in IT budgets are hardware maintenance contracts and the salaries of IT analysts. In an analogous fashion, the purchase of a car is a capital expense. Gasoline and tune-ups are operating expenses. Both capital and operating budgets are prepared for IT initiatives.

Support, Ongoing, and New IT *Support* refers to those IT costs (staff, hardware, and software licenses) necessary to support and maintain the applications and infrastructure that are in place now. Software maintenance contracts ensure that applications receive appropriate upgrades and bug fixes. Staff are needed to run the computer rooms and perform minor enhancements. Disk drives may need to be replaced. Failure to fund support activities can make it much more difficult to ensure the reliability of systems or to evolve applications to accommodate ongoing needs: for example, adding a new test to the dictionary for a laboratory system or introducing a new plan type into the patient accounting system.

Ongoing projects are those application implementations begun in a prior year and still under way. The implementation of a patient accounting system or a computerized provider order entry system can take several years. Hence a capital and operating budget is needed for several years to continue the implementation.

New projects are just that—there is a proposal for a new application or infrastructure application. The IT strategy may call for new systems to support nursing. Concerns over network security may lead to requests for new software to deter the efforts of hackers.

Support Current Operations or Strategic Plan Proposals may be directed to supporting current operations, perhaps by responding to new regulations or streamlining the workflow in a department. Proposals may also be explicitly linked to an aspect of the health care organization's strategic plan—they might call for applications to support a strategic emphasis on disease management, for example.

Budget Targets During the budget process, organizations define targets for the budget overall and for its components. For example, the organization might state that it would like to keep the overall growth in its operating budget to 2 percent but is willing to allow 5 percent growth in the IT operating budget. The organization might also direct that within that overall 5 percent growth, the budget for support should not grow by more than 3 percent but the budget for new projects and ongoing projects combined can grow by 11 percent. Table 13.1 illustrates the application of overall and selective operating budget targets.

Similarly, targets can be set for the capital budget. For example, perhaps it will be decided that the capital budget for support should remain flat but that given the decision to invest in an electronic medical record (EMR) system, the overall capital budget will increase to accommodate the capital required by the EMR investment.

TABLE 13.1. **Target Increases in an IT Operating Budget**

	Support Operations	Strategic Initiatives	Overall Target
Ongoing and new	9%	15%	11%
Support	3%	3%	3%
OVERALL TARGET	4%	7%	5%

Management Development of IT Budget Categories

The management discussion of the IT budget begins with the discussion of its categories and targets. Should the organization develop categories such as support, ongoing, and new? Should it assign selective budget targets by category? What should those targets be? There are no rules for this conversation. There is no optimal outcome.

However, the categories can be used to achieve various objectives. On the one hand, support often accounts for 70 to 80 percent of the IT operating budget and 20 to 30 percent of its capital budget. The organization can decide that support must work well but is of modest strategic value. Hence the budget orientation is to be efficient with support. The budget target should be sufficient to cover salary growth and increases in maintenance contracts but it should also encourage ongoing efforts to be more efficient. Efficiency can be gained, for example, by asking the IT function every year to achieve a 2 percent improvement in efficiency. On the other hand, an IT agenda with several important strategic initiatives may lead the organization to conclude that it will allow a 7 percent growth in the operating budget to support strategic initiatives but a more modest 4 percent growth in initiatives to support operations.

Whatever the outcome of the management discussion, the IT budget categories should remain consistent from year to year so that yearly comparisons of the budget can be made. Moreover, stability in definitions enables the management team to develop a common language and concepts during budget discussions. However, the targets may change annually, depending on the fiscal health of the organization and the strategic importance of the IT agenda.

IT Budget Development

In addition to formulating the categories already discussed, organizational leadership will need to develop the process through which the IT budget is discussed, prioritized, and approved. In other words, it must answer the question, What processes will we use to decide which projects will be approved subject to our targets? An example of a budget process is outlined in this section and illustrated in Figure 13.1.

This process example has five components, and the steps described here use some typical targets.

First, the IT department submits an operating budget to support the applications and infrastructure that will be in place as of the beginning of the fiscal year (the support

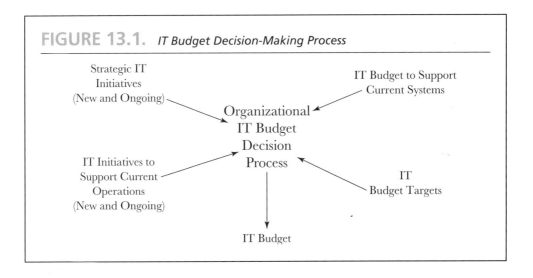

FIGURE 13.1. *IT Budget Decision-Making Process*

budget). This budget might be targeted to a 3 percent increase over the support budget for the prior fiscal year. The 3 percent increase reflects inflation, salary increases, a recognition that new systems were implemented during the fiscal year and will require support, and an acknowledgment that infrastructure (workstations, remote locations, and storage) consumption will increase. A figure for capital to support applications and infrastructure is also submitted, and it should be the same as that budgeted in the prior fiscal year. If the support operating and capital budgets achieve their targets, there is minimal management discussion of those budgets.

Second, IT leadership reviews the strategic IT initiatives (new and ongoing) with the senior leadership of the organization. This review may occur in a forum such as the executive committee. This committee, mindful of its targets, determines which strategic initiatives will be funded. If the budget being sought to support strategic IT initiatives is large or a major increase over the previous year, there will be discussions about the budget with the board.

Third, the organization must decide which new and ongoing initiatives that support current operations—for example, a new clinical laboratory or contract management system—will be funded. These discussions must occur in the forum where the overall operations budget is discussed. The forums in which such discussions occur are generally organizational meetings that routinely discuss operations and that number among their members the managers of major departments and functions. Budget requests for new IT applications are reviewed in the same conversation that discusses budget requests for new clinical services or improvement of the organization's physical plant.

Fourth, both the strategy budget discussion and the operations budget discussion follow a set of ground rules:

■ The IT budget is discussed in the same conversations that discuss non-IT budget requests. This will result in trade-offs between IT expenditures and other expenditures. This integration forces the organization to examine where it believes its monies are best spent, asking, for example, Should we invest in this IT proposal or should we invest in hiring staff to expand a clinical service? Following this process also means that IT requests and other budget requests are treated no differently.

- The level of analytical rigor required of the IT projects is the same as that required of any other requested budget item.

- Where appropriate, a sponsor—for example, a clinical vice president or a CFO— defends the IT requests that support his or her department in front of his or her colleagues. The IT staff or CIO should be asked to defend infrastructure investments—for example, major changes to the network—but should not be asked to defend applications.

The ground rule that sponsors should present their own IT requests deserves a bit more discussion, because the issue of who defends the request has several important ramifications, particularly for initiatives designed to improve current operations. Having this ground rule has the following results:

It forces assessment of trade-offs between IT and non-IT investments. The sponsor will determine whether to present the IT proposal or some other, perhaps non-IT, proposal. Sponsors are choosing which investments are the most important to them.

It forces accountability for investment results. The sponsor and his or her colleagues know that if the IT proposal is approved there will be less money available for other initiatives. The defender also knows that the value being promised must be delivered or his or her credibility in next year's budget discussion will be diminished.

It improves management comfort when dealing with IT proposals. Managers can be more comfortable with the IT proposal if one of their operations colleagues is defending it. The defender also learns how to be comfortable when presenting IT proposals.

It gets IT out of the role of defending other people's operation improvement initiatives. However, the IT function must still support the budget requests of others by providing data on the costs and capabilities of the proposed applications and the time frames and resources required to implement them. If the IT function believes that the proposed initiative lacks merit or is too risky, IT staff need to ensure that this opinion is heard during the budget approval process.

In the fifth and final step of the process, the operations and strategic budget recommendations are reviewed and discussed at an executive committee meeting. The executive committee can accept the recommendations, request further refinement (perhaps cuts) of the budget, or determine that a discussion of the budget is required at an upcoming board meeting.

SUMMARY

The management and leadership of an organization play significant roles in determining the effectiveness of information technology. This chapter discussed the role of developing and maintaining IT governance mechanisms—the processes, procedures, and roles that the organization uses to make IT decisions. These decisions cover diverse terrain: budgets, roles, and responsibility distribution and the process for resolution of IT issues.

Health care executives must also take steps to improve the overall ability of the organization to apply IT. These steps may involve working on improving IT-user relationships, managing IT architecture, developing approaches to IT experimentation, ensuring IT strategic alignment, and developing the skills of the IT staff.

An annual responsibility of the leadership is determining the IT budget. Developing this budget is difficult. Comparing diverse and numerous IT proposals is challenging. However, the budget process can be made easier (although not easy) by establishing clear definitions of budget categories, category targets, and the process for IT proposal review.

KEY TERMS

IT budget

IT effectiveness

IT governance

IT steering committee

IT, user and senior management responsibilities

 ## LEARNING ACTIVITIES

1. Interview a member of the senior leadership team of a health care organization on the subject of IT governance. Describe the organization's approach to IT governance, and assess its effectiveness.

2. Interview a health care CIO and a member of the senior leadership team of the same health care organization separately. Ask each of them to describe the process of preparing the IT budget. Compare and discuss their responses.

3. Interview a health care CIO and a member of the senior leadership team of the same health care organization separately. Ask each of them to describe the distribution of IT and user responsibilities. Compare and discuss their responses.

4. Assume that you are a consultant who has been asked to assess the effectiveness of an organization in applying IT. Construct a questionnaire (twenty questions) to guide the interviews of organizational leaders that you would conduct to determine effectiveness.

CHAPTER

14

MANAGEMENT'S ROLE IN MAJOR IT INITIATIVES

LEARNING OBJECTIVES

- To be able to understand the different types of organizational change associated with IT initiatives.
- To be able to discuss the strategies for effecting organizational change.
- To review the structures and processes used to manage IT projects.
- To review the factors that contribute to IT project failures.

Health care organizations routinely undertake projects or initiatives designed to improve the performance of the organization or advance its strategies through the use of new or existing information technologies. Many of these projects involve the implementation of a major application system, and often these projects are labeled "IT projects." Examples of such projects include implementing computerized provider order entry, streamlining the front-end processes of registration and scheduling, and enhancing the discharge process.

This chapter discusses the role of management in these IT projects. The strategy may have been defined and the IT agenda may have been aligned; now it is time to execute the plan. What role should management play during the execution of IT initiatives? What structures, processes, and roles should be in place to make sure that the initiatives are well managed?

This chapter covers three major topics:

- Managing organizational change due to IT initiatives
- Managing IT projects
- Understanding factors that contribute to IT initiative failures

MANAGING CHANGE DUE TO IT

A majority of IT initiatives involve or require organizational change—change in processes or organizational structure or change in the form of expansion or contraction of roles or services. IT-enabled change and IT-driven change have several possible origins:

- The new IT system has capabilities different from those of the previous system and hence the workflow that surrounds the system has to change and the tasks that staff perform have to change. For example, if a new electronic medical record system automatically generates letters for patients with normal test results, then the individuals who used to generate these letters will no longer have to do this task.

- The discussion surrounding the desired capabilities of a new application can lead to a reassessment of current processes, workflow, and distribution of tasks across staff and a decision to make changes in processes that extend well beyond the computer system. For example, the analysis surrounding a new patient accounting system might highlight problems that occur during registration and scheduling (such as failure to check insurance coverage during appointment check-in) that hinder the optimal performance of patient accounting. In this way a new system becomes a catalyst for a comprehensive set of changes.

- The health care organization's strategy may call for significant changes in the way the organization operates and delivers care. For example, the organization may decide to move aggressively to protocol-driven care. This transformation has extensive ramifications for processes, roles, and workflow and for the design of applications. New IT systems will be critical contributors to the changes needed, but they are not the epicenter of the change discussion.

Change management is an essential skill for the leaders of health care organizations. Although the need for this skill is not confined to situations that involve the implementation of major applications, change management is a facet of virtually all implementations of such applications.

Types of Organizational Change

Keen (1997) identified four categories of organizational change:

- Incremental
- Step-shift
- Radical
- Fundamental

Incremental Change   *Incremental change* occurs through a series (at times continuous) of small to medium-sized changes to processes, tasks, and roles. Each change carries relatively low risk, can be completed quickly, and is often accomplished without the need for substantial analysis or leadership intervention. At times, organizations establish an overall emphasis on continuous change and create groups to help departments make changes and measure change impact. Techniques such as LEAN and Six Sigma emphasize continuous, incremental change. Continuous, incremental change can be seen as plodding and lacking bold vision. However, this perception misses the power of such change over the course of time and the occurrence of such change across many facets of the organization. One should remember that the Grand Canyon was formed from continuous, incremental erosion.

The implementation of an application can involve change that is incremental. This is particularly true when the application is an upgrade of an existing application and has new reports and features that require modest alterations to existing workflow.

One outcome of continuous change may be the recognition that current application systems are progressively becoming a poor fit with the evolving organization. After several years of dealing with a growing gap between the capabilities of an application and the direction of an evolving organization, the organization may decide to purchase a new application; one that is a better fit.

Step-Shift Change   In *step-shift change* the leadership is committed to making significant changes but is not changing the basic direction of the organization or how it generates value. Examples of such change include a focused effort to significantly reduce the cost of care or improve patient safety, the addition of a nonacute business line in an organization that has previously focused on acute care, and a major effort to improve the patient service experience in the outpatient clinics. Step-shift change involves an intense focus on a critical aspect of the organization and, for the areas within that focus, major changes in processes, roles, and tasks. Step-shift change is often driven by a strategic realization that the basis of competition has evolved to the point that in the absence of such change, the organization's success is in some degree of peril.

This type of change invariably leads to the implementation of major new applications. An emphasis on patient safety may lead to the implementation of computerized provider order entry, and an effort to improve the patient experience in outpatient care may result in the implementation of a new registration and scheduling application. At times the leadership responsible for implementing a new application will realize that this implementation creates the opportunity to effect step-shift change, asking, for example, Why don't we take advantage of this new outpatient system to make significant improvements in the service experience?

Radical Change   *Radical change* leaves the organization and its core assumptions intact but significantly alters the way the organization carries out its business. The creation of an integrated delivery system from a collection of previously independent organizations is an example of radical change. The movement from fee-for-service reimbursement to full capitation (that is, fixed fee per patient per year) is radical change. Radical change always requires some changes, at times extensive changes, in the IT application portfolio. Because the way work is done has changed significantly across many facets of the organization, applications that fit the way work was previously done may no longer be helpful.

In health care it is rare that IT will cause or lead to a decision to undergo radical organizational change. The Internet frenzy that occurred in the early part of this century led many health care organizations to wonder whether the Internet would cause radical change. For example, if patients could look up medical information on the Internet would this significantly reduce their need for physicians? This radical change did not occur, although use of the Internet has led to incremental change and some step-shift change.

Fundamental Change   With *fundamental change* the leadership is committed to creating what will in effect be a new organization that is in a different business from the one the current organization engages in. This fundamental change has occurred for some companies. For example, the now deservedly maligned Enron changed its core business from acquiring and managing natural gas pipelines to managing a complex web of businesses that included a global broadband network and the trading of paper products. A health care example would be an acute care provider that closes all its beds and becomes a diagnostic imaging center. Fundamental change is risky, and the failure rate is very high.

Clearly, in these cases the entire IT application suite may need to be jettisoned and replaced with new applications that support the new business.

Effecting Organizational Change

The management strategies required to manage change depend on the type of change. As one moves from incremental to fundamental change, the magnitude and risk of the change increases enormously, as does the uncertainty about the form and success of the outcome.

In this section we will present some normative approaches to managing a blend of step-shift and radical change. Fundamental change is rare in health care. Incremental change carries less risk and hence requires less management. Note, however, that a program of continuous incremental change is in effect a form of step-shift change.

Managing change of this magnitude (step-shift to radical) is deceptively simple and quite hard at the same time. It is the same duality encountered in raising children. At one level it is easy; all you have to do is feed, teach, protect, and love them. At another level, especially during the teenage years, it can be an exceptionally complicated, exasperating, and scary experience.

Managing change has several necessary aspects (Keen, 1997):

- Leadership
- Language and vision
- Connection and trust
- Incentives
- Planning, implementing, and iterating

Leadership   Change must be led. Leadership, often in the form of a committee of leaders, will be necessary to

- Define the nature of the change.
- Communicate the rationale for and approach to the change.
- Identify, procure, and deploy necessary resources.
- Resolve issues, and alter direction as needed.
- Monitor the progress of the change initiative.

This leadership committee needs to be chaired by an appropriate senior leader. If the change affects the entire organization, the CEO should chair the committee. If the change is focused on a specific area, the most senior leader who oversees that area should chair the committee.

Language and Vision   The staff who are experiencing the change must understand the nature of the change. They must know what the world will look like (to the degree that this is clear) when the change has been completed, how their roles and work life will be different, and why making this change is important. The absence of this vision or a failure to communicate the importance of the vision elevates the risk that staff will resist the change and through subtle and not-so-subtle means cause the change to grind to a halt. Change is hard for people. They must understand the nature of the change and why they should go through with what they will experience as a difficult transition.

Leaders might describe the vision, the desired outcome of efforts to improve the outpatient service experience, in this way:

- Patients should be able to get an appointment for a time that is most convenient for them.

- Patients should not have to wait longer than ten minutes in the reception area before a provider can see them.

- We should communicate clearly with patients about their disease and the treatment that we will provide.

- We should seek to eliminate administrative and insurance busywork from the professional lives of our providers.

These examples illustrate a *thoughtful* use of language. They first and foremost focus on *patients*. But the organization also wants to improve the lives of its *providers*. The examples use the word *should* rather than the word *must* because it is thought that staff won't believe the organization can pull off 100 percent achievement of these goals and leaders do not want to establish goals seen as unrealistic. The examples also use the word *we* rather than the word *you*. *We* means that this vision will be achieved through a team effort, rather than implying that those hearing this message have to bear this challenge without leadership's help.

Connection and Trust   Achieving connection means that leadership takes every opportunity to present the vision throughout the organization. Leaders may use department head meetings, medical staff forums, one-on-one conversations in the hallway, internal publications, and e-mail to communicate the vision and to keep communicating the vision. Even when they start to feel ill because they have communicated the vision one thousand times, they have to communicate it another one thousand times. A lot of this communication has to be done in person, where others can see the leaders, rather than hiding behind an e-mail. The communication must invite feedback, criticism, and challenges.

The members of the organization must trust the integrity, intelligence, compassion, and skill of the leadership. Trust is earned or lost by everything that leaders do or don't do. The members must also trust that leaders have thoughtfully come to the conclusion that the difficult change has excellent reasons behind it and represents the best option for the organization. Organizational members are willing to rise to a challenge, often to heroic levels, if they trust their leaders. Trust requires that leaders act in the best interests of the staff and the organization and that leaders listen and respond to the organization's concerns.

Incentives   Organizational members must be motivated to support significant change. At times, excitement with the vision will be sufficient incentive. Alternatively, fear of what will happen if the organization fails to move toward the vision may serve as an incentive. Although important, neither fear nor rapture is necessarily sufficient.

If organizational members will lose their jobs or have their roles changed significantly, education that prepares them for new roles and or new jobs must be offered. Bonuses may be offered to key individuals, awarded according to the success of the change and each person's contribution to the change. At times, frankly, support is obtained through old-fashioned horse-trading—if the other person will support the change, you will deliver something that is of interest to him or her (space, extra staff, a promotion). Incentives may also take the form of awards—for example, plaques and dinners for two—to staff who go above and beyond the call of duty during the change effort.

Planning, Implementing, and Iterating   Change must be planned. These plans describe the tasks and task sequences necessary to effect the change. Tasks can range from redesigning forms to managing the staged implementation of application systems to retraining staff. Tasks must be allotted resources, and staff accountable for task performance must be designated.

Implementation of the plan is obviously necessary. Because few organizational changes of any magnitude will be fully understood beforehand, problems will be encountered during implementation. New forms may fail to capture necessary data. The estimate of the time needed to register a patient may be wrong and long lines may form at the registration desk. The planners may have forgotten to identify how certain information would flow from one department to another.

These problems are in addition to the problems that occur, for example, when task timetables slip and dependent tasks fall idle or are in trouble. The implementation of the application has been delayed and will not be ready when the staff move to the new building—what do we do? Iteration and adjustment will be necessary as the organization handles problems created when tasks encounter trouble, and learns about glitches with the new processes and workflows.

MANAGING IT PROJECTS

Within the overall change agenda, projects will be formed, managed, and completed. In large change initiatives, the IT project may be one of several projects. For several step-shift changes, the change management agenda may be composed almost entirely of the implementation of an application system.

Change management places an emphasis on many of the "softer," although still critical, aspects of management and leadership: communicating vision, establishing trust, and developing incentives. *Project management* is a "harder" aspect of management. Project management centers on a set of management disciplines and practices that when executed well, increase the likelihood that a project will deliver the desired results. Project management has several objectives:

- Clearly define the scope and goals of the project.
- Identify accountability for the successful completion of the project and associated project tasks.
- Define the processes for making project-related decisions.
- Identify the project's tasks and task sequence and interdependencies.
- Determine the resource and time requirements of the project.
- Ensure appropriate communication with relevant stakeholders about project status and issues.

Different projects require different management strategies. Projects that are pilots or experiments require less formal oversight (and are not helped by large amounts of formal oversight) than large, multiyear, multimillion-dollar undertakings. Projects carried out by two or more organizations working together will have decision-making structures different from those found in projects done by several departments in one organization.

In this chapter we discuss a normative approach to managing relatively large projects within one organization. (Much of the following discussion is adapted from Spurr, 2003.) This approach is put in place once the need for the project has been established (through the IT strategy, for example), the project objectives have been defined, the budget has been approved, and the major stakeholders have been identified.

Project Roles

Four roles are important in the management of large projects:

- Business sponsor
- Business owner
- Project manager
- IT manager

Business Sponsor   The *business sponsor* is the individual who holds overall accountability for the project. The sponsor should represent the area of the organization that is the major recipient of the performance improvement that the project intends to deliver. For example, a project that involves implementing a new claims processing system may have the chief financial officer as the business sponsor. A project to improve nursing workflow may ask the chief nursing officer to serve as business sponsor. A project that affects a large portion of the organization may have the chief executive officer as the business sponsor.

The sponsor's management or executive level should be appropriate to the magnitude of the decisions and the support that the project will require. The more significant the undertaking, the higher the organizational level of the sponsor.

The business sponsor has several duties; he or she

- Secures funding and needed business resources: for example, the commitment of people's time to work on the project.

- Has final decision-making and sign-off accountability for project scope, resources, and approaches to resolving project problems.

- Identifies and supports the business owner(s) (discussed in the next section).

- Promotes the project internally and externally, and obtains the buy-in from business constituents.

- Chairs the project steering committee and is responsible for steering committee participation during the life of the project

- Helps define deliverables, objectives, scope, and success criteria with identified business owners and the project manager.

- Helps remove business obstacles to meeting the project timeline and producing deliverables, as appropriate.

Business Owner   A *business owner* generally has day-to-day responsibility for running a function or a department: for example, a business owner might be the director of the clinical laboratories. A project may need the involvement of several business owners. For example, the success of a new patient accounting system may depend on processes that occur during registration and scheduling (and hence the director of outpatient clinics and the director of the admitting department will both be business owners) and may also depend on adequate physician documentation of the care provided (and hence the administrator of the medical group will be another business owner).

Business owners often work on the project team. Among their several responsibilities they

- Represent their department or function at steering committee and project team meetings.

- Secure and coordinate necessary business and departmental resources.

- Remove business obstacles to meeting the project timeline and producing deliverables, as appropriate.

- Work jointly with the project manager on several tasks (as described in the next section).

Project Manager   The *project manager* does just that—manages the project. He or she is the person who provides the day-to-day direction setting, conflict resolution, and communication needed by the project team. The project manager may be an IT staffer or a person in the business, or function, benefiting from the project. Among their several responsibilities, project managers

- Identify and obtain needed resources.

- Deliver the project on time, on budget, and according to specification.

- Communicate progress to sponsors, stakeholders, and team members.

- Ensure that diligent risk monitoring is in place and appropriate risk mitigation plans have been developed.

- Identify and manage the resolution of issues and problems.

- Maintain the project plan.

- Manage project scope.

The project manager works closely with the business owners and business sponsor in performing these tasks. Together they set meeting agendas, manage the meetings, track project progress, communicate project status, escalate issues as appropriate, and resolve deviations and issues related to the project plan.

IT Manager   The *IT manager* is the senior IT person assigned to the project. He or she may be the boss of the project manager. In performing his or her responsibilities, the IT manager

- Represents the IT department.

- Has final IT decision-making authority and sign-off accountability.

- Helps remove IT obstacles to meeting project timelines and producing deliverables.
- Promotes the project internally and externally, and obtains buy-in from IT constituents.

Project Committees

These four roles may employ two or three major committees to provide project guidance and management: a project steering committee, a project team, and a project review committee.

Project Steering Committee   The *project steering committee* provides overall guidance and management oversight of the project. The steering committee has the authority to resolve changes in scope that affect the budget, milestones, and deliverables. This committee is expected to resolve issues and address risks that cannot be handled by the project team. It also manages communications with the leadership of the organization and the project team. The project steering committee may be the same committee that leads the overall change process or a subcommittee of that group.

The business sponsor should chair this committee. Its members should be representatives of the major areas of the organization that will be affected by the project and whose efforts are necessary if the project is to succeed. Returning to an earlier example, a steering committee overseeing the implementation of a new patient accounting system might include the director of outpatient clinics, the director of the admitting department, and the medical group administrator as members. The senior IT manager should also be on this committee. Depending on the size and importance of the project, this person could be the CIO. It is rare for the chair of the steering committee to be an IT person although having an IT person as a cochair is not uncommon.

Project Team   The *project team* may not be called a committee, but it will meet regularly and it does have responsibilities. The project manager chairs the project team. This team

- Manages the performance of the project work.
- Resolves day-to-day project issues.
- Manages and allocates resources as necessary to do the work.
- Works with the steering committee and business owners, as necessary, to resolve problems; assess potential changes in scope, timeline, or budget; and communicate the status of the project.

Project team members may be business owners, business owners' staff, IT managers, or IT managers' staff.

Project Review Committee   If the organization has a relatively large number of simultaneously active IT projects (say, fifty or so), a *project review committee* can be helpful. The project review committee focuses on a subset of all IT projects, those deemed to be the most important to the organization or the riskiest, or both. The review committee checks the status of each project in this subset to determine if the project is proceeding well or likely to be heading into trouble. If trouble is on the horizon, the committee discusses ways to reduce the threats to the project. The committee also looks for opportunities to leverage the work from one project across other projects and checks for areas where redundant work or work at cross-purposes may be occurring. For example, two projects may need large numbers of workstations deployed during the same interval of time. The IT group that deploys workstations cannot handle this volume. The project review committee would discuss ways to resolve this problem.

The review committee serves as a second pair of eyes on critical projects and has the ability to move resources between projects. For example, if Project A is experiencing instability with its core infrastructure, the review committee can pull network engineers and database server team members from Project B to help out on Project A. The review committee is often chaired by a senior IT person and is composed largely of IT project managers.

Key Project Elements

Over the course of decades and millions of projects, a set of management disciplines and processes has been developed to help ensure that projects succeed. This collected set of practices is referred to as *project management*. One will see these disciplines and processes in action in any well-run project. Excellent project management does not ensure project success. However, without such project management the risks of failure skyrocket, particularly for large projects. The elements of project management (above and beyond the roles just described) are reviewed in the following sections. These elements are created or established after the project proposal has been approved.

Project Charter   The *project charter* is a document that describes the purpose, scope, objectives, costs, and schedule for the project. This document also discusses the roles and responsibilities of the individuals and functions that must contribute to the project. The project charter serves three basic objectives:

- It ensures that planning assumptions or potentially ambiguous objectives are discussed and resolved (this occurs during development of the charter).
- It prevents participants from developing different understandings of the project intent, timeline, or cost.
- It enables the project leadership to communicate as necessary with the organization about the project.

The project charter sets out these project elements:

- Project overview and objectives
- Application features and capabilities (vision of the solution)
- Project scope and limitations
- Metrics for determining project success
- Budget and overall timetable

- Project organization
- Project management strategies

Appendix B contains an example of a project charter.

Project Plan   The project charter provides an overview of the project. The *project plan* provides the details of the tasks, phases, and resources needed, by task and phase and timeline. The project plan is the tool used by the project team during the day-to-day management of the project. The project plan has several components:

- Project phases and tasks. A phase may have multiple tasks. For example, there may be a phase called "conduct analysis," and it may involve such tasks as "review admitting department forms," "document the admitting workflow," and "document the discharge workflow."
- The sequence of phases and tasks.
- Interdependencies between phases and tasks.
- The duration of phases and tasks.
- Staff resources needed, by phase and task.

Several software tools are available that assist project managers in developing project plans. These tools enable the project manager to develop the plan (as described earlier), prepare plan charts and resource use by phase and task, and model the impact on the plan if timelines change or resource availability alters.

Figure 14.1 is an example of a project timeline with project phases. Table 14.1 illustrates an analysis of project resources (staff) that shows project team members' time commitment by activity.

Project Plan and Charter Considerations   Developing project plans and charters requires skill and experience. Managers are often in forums (such as project steering committee meetings) where they are asked to review, critique, and approve a project plan. What should they look for in these plans?

To a large degree, the reputations of project managers precede them. If project managers have proven themselves over the course of many projects, then their plans are likely to be generally sound. If project managers are novices or have an uneven track record, their plans may require greater scrutiny. Regardless of track record, there are several cues that a project plan is as solid as one can make it at the inception of the project:

- The project charter is clear and explicit. Fuzzy objectives and vague understandings of resource needs indicate that the plan needs further discussion and development.
- The leaders of the departments and functions that will be affected by the plan or that need to devote resources to the plan have reviewed the charter and plan, their concerns have been heard and addressed, and they have publicly committed to performing the work needed in the plan.
- The project timelines have been reviewed by multiple parties for reasonableness, and these timelines have taken into consideration factors that will affect the plan—for example, key staff going on vacation or organizational energies being

FIGURE 14.1. Project Timeline with Project Phases

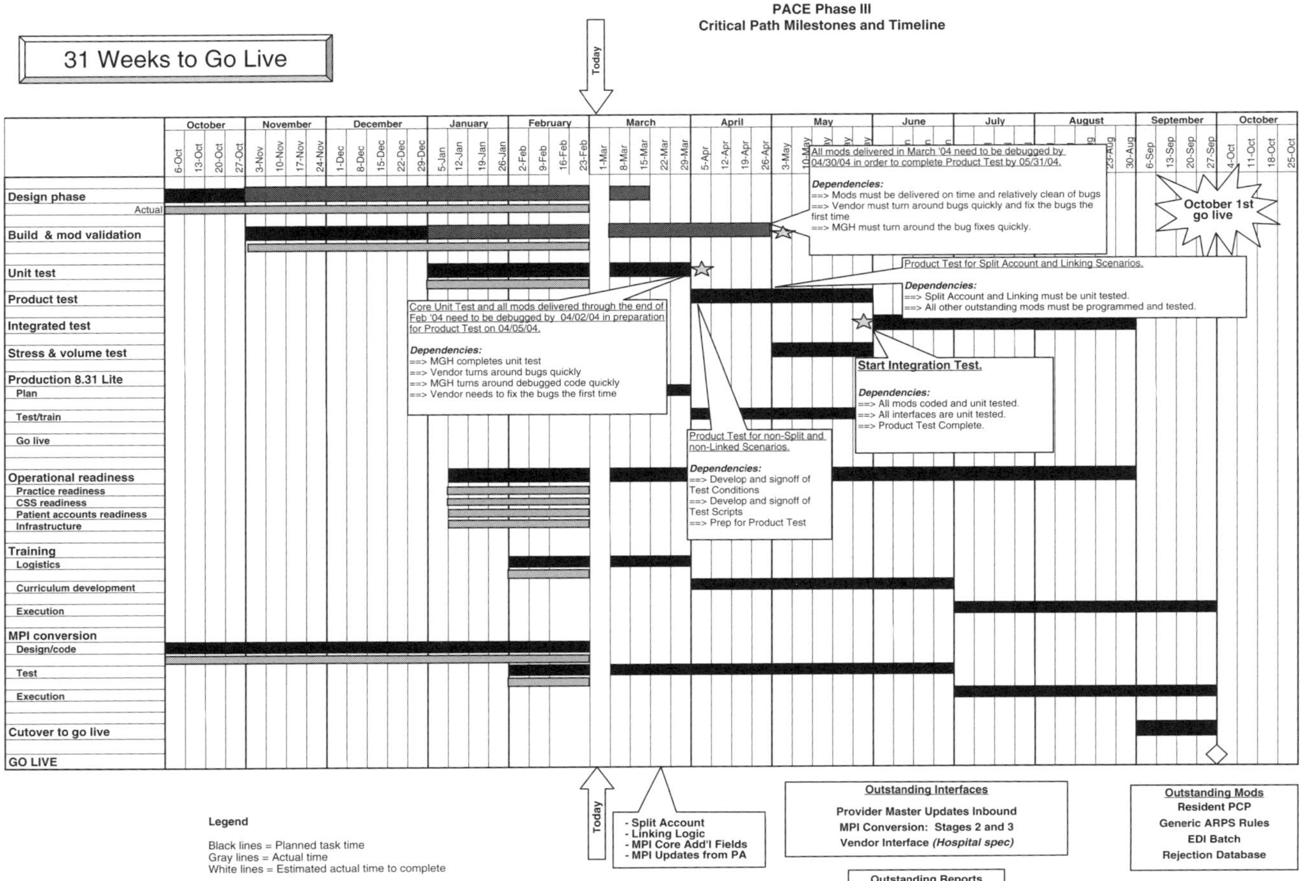

TABLE 14.1. Project Resource Analysis

Analysis Project	Activity	Start Activity	Finish Activity	% Allocated*
Susan Smith				
DFCI - CRIS --> Cancer Registry Data Load	Application design	11/3/2008	11/10/2008	18.95%
DFCI - CRIS --> Cancer Registry Data Load	Application testing	11/3/2008	12/12/2008	25.38%
DFCI - CRIS --> Cancer Registry Data Load	Data mapping specification	11/3/2008	11/19/2008	17.25%
DFCI - CRIS --> Cancer Registry Data Load	Functional analysis	11/3/2008	11/14/2008	35.00%
DFCI - CRIS Minor Enhancements	CRIS breast minor enhancements analysis	11/3/2008	11/2/2009	4.75%
DFCI - CRIS Minor Enhancements	CRIS breast minor enhancements testing	11/3/2008	11/2/2009	4.75%
DFCI CRIS/STIP GI Development and Implementation	GI CRA form design/analysis	11/3/2008	1/29/2009	5.38%
DFCI CRIS/STIP GI Development and Implementation	GI follow-up form design/analysis	11/3/2008	2/6/2009	5.75%
DFCI Renal STIP/CRIS	Renal CRIS analysis	11/3/2008	2/5/2009	
	Administration	11/3/2008	9/30/2009	12.63%
	Support work	11/3/2008	9/30/2009	55.50%
James Jones				
BICS Modernization	Background research	11/3/2008	10/28/2009	19.50%
BICS Modernization	Develop overall project plan	11/3/2008	12/13/2009	8.50%
BICS Modernization	E-mail coding	11/3/2008	1/15/2009	10.00%
Gartner TCO Analysis	Collect data and Input into template—Rd 1	11/3/2008	11/11/2008	8.55%
LDRPS Implementation	Plan building pilot group	11/3/2008	12/1/2008	11.00%
PHS Document Management	VDRNETS security testing	11/3/2008	11/11/2008	
	Administration	11/3/2008	9/30/2009	19.50%
	Support work	11/3/2008	9/30/2009	24.40%

*Percentage of employee's time devoted to a project during the interval bounded by the "start activity" date and the "finish activity" date.

diverted to develop the annual budget—and any uncertainties that might exist for particular phases or tasks—for example, if it is not fully clear how a specific task will be performed, that task timeline should have some "slack" built into it.

- The resources needed have been committed. The budget has been approved. Staff needed by the plan can be named, and their managers have taken steps to free up the staff time needed by the plan.

- The accountabilities for the plan and for each plan phase and task are explicit.

- Project risks have been comprehensively assessed, and thoughtful approaches to addressing each risk developed. Some examples of project risks are unproven information technology, a deterioration in the organization's financial condition, and turnover of project staff.

- A reasonable amount of contingency planning has addressed inevitable problems and current uncertainties. In general, projects should add 10 percent to the timeline and 10 percent to the budget to reflect the time and dollar cost of inevitable problems. For very complex projects, it is not unusual to see 20 to 25 percent of the budget and the duration of some tasks labeled "unknown" or "unclear."

Project Status Report   The *project status report* documents and communicates the current condition of the project. This report is generally prepared monthly and distributed to project participants and stakeholders. The status report often provides matter for discussion at steering committee meetings. It typically covers recent accomplishments and decisions, work in progress, upcoming milestones, and issues that require resolution (see the example in Exhibit 14.1). It may use a green (task or phase proceeding well), yellow (task or phase may be facing a timeline or other problem), and red (task or phase is in trouble and requires attention) color scheme when graphically depicting the status of a project. When a plethora of tasks and phases are tagged with red, then the project is experiencing significant difficulty. Conversely, a sea of green indicates that the project is going well.

The preparation, distribution, and discussion of the project status report are part of the overall project communication plan. Other important communications might include quarterly project presentations at meetings of the organization's department heads, articles about the project in the organization's internal newsletter, and presentations at specific leadership forums: for example, at a medical staff forum or at a meeting of the board or of the executive committee.

UNDERSTANDING IT INITIATIVE FAILURES

The failure rate of IT initiatives is surprisingly high. Project failure occurs when a project is significantly over budget, takes much longer than the estimated timeline, or has to be terminated because so many problems have occurred that proceeding

EXHIBIT 14.1. *Sample Project Status Report*

Electronic Medication Administration Record (e-MAR) - Status Report
Reporting Period: July 2008

Business Sponsor: Sally Salisbury, RN, Vice President Patient Care Services

Business Owners: Amy Leron RN, Director of Nursing Quality and Practice; William Farnsworth RPh, Director of Pharmacy

Information Systems Sponsors: Cindy Mason RNC, Corporate Director of Clinical Systems Management; Sue Kimit, CIO-BWH

PROJECT SCHEDULE

Activity	Planned	Revised	Actual Delivery
Functional specification requirements completed	• 01/08	• 07/08	• 07/08
Technical Specifications completed	• 02/08	• 11/28/08	•
Wireless Infrastructure in place for pilot pods	• 02/08	• 9/15/08	•
Wireless Infrastructure in place for training room (Ledge Site)	• 02/08	• 07/08	• 07/08
Wireless Infrastructure in place for pharmacy	• 02/08	• 05/08	• 06/08
Wireless Infrastructure in place for all adult inpatient pods	• 03/08	• 09/26/08	•
Bar Code development – Medications	• 06/08	• 08/29/08	•
Bar Code development – Patient ID band Implementation	• 05/08	• 08/15/08	•
Bar Code development – Clinical Staff Implementation (employee ID)	• 05/08	• 08/15/08	•
Bar Code Imager Selection	• 02/08	• 04/08	• 04/08
Adult Pharmacy development	• 06/08	• 08/08	•
Adult Pharmacy application pilot	• 08/05	• 08/25	•
Code Freeze (pilot)	• 04/08	• 09/15/08	•
Integrated Testing (pilot)	• 04/08	• 9/15/08 – 10/25/08	•
PILOT			
Hardware Purchase (notebook, imager)	• 06/08	• 07/08	• 07/08
Create Image/Test Fujitsu Lifebook	• 06/08	• 07/08	• 07/08
Hiring/Training Support Staff	• 07/08	• 09/26/08	•
Hardware Deployment	• 08/08	• 10/27/08	•
Training – Planning complete	• 06/08	• 07/08	• 07/08
Training – Development complete	• 07/08	• 10/01/08	•
Training- Conduct Classes	• 08/08	• 10/14 – 10/25	•
Implementation	• 06/08	• 10/27	•
Evaluation of pilot	• 07/08	• 12/08	•
ROLLOUT			
Rollout Implementation Plan	• 09/08	• 08/29/08	•
Hiring Support Staff	• 12/08	• 01/ 04	•
Training Support Staff	• 01/09	• 01/ 04	•
Hardware Deployment	• 07/08	• 2/09 – 5/09	•
Training – Planning	• 08/08	• 12/09	•
Training- Development	• 09/08	• 01/ 04	•
Training- Conduct Classes	• 09/08	• 02/01/09 – 05/08/09	•
Implementation Begin	• 10/08	• 02/16/09	•
Implementation End	• 04/09	• 05/21/09	•

ACCOMPLISHMENTS

- The functional requirements for the pilot have been agreed upon and finalized

DECISIONS

- The pilot date was revised to 10/27 – 11/21. The additional time is needed to complete the application development for upcoming changes to OE, such as the new KCL scales and PCA templates
- The format for the Medical Record Copy of the eMAR was approved by Health Information Systems

WORK IN PROGRESS

- Completing the bar coded Employee ID badge. This should be ready for testing during the second week in August
- Completing the bar coded patient ID band, which can be finalized when the font software arrives

---

EXHIBIT 14.1.   *(Continued)*

- Programming for recently finalized eMAR specifications – scales, tapers, various templates, downtime procedures, reports, etc.
- Programming for BICS changes necessary for eMAR
- Anne Bane is working with several cart vendors to secure carts for the pilot
- Wiring/cabling for the wireless network on the inpatient pods begins 8/4 and continues through 9/26
- Planning for integration testing
- Unit testing

ISSUES

- Accessing BICS from the web pod monitor is inconsistent and slow. The platform architecture specialists are investigating a solution, and it's being tested now
- The font software for patient ID bands has been delayed. Joanne Johnson is working to expedite this so that final development can occur

Upcoming Activities

- ID badge replacement scheduled for RNs and pharmacists 8/14 – 8/22
- The pharmacy will conduct a pilot of its new web system beginning on 8/25

---

is no longer judged to be viable. Cook (2007) finds that 35 percent of IT projects were successful whereas 19 percent failed. The remaining 46 percent delivered a useful product but suffered from budget overruns, prolonged timetables, and application feature shortfalls.

Cash, McFarlan, and McKenney (1992) note that two major categories of risk confront significant IT investments: strategy failures and implementation failures. The project failure rates suggest that management should be more worried about IT implementation than IT strategy. IT strategy is sexier and more visionary than implementation. However, a very large number of strategies and visions go nowhere or are diminished because the organization is unable to implement them.

Why is this failure rate so high? What happens?

In the sections that follow, we will examine several classes of barriers that hinder large IT projects.

Lack of Clarity of Purpose

Any project or initiative is destined for trouble if its objectives and purpose are unclear. Sometimes the purpose of a project is only partially clear. For example, an organization may have decided that it should implement an electronic health record in an effort to "improve the quality and efficiency of care." However, it is not really clear to the leadership and staff *how* the EHR will be used to improve care. Will problems associated with finding a patient's record be solved? Will the record be used to gather data about care quality? Will the record be used to support outpatient medication ordering and reduce medication error rates?

All these questions can be answered yes, but if the organization never gets beyond the slogan of "improve the quality and efficiency of care." the scope of the project will be murky. The definition of care improvement is left up to the project participant to interpret. And the scope and timetable of the project cannot possibly be precise because project objectives are too fuzzy.

Lack of Belief in the Project

At times the objectives are very clear, but the members of the organization are not convinced that the project is worth doing at all. Because the project will change the work life of many members and require that they participate in design and implementation, they need to be sufficiently convinced that the project will improve their lives or is necessary if the organization is to thrive. They will legitimately ask, What's in it for me? Unconvinced of the need for the project, they will resist it. A resistant organization will likely doom any project. Projects that are viewed as illegitimate by a large portion of the people in an organization rarely succeed.

Insufficient Leadership Support

The organization's leaders may be committed to the undertaking yet not demonstrate that commitment. For example, leaders may not devote sufficient time to the project or may decide to send subordinates to meetings. This broadcasts a signal to the organization that the leaders have other, "more important" things to do. Tough project decisions may get made in a way that shows the leaders are not as serious as their rhetoric, because when push came to shove, they caved in.

Members of the leadership team may have voted yes to proceed with a project, but their votes may not have included their reservations about the utility of the project or the way it was put together. Once problems are encountered in the project (and all projects encounter problems), this qualified leadership support evaporates, and the silent reservations become public statements such as, "I knew that this would never work."

Organizational Inertia

Even when the organization is willing to engage in a project, inertia can hinder it. People are busy. They are stressed. They have jobs to do. Some of the changes are threatening. Staff may believe these changes leave them less skilled or less instrumental or with reduced power. Or they may not have a good understanding of their work life after the change, and they may imagine that an uncertain outcome cannot be a good outcome.

Projects add work on top of the workload of often already overburdened people. Projects add stress for often already stressed people. As a result, despite the valiant efforts of leadership and the expenditure of significant resources, a project may slowly grind to a halt because too many members find ways to avoid or not deal with the efforts and changes the initiative requires. Bringing significant change to a large portion of the organization is very hard because, if nothing else, there is so much inertia to overcome.

Organizational Baggage

Organizations have baggage. Baggage comes in many forms. Some organizations have no history of competence in making significant organizational change. They have never learned how to mobilize the organization's members. They do not know how to handle conflict. They are unsure how to assemble and leverage multidisciplinary teams. They have never mastered staying the course over years during the execution of complex agendas. These organizations are "incompetent," and this incompetence extends well beyond IT, although it clearly includes IT initiatives.

An organization may have tried initiatives "like this" before and failed. The proponents of the initiative may have failed at other initiatives. Organizations have very long memories, and their members may be thinking something like, "The same clowns who brought us that last fiasco are back with an even better idea." The odor from prior failures significantly taints the credibility of newly proposed initiatives and helps to ensure that organizational acceptance will be weak.

Lack of an Appropriate Reward System

Aspects of organizational policies, incentives, and practices can hinder a project. The organization's incentive system may not be structured to reward multidisciplinary behavior: for example, physicians may be rewarded for research prowess or clinical excellence but not for sitting on committees to design new clinical processes. An integrated delivery system may have encouraged its member hospitals to be self-sufficient. As a result, management practices that involve working across hospitals never matured, and the organization does not know how (even if it is willing) to work across hospitals.

Lack of Candor

Organizations can create environments that do not encourage healthy debate. Such environments can result when leadership is intolerant of being challenged or has an inflated sense of its worth and does not believe that it needs team effort to get things done. The lack of a climate that encourages conflict and can manage conflict means that initiative problems will not get resolved. Moreover, organizational members, not having had their voices heard, will tolerate the initiative only out of the hope that they will outlast the initiative and the leadership.

Sometimes the project team is uncomfortable delivering bad news. Project teams will screw up and make mistakes. Sometimes they really screw up and make really big mistakes. Because they may be embarrassed, or worried that they will get beaten up, they hide the mistakes from the leadership and attempt to fix the problems without "anyone having to know." This attempt to hide bad news is a recipe for disaster. It is unrealistic to expect problems to go unnoticed; invariably the leadership team finds out about the problem and its trust in the project team erodes. At times leadership has to look in the mirror to see if its own intolerance for bad news in effect created the problem.

Project Complexity

Project complexity is determined by many factors:

- The number of people whose work will be changed by the project and the depth of those changes

- The number of organizational processes that will be changed and the depth of those changes

- The number of processes linking the organization and other organizations that will be changed and the depth of those changes

- The interval over which all this change will occur: for example, will it occur quickly or gradually?

If the change is significant in scale, scope, and depth, then it becomes very difficult (often impossible) for the people managing the project to truly understand what the project needs to do. The design will be imperfect. The process changes will not integrate well. And many curves will be thrown the project's way as the implementation unfolds and people realize their mistakes and understand what they failed to understand initially.

Sometimes complex projects disappear in an organizational mushroom cloud. The complexity overwhelms the organization and causes the project to crash suddenly. More common is the "death by ants"—no single bite (or project problem) will kill the project, but a thousand will. The organization is overwhelmed by the thousand small problems and inefficiencies and terminates the undertaking.

Managers should remember that complexity is relative. Organizations generally have developed a competency to manage projects up to a certain level and type of complexity. Projects that require competency beyond that level are inherently risky. A project that is risky for one organization may not be risky for another. For example, an organization that typically manages projects that cost $2 million, take ten person-years of effort, and affect 300 people will struggle with a project that costs $20 million and takes one hundred person-years of effort (Cash et al., 1992).

Failure to Respect Uncertainty

Significant organizational change brings a great deal of uncertainty with it. The leadership may be correct in its understanding of where the organization needs to go and the scope of the changes needed. However, it is highly unlikely that anyone really understands the full impact of the change and how new processes, tasks, and roles will really work. At best, leadership has a good approximation of the new organization. The belief that a particular outcome is certain can be a problem in itself.

Agility and the ability to detect when a change is not working and to alter its direction are very important. Detection requires that the organization listens to the feedback of those who are waist deep in the change, and is able to discern the difference between the organizational noise that comes with any change and the organizational noise that reflects real problems. Altering direction requires that the leadership not cling to ideas that cannot work and also be willing to admit to the organization that it was wrong about some aspects of the change.

Initiative Undernourishment

There may be a temptation, particularly as the leadership tries to accomplish as much as it can with a constrained budget, to tell a project team, "I know you asked for ten people, but we're going to push you to do it with five." The leadership may believe that such bravado will make the team work extra hard and, through heroic efforts, complete the project in a grand fashion. However, bravado may turn out to be bellicose stupidity. This approach may doom a project, despite the valiant efforts of the team to do the impossible.

Another form of undernourishment involves placing staff other than the best staff on the initiative. If the initiative is very important, then it merits using the best staff possible and freeing up their time so they can focus on the initiative. An organization's best staff are always in demand, and there can be a temptation to say that it would be too difficult to pull them away from other pressing issues. They are needed elsewhere and this decision is difficult. However, if the initiative is critical to the organization, then those other demands are less important and can be given to someone else. Critical organizational initiatives should not be staffed with the junior varsity.

Failure to Anticipate Short-Term Disruptions

Any major change will lead to short-term problems and disruptions in operations. Even though current processes can be made better, they are working and staff know how to make them work. When processes are changed, there is a shakeout period as staff adjust and learn how to make the new processes work well. At times, adjusting to the new application system is the core of the disruption. A shakeout can go on for months and degrade organizational performance. Service will deteriorate. Days in accounts receivable will climb. Balls will be dropped in many areas. The organization can misinterpret these problems as a sign that the initiative is failing.

Listening closely to the issues and suggestions of the front line is essential during this time. These staff need to know that their problems are being heard and that their ideas for fixing these problems are being acted upon. People often know exactly what needs to be done to remove system disruptions. Listening to and acting on their advice also improves their buy-in to the change.

While working hard to minimize the duration and depth of disruption, the organization also needs to be tolerant during this period and to appreciate the low-grade form of hell that staff are enduring. It is critical that this period be kept as short and as pain free as possible. If the disruption lasts too long, staff may conclude that the change is not working and abandon their support.

Invisible Progress

Sometimes initiatives are launched with great fanfare. Speeches are made outlining the rationale for the initiative. Teams are formed. Budgets are established. The organization is ready to move. Then nothing seems to be happening.

Large, complex initiatives often involve large amounts of preparatory analysis and work. These initiatives may also involve implementing a significant IT foundation of new networks and databases. And even though the project teams are busy, the rest of the organization sees no progress and comes to believe that the initiative is being held hostage. Action-oriented managers want to know what happened to the action.

Change initiatives and IT projects need to communicate their progress regularly, even when that progress is largely unseen by the organization. In a similar fashion the progress made in digging a new tunnel might be invisible to the motorist until the tunnel is open, but the tunnel diggers can report regularly on the work that is being done underground.

If possible, the project should seek to produce a series of short-term deliverables, even if they are small. For example, while the IT team is performing foundational work, the organization might go ahead and make some process changes without waiting for the implementation of the application. Deliverables demonstrate that progress is being made and help to sustain organizational commitment to the initiative. Organizational commitment is like a slowly leaking balloon; it must be constantly reinflated.

Lack of Technology Stability and Maturity

Information technology may be obviously immature. New technologies are being introduced all the time, and it takes time for them to work through their kinks and achieve an acceptable level of stability, supportability, and maturity. Some forms of Web 2.0 are current examples of information technologies that are in their youth.

Organizations can become involved in projects that require immature technology to play a critical role. This clearly elevates the risk of the project. The technology will suffer from performance problems, and the organization's IT staff and the technology supplier may have a limited ability to identify and resolve technology problems. Organizational members, tired of the instability, become tired of the project and it fails.

In general it is not common, nor should it be often necessary, for a project to hinge on the adequate performance of new technology. A thoughtful assessment that a new technology has potentially extraordinary promise and that the organization can achieve differential value by being an early adopter should precede any such decision. Even in these cases, pilot projects that provide experience with the new technology while limiting the scope of its implementation (which minimizes potential damage) are highly recommended.

The organization should remember that technology maturity is also relative. Even if the rest of the world has used a technology, if it is new to your vendor and new to your IT staff, then it should be considered immature. Your vendor and staff will need to learn, often the hard way, how to manage and support this technology.

Projects can also get into trouble when the amount of technology change is extensive. For example, the organization may be attempting to implement, over a short period of time, applications from several different vendors that involve different operating systems, network requirements, security models, and database management systems. This broad scope can overwhelm the IT department's ability to respond to technology misbehavior.

PERSPECTIVE

CRITICAL SUCCESS FACTORS

Jay Toole outlines several critical success factors for successful clinical information system (CIS) implementation and transformation of clinical processes.

- Set realistic and clear expectations for the outcomes that will result from implementing the CIS.

- Recognize that implementing a CIS and transforming care processes is an operational initiative and not an IT initiative.

- Operational executives must take ownership of the implementation and related transformation and must be held accountable for its success.

- Clinicians must actively participate in the CIS design and implementation.

- A liaison person knowledgeable in both IT and medical issues should be designated to keep the physicians engaged in the implementation process.

- A strong project manager with CIS implementation experience needs to be dedicated to the initiative. [He or she] must have dedicated staff resources with the right mix of clinical, operational and technical expertise.

- A well-defined implementation plan and the ability to monitor and track results against the plan is crucial.

- Incentives must be aligned and these incentives should reward all participants for successful implementation and achievement of predefined outcomes.

Source: Toole, 2003, p. 157.

How to Avoid These Mistakes

Major IT projects fail in many ways. However, a large number of these failures involve management action or inaction. Few management teams and senior leaders start IT projects hoping that failure is the outcome. Summarizing our discussion in this chapter produces a set of recommendations that can help organizations reduce the risk of failure:

- Ensure that the objectives of the IT initiative are clear.

- Communicate the objectives and the initiative, and test the degree to which organizational members have bought into them.

- Publicly demonstrate conviction by "being there" and showing resolve during tough decisions.

- Respect organizational inertia, and keep hammering away at it.

- Distance the project from any organizational baggage, perhaps through a thoughtful choice of project sponsors and managers.

- Change the reward system if necessary to create incentives for participants to work toward project success.

- Accept and welcome the debate that surrounds projects, invite bad news, and do not hang those who make mistakes.

- Address complexity by breaking the project into manageable pieces, and test for evidence that the project might be at risk from trying to do too much all at once.

- Realize that there is much you do not know about how to change the organization or the form of new processes; be prepared to change direction and listen and respond to those who are on the front line.

- Supply resources for the project appropriately, and assign the project to your best team.

- Try to limit the duration and depth of the short-term operational disruption, but accept that it will occur.

- Ensure and communicate regular, visible progress.

- Be wary of new technology and projects that involve a broad scope of information technology change.

These steps, along with solid project management, can dramatically reduce the risk that an IT project will fail. However, these steps are not foolproof. Major IT projects, particularly those accompanied by major organizational change, will always have a nontrivial level of risk.

There will also be times when a review of the failure factors indicates that a project is too risky. The organization may not be ready; there may be too much baggage, too much inertia to overcome; the best team may not be available; the organization may not be good at handling conflict; or the project may require too much new information technology. Projects with considerable risk should not be undertaken until progress has been made in addressing the failure factors. Management of IT project risk is a critical contributor to IT success.

PERSPECTIVE

IT PROJECT IMPLEMENTATION CHECKLIST

Andrew McAfee has developed a short checklist for managers who are overseeing the implementation of IT projects. This checklist covers critical project management actions necessary to avoid disaster:

- Treat the implementation as a business change effort and not as a technology installation. Project leadership should come from the business side, and the business sponsor should be given the authority to make project decisions and be held accountable for project outcomes.

- Devote the necessary resources to the project. This means putting your best people on the project and avoiding cutting corners on budgets and the use of outside expertise.

- Make sure that goals, scope, and expectations are clear from the outset. Projects get in trouble when they are overhyped, scope is allowed to expand without discipline, and goals are fuzzy.

- Track the project's progress, results, and scope. Sound project management— for example, status reports, milestones, methodical reviews of proposals to change scope, and budget tracking—must be in place.

- Test the new system every way that you can before you go live. Testing and retesting helps minimize unpleasant surprises, technology problems, and poor fit with workflow.

- Secure top management commitment. The leadership must believe in the project—its goals, scope, and the project team. Leadership must also soberly understand the magnitude and difficulty of the undertaking.

Source: Adapted from McAfee, 2003, p. 85.

SUMMARY

The leadership of health care organizations plays an essential role in managing the change that invariably accompanies the implementation of an IT application. This role is particularly important in step-shift, radical, and fundamental change. The leadership must lead, establish a vision, communicate, manage trust, plan the change, implement the change, and iterate as the organization experiences the change.

The hard science of implementation requires the creation of roles such as the business sponsor and project managers and committees such as the project steering committee and project teams. Solid project management techniques must be in place: for example, project charters and project plans must be created, and project communication must be carried out.

There are many ways that a project failure can occur; unclear objectives, embryonic information technology, or neglecting to anticipate short-term operational disruptions may lead to failure, for example. It is the responsibility of the organization's leadership to minimize the occurrence and severity of factors that threaten to undermine the change.

KEY TERMS

IT initiative failures
Managing IT projects
Organizational change
Project charter

Project committees
Project plan
Project roles
Project status report

LEARNING ACTIVITIES

1. Attend a project team meeting for each of two different projects. Describe the project and the challenges facing the project teams. Comment on the differences between the teams and the projects.

2. Interview the business sponsor of a major project. Describe the role of this business sponsor. Discuss the scope of the project and its objectives. Describe the change strategy for the project.

3. Interview a project manager. Describe the factors and skills that he or she associates with successful projects.

CHAPTER

15

ASSESSING AND ACHIEVING VALUE IN HEALTH CARE INFORMATION SYSTEMS

LEARNING OBJECTIVES

- To be able to discuss the nature of IT-enabled value.
- To review the components of the IT project proposal.
- To be able to understand steps to improve IT project value realization.
- To be able to discuss why IT investments can fail to deliver returns.
- To review factors that challenge the realization of IT value.

Virtually all the discussion in this book has focused on the knowledge and management processes necessary to achieve one fundamental objective: organizational investments in IT resulting in a desired value. That value might be the furtherance of organizational strategies, improvement in the performance of core processes, or the enhancement of decision making. Achieving value requires the alignment of IT with overall strategies, thoughtful governance, solid information system selection and implementation approaches, and effective organizational change.

Failure to achieve desired value can result in significant problems for the organization. Money is wasted. Execution of strategies is hamstrung. Organizational processes can be damaged.

This chapter carries the IT value discussion further. Specifically, it covers the following topics:

- The definition of IT-enabled value
- The IT project proposal
- Steps to improve value realization
- Why IT investments may fail to deliver returns
- Analyses of the IT value challenge

DEFINITION OF IT-ENABLED VALUE

We can make several observations about IT-enabled value:

- IT value can be both tangible and intangible.
- IT value can be significant.
- IT value can be diverse across IT proposals.
- A single IT investment can have a diverse value proposition.
- Different IT investments have different objectives and hence different value propositions and value assessment techniques.

These observations will be discussed in more detail in the following sections.

Both Tangible and Intangible

Tangible value can be measured whereas intangible value is very difficult, perhaps practically impossible, to measure.

Some tangible value can be measured in terms of dollars:

- Increases in revenue.
- Reductions in labor costs: for example, through staff layoffs, overtime reductions, or shifting work to less expensive staff.
- Reductions in supplies needed: for example, paper.
- Reductions in maintenance costs for computer systems.

■ Reductions in use of patient care services: for example, fewer lab tests are performed or care is conducted in less expensive settings.

Some tangible value can be measured in terms of process improvements:

■ Fewer errors

■ Faster turnaround times for test results

■ Reductions in elapsed time to get an appointment

■ A quicker admissions process

■ Improvement in access to data

Some tangible value can be measured in terms of strategically important operational and market outcomes:

■ Growth in market share

■ Reduction in turnover

■ Increase in brand awareness

■ Increase in patient and provider satisfaction

■ Improvement in reliability of computer systems

In contrast, intangible value can be very difficult to measure. The organization is trying to measure such things as

■ Improving in decision making

■ Improving in communication

■ Improving in compliance

■ Improving in collaboration

■ Increasing in agility

■ Becoming more state of the art

■ Improving in organizational competencies—for example, becoming better at managing chronic disease

■ Becoming more customer friendly

Significant

Glaser, DeBor, and Stuntz (2003) describe the return achieved by replacing the manual approach to determining patient eligibility for coverage with an electronic data interchange (EDI) based approach. One hospital estimated that for an initial investment of $250,000 in eligibility interface development and rollout effort, plus an annual maintenance fee of $72,000, it could achieve ongoing annual savings of approximately $485,000. This return on its EDI investment was achieved within one year of operation.

Wang et al. (2003) performed an analysis of the costs and benefits of the electronic medical record (EMR) system in primary care. This sophisticated analysis explored the return over a range of EMR capabilities (from basic to advanced), practice sizes (small to large), and reimbursement structures (from entirely fee-for-service to extensive risk-sharing arrangements). On average the net estimated benefit was $86,000 per provider over five years.

Bates et al. (1998) found that a 55 percent reduction in serious medication errors resulted from implementing inpatient provider order entry at the Brigham and Women's Hospital. This computerized order entry system highlighted, at the time of ordering, possible drug allergies, drug-drug interactions, and drug–lab result problems.

Bu et al. (2007) estimated that the implementation of a range of telehealth technologies nationwide would save $14.5 billion in diabetes-related costs over ten years.

Diverse Across Proposals

Consider three proposals (real ones from a large integrated delivery system) that might be in front of organizational leadership for review and approval: a disaster notification system, a document imaging system, and an e-procurement system. Each offers a different type of value to the organization.

The disaster notification system would enable the organization to page critical personnel, inform them that a disaster—for example, a train wreck or biotoxin outbreak—had taken place, and tell them the extent of the disaster and the steps they would need to take to help the organization respond to the disaster. The system would cost $520,000. The value would be "better preparedness for a disaster."

The document imaging system would be used to electronically store and retrieve scanned images of paper documents, such as payment reconciliations, received from insurance companies. The system would cost $2.8 million, but would save the organization $1.8 million per year ($9 million over the life of the system) due to reductions in the labor required to look for paper documents and in the insurance claim write-offs that occur because a document cannot be located.

The e-procurement system would enable users to order supplies, ensure that the ordering person had the authority to purchase supplies, transmit the order to the supplier, and track the receipt of the supplies. Data from this system could be used to support the standardization of supplies: that is, to reduce the number of different supplies used. Such standardization might save $500,000 to $3 million per year. The actual savings would depend on physician willingness to standardize. The system would cost $2.5 million.

These proposals reflect a diversity of value, ranging from "better disaster response" to a clear financial return (document imaging) to a return with such a wide potential range (e-procurement) that it could be a great investment (if you really could save $3 million a year) or a terrible investment (if you could save only $500,000 a year).

Diverse in a Single Investment

Picture archiving and communication systems (PACS) are used to store radiology (and other) images, support interpretation of images, and distribute the information to the physician providing direct patient care. A PACS can

- Reduce costs for radiology film and the need for film librarians.
- Improve service to the physician delivering care, through improved access to images.
- Improve productivity for the radiologists and for the physicians delivering care (both groups reduce the time they spend looking for images).
- Generate revenue, if the organization uses the PACS to offer radiology services to physician groups in the community.

This one investment has a diverse value proposition; it has the potential to deliver cost reduction, productivity gains, service improvements, and revenue gains.

Different for Different Objectives

The Committee to Study the Impact of Information Technology on the Performance of Service Activities (1994), organized by the National Research Council, has identified six categories of IT investments, reflecting different objectives. The techniques used to assess IT investment value should vary by the type of objective that the IT investment intends to support. One technique does not fit all IT investments.

PERSPECTIVE

FOUR TYPES OF IT INVESTMENT

Jeanne Ross and Cynthia Beath studied the IT investment approaches of thirty companies from a wide range of industries. They identified four classes of investment:

- *Transformation.* These IT investments had an impact that would affect the entire organization or a large number of business units. The intent of the investment was to effect a significant improvement in overall performance or change the nature of the organization.

- *Renewal.* Renewal investments were intended to upgrade core IT infrastructure and applications or reduce the costs or improve the quality of IT services. Examples of these investments include application replacements, upgrades of the network, or expansion of data storage.

- *Process improvement.* These IT investments sought to improve the operations of a specific business entity—for example, to reduce costs and improve service.

- *Experiments.* Experiments were designed to evaluate new information technologies and test new types of applications. Given the results of the experiments, the organization would decide whether broad adoption was desirable.

(Continued)

PERSPECTIVE (*Continued*)

Different organizations will allocate their IT budgets differently across these classes. An office products company had an investment mix of experiments (15 percent), process improvement (40 percent), renewal (25 percent), and transformation (20 percent). An insurance firm had an investment mix of experiments (3 percent), process improvement (25 percent), renewal (18 percent), and transformation (53 percent).

The investment allocation is often an after-the-fact consideration—the allocation is not planned, it just "happens." However, ideally, the organization decides its desired allocation structure and does so before the budget discussions. An organization with an ambitious and perhaps radical strategy may allocate a very large portion of its IT investment to the transformation class whereas an organization with a conservative, stay-the-course strategy may have a large process improvement portion to its IT investments.

Source: Ross & Beath, 2002, p. 54.

Infrastructure   IT investments may be for infrastructure that enables other investments or applications to be implemented and deliver desired capabilities. Examples of infrastructure are data communication networks, workstations, and clinical data repositories. A delivery system–wide network enables a large organization to implement applications to consolidate clinical laboratories, implement organization-wide collaboration tools, and share patient health data between providers.

It is difficult to quantitatively assess the impact or value of infrastructure investments because

- They enable applications. Without those applications, infrastructure has no value. Hence infrastructure value is indirect and depends on application value.

- The allocation of infrastructure value across applications is complex. When millions of dollars are invested in a data communication network, it may be difficult or impossible to determine how much of that investment should be allocated to the ability to create delivery system–wide EMRs.

- A good IT infrastructure is often determined by its agility, its potency, and its ability to facilitate integration of applications. It is very difficult to assign return on investment numbers or any meaningful numerical value to most of these characteristics. What, for instance, is the value of being agile enough to speed up the time it takes to develop and enhance applications?

Information system infrastructure is as hard to evaluate as other organizational infrastructure, such as having talented, educated staff. As with other infrastructure:

- Evaluation is often instinctive and experientially based.

- In general, underinvesting can severely limit the organization.

■ Investment decisions involve choosing between alternatives that are assessed based on their ability to achieve agreed-upon goals. For example, if an organization wishes to improve security, it might ask whether it should invest in network monitoring tools or enhanced virus protection. Which of these investments would enable it to make the most progress toward its goal?

Mandated Information system investment may be necessary because of mandated initiatives. Mandated initiatives might involve reporting quality data to accrediting organizations, making required changes in billing formats, or improving disaster notification systems. Assessing these initiatives is generally approached by identifying the least expensive and the quickest to implement alternative that will achieve the needed level of compliance.

Cost Reduction Information system investments directed to cost reduction are generally highly amenable to return on investment (ROI) and other quantifiable dollar-impact analyses. The ability to conduct a quantifiable ROI analysis is rarely the question. The ability of management to effect the predicted cost reduction or cost avoidance is often a far more germane question.

Specific New Products and Services IT can be critical to the development of new products and services. At times the information system delivers the new service, and at other times it is itself the product. Examples of information system–based new services include bank cash-management programs and programs that award airline mileage for credit card purchases. A new service offered by some health care providers is a personal health record that enables a patient to communicate with his or her physician and to access care guidelines and consumer-oriented medical textbooks. The value of some of these new products and services can be quantifiably assessed in terms of a monetary return. These assessments include analyses of potential new revenue, either directly from the service or from service-induced use of other products and services. A return-on-investment analysis will need to be supplemented by techniques such as sensitivity analyses of consumer response. Despite these analyses the value of this IT investment usually has a speculative component. This component involves consumer utilization, competitor response, and impact on related businesses.

Quality Improvement Information system investments are often directed to improving the quality of service or medical care. These investments may be intended to reduce waiting times, improve the ability of physicians to locate information, improve treatment outcomes, or reduce errors in treatment. Evaluation of these initiatives, although quantifiable, is generally done in terms of service parameters that are known or believed to be important determinants of organizational success. These parameters might be measures of aspects of organizational processes that customers encounter and then use to judge the organization: for example, waiting times in the physician's office. A quantifiable dollar outcome for the service of care quality improvement can be very difficult to predict. Service quality is often necessary to protect current business and the effect of a failure to continuously improve service or medical care can be difficult to project.

Major Strategic Initiative   Strategic initiatives in information technology are intended to significantly change the competitive position of the organization or redefine the core nature of the enterprise. In health care it is rare that information systems are the centerpiece of a redefinition of the organization. However, other industries have attempted IT-centric transformations. Amazon.com is an effort to transform retailing. Schwab.com is an undertaking intended to redefine the brokerage industry through the use of the Internet. There can be an ROI core or component to analyses of such initiatives, because they often involve major reshaping or reengineering of fundamental organizational processes. However, assessing the ROIs of these initiatives and their related information systems with a high degree of accuracy can be very difficult. Several factors contribute to this difficulty:

- These major strategic initiatives usually recast the organization's markets and its roles. The outcome of the recasting, although visionary, can be difficult to see with clarity and certainty.

- The recasting is evolutionary; the organization learns and alters itself as it progresses, over what are often lengthy periods of time. It is difficult to be prescriptive about this evolutionary process. Most integrated delivery systems (IDS) are confronting this phenomenon.

- Market and competitor responses can be difficult to predict.

IT value is diverse and complex. This diversity indicates the power of IT and the diversity of its use. Nonetheless, the complexity of the value proposition means that it is difficult to make choices between IT investments and also difficult to assess whether the investment ultimately chosen delivered the desired value or not.

THE IT PROJECT PROPOSAL

The IT project proposal is a cornerstone in examining value. Clearly, ensuring that all proposals are well crafted does not ensure value. To achieve value, alignment with organizational strategies must occur, factors for sustained IT excellence must be managed, budget processes for making choices between investments must exist, and projects must be well managed. However, the proposal (as discussed in Chapter Thirteen) does describe the intended outcome of the IT investment. The proposal requests money and an organizational commitment to devote management attention and staff effort to implementing an information system. The proposal describes why this investment of time, effort, and money is worth it—that is, the proposal describes the value that will result.

In Chapter Thirteen we also discussed budget meetings and management forums that might review IT proposals and determine whether a proposal should be accepted. In this section we discuss the value portion of the proposal and some common problems encountered with it.

Sources of Value Information

As project proponents develop their case for an IT investment they may be unsure of the full gamut of potential value or of the degree to which a desired value can be truly realized. The organization may not have had experience with the proposed application and may have insufficient analyst resources to perform its own assessment. It may not be able to answer such questions as, What types of gains have organizations seen as a result of implementing an electronic health record (EHR) system? To what degree will IT be a major contributor to our efforts to streamline operating room throughput?

Information about potential value can be obtained from several sources (discussed in Appendix A). Conferences often feature presentations that describe the efforts of specific individuals or organizations in accomplishing initiatives of interest to many others. Industry publications may offer relevant articles and analyses. Several industry research organizations—for example, Gartner and Forrester—can offer advice. Consultants can be retained who have worked with clients who are facing or have addressed similar questions. Vendors of applications can describe the outcomes experienced by their customers. And colleagues can be contacted to determine the experiences of their organizations.

Garnering an understanding of the results of others is useful but insufficient. It is worth knowing that Organization Y adopted computerized provider order entry (CPOE) and reduced unnecessary testing by X percent. However, one must also understand the CPOE features that were critical in achieving that result and the management steps taken and the process changes made in concert with the CPOE implementation.

Formal Financial Analysis

Most proposals should be subjected to formal financial analyses regardless of their value proposition. Several types of financial measures are used by organizations. An organization's finance department will work with leadership to determine which measures will be used and how these measures will be compiled.

Two common financial measures are net present value and internal rate of return:

- *Net present value* is calculated by subtracting the initial investment from the future cash flows that result from the investment. The cash can be generated by new revenue or cost savings. The future cash is discounted, or reduced, by a standard rate to reflect the fact that a dollar earned one or more years from now is worth less than a dollar one has today (the rate depends on the time period considered). If the cash generated exceeds the initial investment by a certain amount or percentage, the organization may conclude that the IT investment is a good one.

- *Internal rate of return* (IRR) is the discount rate at which the present value of an investment's future cash flow equals the cost of the investment. Another way to look at this is to ask, Given the amount of the investment and its promised cash, what rate of return am I getting on my investment? On the one hand a return of 1 percent is not a good return (just as one would not think that a 1 percent return on one's savings was good). On the other hand a 30 percent return is very good.

Table 15.1 shows the typical form of a financial analysis for an IT application.

TABLE 15.1. Financial Analysis of a Patient Accounting Document Imaging System

	Current Year	Year 1	Year 2	Year 3	Year 4	Year 5	Year 6	Year 7
COSTS								
One-time capital expense	$1,497,466	$1,302,534						
System operations								
System maintenance	-	288,000	$288,000	$288,000	$288,000	$288,000	$288,000	$288,000
System maintenance (PHS)	-	152,256	152,256	152,256	152,256	152,256	152,256	152,256
TOTAL COSTS	1,497,466	1,742,790	440,256	440,256	440,256	440,256	440,256	440,256
BENEFITS								
Revenue gains								
Rebilling of small secondary balances	-	651,000	868,000	868,000	868,000	868,000	868,000	868,000
Medicaid billing documentation	-	225,000	300,000	300,000	300,000	300,000	300,000	300,000
Disallowed Medicare bad debt audit	-	-	-	-	100,000	100,000	100,000	100,000
Staff savings								
Projected staff savings	-	36,508	136,040	156,504	169,065	169,065	169,065	171,096
Operating savings								
Projected operating savings	-	64,382	77,015	218,231	222,550	226,436	226,543	229,935
TOTAL BENEFITS	-	976,891	1,381,055	1,542,735	1,659,615	1,663,502	1,663,608	1,669,031
CASH FLOW	(1,497,466)	(765,899)	940,799	1,102,479	1,219,359	1,223,246	1,223,352	1,228,775
CUMULATIVE CASH FLOW	(1,497,466)	(2,263,365)	(1,322,566)	(220,087)	999,272	2,222,517	3,445,869	4,674,644
NPV (12% discount)	1,998,068							
IRR	33%							

Comparing Different Types of Value

Given the diversity of value, it is very challenging to compare IT proposals that have different value propositions. How does one compare a proposal that promises to increase revenue and improve collaboration to one that offers improved compliance, faster turnaround times, and reduced supply costs?

At the end of the day, judgment is used to choose one proposal over another. Health care executives review the various proposals and associated value statements and make choices based on their sense of organizational priorities, available monies, and the likelihood that the proposed value will be seen. These judgments can be aided by developing a scoring approach that allows leaders to apply a common metric across proposals. For example, the organization might decide to score each proposal according to how much value it promises to deliver in each of the following areas:

- Revenue impact
- Cost reduction
- Patient or customer satisfaction
- Quality of work life
- Quality of care
- Regulatory compliance
- Potential learning value

In this approach, each of these areas in each proposal is assigned a score, ranging from 5 (significant contribution to the area) to 1 (minimal or no contribution). The scores are then totaled for each proposal, and in theory, one picks those proposals with the highest aggregate scores. In practice, IT investment decisions are rarely that purely algorithmic. However, such scoring can be very helpful in sorting through complex and diverse value propositions:

- Scoring forces the leadership team to discuss why different members of the team assigned different scores—why, for example, did one person assign a score of 2 for the revenue impact of a particular proposal and another person assign a 4? These discussions can clarify people's understandings of proposal objectives and help the team arrive at a consensus on each project.
- Scoring means that the leadership team will have to defend any decision not to fund a project with a high score or to fund one with a low score. In the latter case, team members will have to discuss why they are all in favor of a project when it has such a low score.

The organization can decide which proposal areas to score and which not to score. Some organizations give different areas different weights: for example, reducing costs might be considered twice as important as improving organizational learning. The resulting scores are not binding, but they can be helpful in arriving at a decision about which projects will be approved and what value is being sought. (A form of this scoring process was displayed earlier in Figure 12.1).

Tactics for Reducing the Budget

Proposals for IT initiatives may originate from a wide variety of sources in an organization. The IT group will submit proposals as will department directors and physicians. Many of these proposals will not be directly related to an overall strategy but may nevertheless be "good ideas" that if implemented would lead to improved organizational performance. So it is common for an organization to have more proposals than it can fund. For example, during the IT budget discussion the leadership team may decide that although it is looking at $2.2 million in requests, the organization can afford to spend only $1.7 million, so $500,000 worth of requests must be denied. Table 15.2 presents a sample list of requests.

TABLE 15.2. **Requests for New Information System Projects**

Community General Hospital

Project Name	Operating Cost
TOTAL	$2,222,704
Clinical portfolio development	38,716
Enterprise monitoring	70,133
HIPAA security initiative	36,950
Accounting of disclosure—HIPAA	35,126
Ambulatory Center patient tracking	62,841
Bar-coding infrastructure	64,670
Capacity management	155,922
Chart tracking	34,876
Clinical data repository—patient care information system (PCIS) retirement	139,902
CRP research facility	7,026
Emergency Department data warehouse	261,584
Emergency Department order entry	182,412
Medication administration system	315,323
Order communications	377,228
Transfusion services replacement system	89,772
Wireless infrastructure	44,886
Next generation order entry	3,403
Graduate medical education duty hours	163,763

Reducing the budget in situations like this requires a value discussion. The leadership is declaring some initiatives to have more value than others. Scoring initiatives according to criteria is one approach to addressing this challenge.

In addition to such scoring, other assessment tactics can be employed, prior to the scoring, to assist leaders in making reduction decisions.

- Some requests are mandatory. They may be mandatory because of a regulation requirement (such as the HIPAA Security Rule) or because a current system is so obsolete that it is in danger of crashing—permanently—and it must be replaced soon. These requests must be funded.

- Some projects can be delayed. They are worthwhile, but a decision on them can be put off until next year. The requester will get by in the meantime.

- Key groups within IT, such as the staff who manage clinical information systems, may already have so much on their plate that they cannot possibly take on another project. Although the organization wants to do the project, it would be ill advised to do so now, and so the project can be deferred to next year.

- The user department proposing the application may not have strong management or may be experiencing some upheaval; hence implementing a new system at this time would be risky. The project could be denied or delayed until the management issues have been resolved.

- The value proposition or the resource estimates, or both, are shaky. The leadership team does not trust the proposal, so it could be denied or sent back for further analysis. Further analysis means that the proposal will be examined again next year.

- Less expensive ways may exist of addressing the problems cited in the proposal, such as a less expensive application or a non-IT approach. The proposal could be sent back for further analysis.

- The proposal is valuable, and the leadership team would like to move it forward. However, the team may reduce the budget, enabling progress to occur but at a slower pace. This delays realizing the value but ensures that resources are devoted to making progress.

These tactics are routinely employed during budget discussions aimed at trying to get as much value as possible given finite resources.

Common Proposal Problems

During the review of IT investment proposals, organizational leadership might encounter several problems related to the estimates of value and the estimates of the resources needed to obtain the value. If undetected, these problems might lead to a significant overstatement of potential return. An overstatement, obviously, may result in significant organizational unhappiness when the value that people thought they would see never materializes and never could have materialized.

Fractions of Effort Proposal analyses might indicate that the new IT initiative will save fractions of staff time, for example, that each nurse will spend fifteen minutes less per shift on clerical tasks. To suggest a total value, the proposal might multiply as follows (this example is highly simplified): 200 nurses × 15 minutes saved per 8-hour shift × 250 shifts worked per year = 12,500 hours saved. The math might be correct, and the conclusion that 12,500 hours will become available for doing other work such as direct patient care might also be correct. But the analysis will be incorrect if it then concludes that the organization would thus "save" the salary dollars of six nurses (assuming 2,000 hours worked per year per nurse).

Saving fractions of staff effort does not always lead to salary savings, even when there are large numbers of staff, because there may be no practical way to realize the savings—to, for example, lay off six nurses. If, for example, there are six nurses working each eight-hour shift in a particular nursing unit, the fifteen minutes saved per nurse would lead to a total savings of 1.5 hours per shift. But if one were then to lay off one nurse on a shift, it would reduce the nursing capacity on that shift by eight hours, damaging the unit's ability to deliver care. Saving fractions of staff effort does not lead to salary savings when staff are geographically highly fragmented or when they work in small units or teams. It leads to possible salary savings only when staff work in very large groups and some work of the reduced staff can be redistributed to others.

Reliance on Complex Behavior   Proposals may project with great certainty that people will use systems in specific ways. For example, several organizations expect that consumers will use Internet-based quality report cards to choose their physicians and hospitals. However, few consumers actually rely on such sites. Organizations may expect that nurses will readily adopt systems that help them discharge patients faster. However, nurses often delay entering discharge transactions so that they can grab a moment of peace in an otherwise overwhelmingly busy day.

System use is often not what was anticipated. This is particularly true when the organization has no experience with the relevant class of users or with the introduction of IT into certain types of tasks. The original value projection can be thrown off by the complex behaviors of system users. People do not always behave as we expect or want them to. If user behavior is uncertain, the organization would be wise to pilot an application and learn from this demonstration.

Unwarranted Optimism   Project proponents are often guilty of optimism that reflects a departure from reality. Proponents may be guilty of any of four mistakes:

- They assume that nothing will go wrong with the project.
- They assume that they are in full control of all variables that might affect the project—even, for example, quality of vendor products and organizational politics.
- They believe that they know exactly what changes in work processes will be needed and what system features must be present, when what they really have, at best, are close approximations of what must happen.
- They believe that everyone can give full time to the project and forget that people get sick or have babies and that distracting problems unrelated to the project will occur, such as a sudden deterioration in the organization's fiscal performance, and demand attention.

Decisions based on such optimism eventually result in overruns in project budgets and timetables and compromises in system goals. Overruns and compromises change the value proposition.

Shaky Extrapolations Projects often achieve gains in the first year of their implementation, and proponents are quick to project that such gains will continue during the remaining life of the project. For example, an organization may see 10 percent of its physicians move from using dictation when developing a progress note to using structured, computer-based templates. The organization may then erroneously extrapolate that each year will see an additional 10 percent shift. In fact the first year might be the only year in which such a gain will occur. The organization has merely convinced the more computer facile physicians to change, and the rest of the physicians have no interest in ever changing.

Phantom Square Feet Project proposals often state that the movement to digital records removes or reduces the need for space to house paper records. At the least, they say, the paper records could be moved off site. This in turn can lead to the claim that the money once spent on that storage space—for example, $40 per square foot—can be considered a fiscal return. In fact, such space "savings" occur only when the building of new space (for any purpose) does not occur because the organization used the freed-up records space instead. Space, like labor, represents a savings only when reducing the need for it truly does prevent further expenditure on space. If the organization uses the freed-up space but never had any intention of spending money to build more space, then any apparent savings are phantom savings.

Underestimating the Effort Project proposals might count the IT staff effort in the estimates of project costs but not count the time that users and managers will have to devote to the project. A patient care system proposal, for instance, may not include the time that will be spent by dozens of nurses working on system design, developing workflow changes, and attending training. These efforts are real costs. They often lead to the need to hire temporary nurses to provide coverage on the inpatient care units, or they might lead to a reduced patient census because there are fewer nursing hours available for patient care. Such miscounting of effort understates the cost of the project.

Fairy-Tale Savings IT project proposals may note that the project can reduce the expenses of a department or function, including costs for staff, supplies, and effort devoted to correcting mistakes that occur with paper-based processes. Department managers will swear in project approval forums that such savings are real. However, when asked if they will reduce their budgets to reflect the savings that will occur, these same managers may become significantly less convinced that the savings will result. They may comment that the freed-up staff effort or supplies budgets can be redeployed to other tasks or expenses. The managers may be right that the expenses should be redeployed, and all managers are nervous when asked to reduce their budgets and still do the same amount of work. However, the savings expected have now disappeared.

Failure to Account for Postimplementation Costs After a system goes live the costs of the system do not go away. System maintenance contracts are necessary. Hardware upgrades will be required. Staff may be needed to provide enhancements to the application. These support costs may not be as large as the costs of implementation. But they are costs that will be incurred every year, and over the course of several years they can add up to some big numbers. Proposals often fail to adequately account for support costs.

STEPS TO IMPROVE VALUE REALIZATION

Achieving value from IT investments requires management effort. There is no computer genie that descends on the organization once the system is live and waves its wand and—shazzam!—value has occurred. Achieving value is hard work but doable work. Management can take several steps to realize value (Dragoon, 2003; Glaser, 2003a, 2003b). These steps are discussed in the sections that follow.

Make Sure the Homework Was Done

IT investment decisions are often based on proposals that are not resting on solid ground. The proposer has not done the necessary homework, and this elevates the risk of a suboptimal return.

Clearly, the track record of the investment proposer will have a significant influence on the investment decision and on leaders' thinking about whether or not the investment will deliver value. However, regardless of the proposer's track record, an IT proposal should enable the leadership team to respond with a strong yes to each of the following questions:

- Is it clear how the plan advances the organization's strategy?
- Is it clear how care will improve, costs will be reduced, or service will be improved? Are the measures of current performance and expected improvement well researched and realistic? Have the related changes in operations, workflow, and organizational processes been defined?
- Are the senior leaders whose areas are the focus of the IT plan clearly supportive? Could they give the presentation?
- Are the resource requirements well understood and convincingly presented? Have these requirements been compared to those experienced by other organizations undertaking similar initiatives?
- Have the investment risks been identified, and is there an approach to addressing these risks?
- Do we have the right people assigned to the project, have we freed up their time, and are they well organized?

Answering with a no, a maybe, or an equivocal yes to any of these questions should lead one to believe that the discussion is perhaps focusing on an expense rather than an investment.

Require Formal Project Proposals

It is a fact of organizational life that projects are approved as a result of hallway conversations or discussions on the golf course. Organizational life is a political life. While recognizing that reality, the organization should require that every IT project be written up in the format of a proposal and that each proposal should be reviewed and subjected to scrutiny before the organization will commit to supporting it. However, an organization may also decide that small projects—for example, those that involve less than $25,000 in costs and less than 120 person-hours—can be handled more informally.

Increase Accountability for Investment Results

Few meaningful organizational initiatives are accomplished without establishing appropriate accountability for results. Accountability for IT investment results can be improved by taking three major steps.

First, the business owner of the IT investment should defend the investment: for example, the director of clinical laboratories should defend the request for a new laboratory system and the director of nursing should defend the need for a new nursing system. The IT staff will need to work with the business owner to define IT costs, establish likely implementation time frames, and sort through application alternatives. The IT staff should never defend an application investment.

Second, as was discussed in Chapter Fourteen, project sponsors and business owners must be defined, and they must understand the accountability that they now have for the successful completion of the project.

Third, the presentation of these projects should occur in a forum that routinely reviews such requests. Seeing many proposals, and their results, over the course of time will enable the forum participants to develop a seasoned understanding of good versus not-so-good proposals. Forum members are also able to compare and contrast proposals as they decide which ones should be approved. A manager might wonder (and it's a good question), "If I approve this proposal, does that mean that we won't have resources for another project that I might like even better?" Examining as many proposals together as possible enables the organization to take a portfolio view of its potential investments.

Figure 15.1 displays an example of a project investment portfolio represented graphically. The size of each bubble reflects the magnitude of a particular IT investment. The axes are labeled "reward" (the size of the expected value) and "risk" (the relative risk that the project will not deliver the value). Other axes may be used. One commonly used set of axes consists of "support of operations" and "support of strategic initiatives."

Diagrams such as this serve several functions:

- They summarize IT activity on one piece of paper, allowing leaders to consider a new request in the context of prior commitments.
- They help to ensure a balanced portfolio, promptly revealing imbalances such as a clustering of projects in the high-risk quadrant.

FIGURE 15.1. *IT Investment Portfolio*

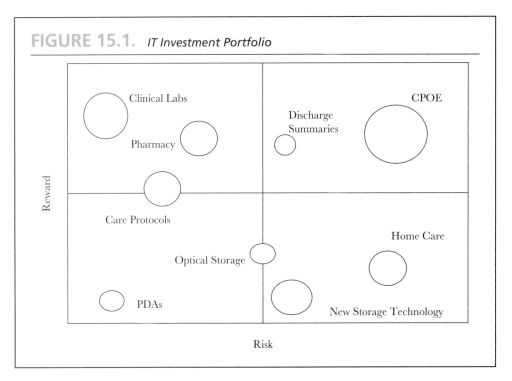

Source: Adapted from Arlotto & Oakes, 2003.

- They help to ensure that the approved projects cover an appropriate spectrum of organizational needs—for example, that projects are directed to revenue cycle improvement, to operational improvement, and to patient safety.

Conduct Postimplementation Audits

Rarely do organizations revisit their IT investments to determine if the promised value was actually achieved. They tend to believe that once the implementation is over and the change settles in, value will have been automatically achieved. This is unlikely.

Postimplementation audits can be conducted to identify value achievement progress and the steps still needed to achieve maximum gain. An organization might decide to audit two to four systems each year, selecting systems that have been live for at least six months. During the course of the audit meeting, these five questions can be asked:

1. What goals were expected at the time the project investment was approved?

2. How close have we come to achieving those original goals?

3. What do we need to do to close the goal gap?

4. How much have we invested in system implementation, and how does that compare to our original budget?

5.   If we had to implement this system again, what would we do differently?

Postimplementation audits assist value achievement by

- Signaling leadership interest in ensuring the delivery of results
- Identifying steps that still need to be taken to ensure value
- Supporting organizational learning about IT value realization
- Reinforcing accountability for results

Celebrate Value Achievement

Business value should be celebrated. Organizations usually hold parties shortly after applications go live. These parties are appropriate; a lot of people worked very hard to get the system up and running and used. However, up and running and used does not mean that value has been delivered. In addition to go-live parties, organizations should consider business value parties; celebrations conducted once the value has been achieved: for example, a party that celebrates the achievement of service improvement goals. Go-live parties alone risk sending the inappropriate signal that implementation is the end point of the IT initiative. Value delivery is the end point.

Leverage Organizational Governance

The creation of an IT committee of the board of directors can enhance organizational efforts to achieve value from IT investments. At times the leadership team of an organization is uncomfortable with some or all of the IT conversation. Team members may not understand why infrastructure is so expensive or why large implementations can take so long and cost so much. They may feel uncomfortable with the complexity of determining the likely value to be obtained from IT investments. The creation of a subcommittee made up of the board members most experienced with such discussions can help to ensure that hard questions are being asked and that the answers are sound.

Shorten the Deliverables Cycle

When possible, projects should have short deliverable cycles. In other words, rather than asking the organization to wait twelve or eighteen months to see the first fruits of its application implementation labors, make an effort to deliver a sequence of smaller implementations. For example, one might conduct pilots of an application in a subset of the organization, followed by a staged rollout. Or one might plan for serial implementation of the first 25 percent of the application features.

Pilots, staged rollouts, and serial implementations are not always doable. Where they are possible, however, they enable the organization to achieve some value earlier rather than later, support organizational learning about which system capabilities are really important and which were only thought to be important, facilitate the development of reengineered operational processes, and create the appearance (whose importance is not to be underestimated) of more value delivery.

Benchmark Value

Organizations should benchmark their performance in achieving value against the performance of their peers. These benchmarks might focus on process performance: for example, days in accounts receivables or average time to get an appointment. An important aspect of value benchmarking is the identification of the critical IT application capabilities and related operational changes that enabled the achievement of superior results. This understanding of how other organizations achieved superior IT-enabled performance can guide an organization's efforts to continuously achieve as much value as possible from its IT investments.

Communicate Value

Once a year the information technology department should develop a communication plan for the twelve months ahead. This plan should indicate which presentations will be made in which forums and how often IT-centric columns will appear in organizational newsletters. The plan should list three or so major themes—for example, specific regional integration strategies or efforts to improve IT service—that will be the focus of these communications. Communication plans try to remedy the fact that even when value is being delivered, most people in the organization may not be fully aware of it.

WHY IT FAILS TO DELIVER RETURNS

It is not uncommon to hear leaders of health care organizations complain about the lack of value obtained from IT investments. These leaders may see IT as a necessary expense that must be tightly controlled rather than as an investment that can be a true enabler. New health care managers often walk into organizations where the leadership mind-set features this set of conclusions:

The magnitude of the organization's IT operating and capital budgets is large. IT operating costs may consume 3 percent of the total operating budget, and IT capital may claim 15 to 30 percent of all capital. Although 3 percent may appear small, it can be the difference between a negative operating margin and a positive margin. A 15 to 30 percent IT consumption of capital invariably means that funding for biomedical equipment (which can mean new revenue) and buildings (which can help the organization appear patient and staff friendly and can support the growth of clinical services) is diminished. IT can be seen as taking money away from "worthwhile initiatives."

The projected growth in IT budgets exceeds the growth in other budget categories. Provider organizations may permit overall operating budgets to increase at a rate close to the inflation rate (recently 3 to 4 percent). However, expenditures on IT often experience growth rates of 10 to 15 percent. At some point an organization will note that the IT budget growth rate may single-handedly lead to insolvency.

Regardless of the amount spent, some members of the leadership team feel that not enough is being spent. Worthwhile proposals go unfunded every year. Infrastructure replacement and upgrades seem never ending: "I thought we upgraded our network two years ago. Are you back already?"

It is difficult to evaluate IT capital requests. At times this difficulty is a reflection of a poorly written or fatuous proposal. However, it can be genuinely difficult to compare a proposal directed at improving service to one directed at improving care quality to one directed at increasing revenue to one needed to achieve some level of regulatory compliance.

When asked to "list three instances over the last five years where IT investments have resulted in clear and unarguable returns to the organization," leaders may return blank stares. However, the conversation may be difficult to stop when they are asked to "list three major IT investment disappointments that have occurred over the last five years."

If the value from information technology can be significant, why does one hear these management concerns? There are several reasons why IT investments become simply IT expenses. The organization

- Fails to clearly link IT investments and organizational strategy.
- Asks the wrong question.
- Conducts the wrong analysis.
- Does not state its investment goals.
- Does not manage outcomes.
- Leaps to an inappropriate solution.
- Mangles the project management.
- Fails to learn from studies of IT effectiveness.

Failing to Clearly Link IT Investments and Organizational Strategy

The linkage between IT investments and the organization's strategy was discussed in Chapter Twelve. When strategies and investments are not aligned, the IT department, even if it is executing well, may be working on the wrong things or trying to support a flawed overall organizational strategy.

Linkage failures can occur because

- The organizational strategy is no more than a slogan or a buzzword with the depth of a bumper sticker, making any investment toward achieving it ill considered.
- The IT department thinks it understands the strategy but it does not, resulting in implementation of the IT version of the strategy rather than the organization's version.
- The strategists (for a variety of reasons) will not engage in the IT discussion, forcing IT leaders to be mind readers.
- The linkage is superficial: for example, "Patient care systems can reduce nursing labor costs but we haven't thought through how that will happen."

■ The IT strategy conversation is separated from the organizational strategy conversation, perhaps as a result of the creation of an information systems steering committee, reducing the likelihood of alignment.

■ The organizational strategy evolves faster than IT can respond.

Asking the Wrong Question

Rarely should one ask the question, What is the ROI of a computer system? This makes as much sense as asking, What is the ROI of a chain saw? If one wants to make a dress, a chain saw is a waste of money. If one wants to cut down some trees, one can begin to think about the return on a chain saw investment. One will want to compare that investment to other investments, such as an investment in an ax. One will also want to consider the user. If the chain saw is to be used by a ten-year-old child, the investment might be ill advised. If the chain saw is to be used by a skilled lumberjack, the investment might be worth it.

An organization can determine the ROI of an investment in a tool only if it knows the task to be performed and the skill level of the participants who are to perform the task. Moreover, a positive ROI is not an inherent property of an IT investment. The organization has to manage a return into existence.

Hence, instead of asking, What is the ROI of a computer system? organizational leaders should ask questions such as these:

■ What are the steps and investments, including IT steps and investments, that we need to take or make in order to achieve our goals?

■ Which business manager owns the achievement of these goals? Does this person have our confidence?

■ Do the cost, risk, and time frame associated with implementing this set of investments, including the IT investment, seem appropriate given our goals?

■ Have we assessed the trade-offs and opportunity costs?

■ Are we comfortable with our ability to execute?

Conducting the Wrong Analysis

There are times when determining ROI is the appropriate investment analysis technique. If a set of investments is intended to reduce clerical staff, an ROI can be calculated. However, there are times when an ROI calculation is clearly inappropriate. What is the ROI of software that supports collaboration? One could calculate the ROI, but it is hard to imagine an organization basing its investment decision on that analysis. Would an ROI analysis have captured the strategic value of the Amazon.com system or the value of automated teller machines? Few strategic IT investments have impacts that are fully captured by an ROI analysis. Moreover, strategic impact is rarely fully understood until years after implementation. Whatever ROI analysis might have been done would have invariably been wrong.

As was discussed earlier, the objective of the IT investment points to the appropriate approach to the analysis of its return. Sometimes organizations apply financial techniques such as internal rate of return in a manner that is overzealous and ignores other analysis approaches. This misapplication of technique can clearly lead to highly worthwhile initiatives being deemed unworthy of funding.

Not Stating Investment Goals

Statements about the positive contributions the investment will make to organizational performance often accompany IT proposals. Statements about specific numerical goals for this improvement are less common. If the investment is intended to reduce medical errors, will it reduce errors by 50 percent or 80 percent or some other number? If it is intended to reduce claim denials, will it reduce them to 5 percent or 2 percent, and how much revenue will be realized as a result of this reduction?

Failure to be numerically explicit about goals can create three fundamental value problems.

- The organization may not know how well it performs now. If the current error rate or denial rate is not known, it is hard to believe that the leadership has studied the problem well enough to be fairly sure that an IT investment will achieve the desired gains. The IT proposal sounds more like a guess about what is needed.

- The organization may never know whether it got the desired value or not. If the proposal does not state a goal, the organization will never know whether the 20 percent reduction in errors it has achieved is as far as it can go or whether it is only halfway to its desired goal. It does not know whether it should continue to work on the error problem or whether it should move on to the next performance issue.

- It will be difficult to hold someone accountable for performance improvement when the organization is unable to track how well he or she is doing.

Not Managing Outcomes

Related to the failure to state goals is the failure to manage outcomes into existence. Once the project is approved and the system is up, management goes off to the next challenge, seemingly unaware that the work of value realization has just begun.

Figure 15.2 depicts a reduction in days in accounts receivable (AR) at a Partners HealthCare physician practice. During the interval depicted, a new practice management system was implemented. The practice did not see a precipitous decline in days in AR (a sign of improved revenue performance) in the time immediately following the implementation in the second quarter of 1997. The practice did see a progressive improvement in days in AR because someone was managing that improvement.

If the gain in revenue performance had been an "automatic" result of the information system implementation, the practice would have seen a sharp drop in days in AR. Instead it saw a gradual improvement over time. This gradual change reflects that

- The gain occurred through day in, day out changes in operational processes, fine-tuning of system capabilities, and follow-ups in staff training.

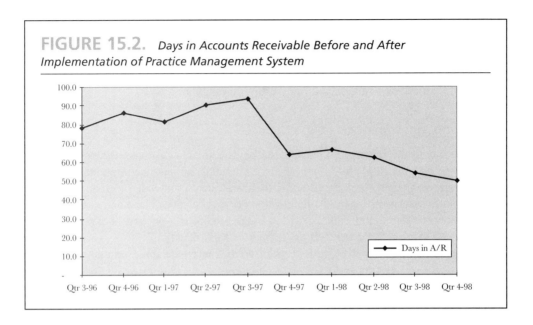

FIGURE 15.2. *Days in Accounts Receivable Before and After Implementation of Practice Management System*

■ A person had to be in charge of obtaining this improvement. Someone had to identify and make operational changes, manage changes in system capabilities, and ensure that needed training occurred.

Leaping to an Inappropriate Solution

At times the IT discussion of a new application succumbs to advanced states of technical arousal. Project participants become overwhelmed by the prospect of using sexy new technology and state-of-the-art gizmos and lose their senses and understanding of why they are having this discussion in the first place. Sexiness and state-of-the-art-ness become the criteria for making system decisions.

In addition the comparison of two alternative vendor products can turn into a features war. The discussion may focus on the number of features as a way of distinguishing products and fail to ask whether this numerical difference has any real impact on the value that is desired.

Both sexiness and features have their place in the system selection decision. However, they are secondary to the discussion that centers on the capabilities needed to effect specific performance goals. Sexiness and features may be irrelevant to the performance improvement discussion.

Mangling the Project Management

One guaranteed way to reduce value is to mangle the management of the implementation project. Implementation failures or significant budget and timetable overruns or really unhappy users, any of these can dilute value.

Among the many factors that can lead to mangled project management are these:

- The project's scope is poorly defined.
- The accountability is unclear.
- The project participants are marginally skilled.
- The magnitude of the task is underestimated.
- Users feel like victims rather than participants.
- All the world has a vote and can vote at any time.

Many of these factors were discussed in Chapters Seven and Fourteen.

Failing to Learn from Studies of IT Effectiveness

Organizations may fail to invest in the IT abilities discussed in Chapter Thirteen, such as good relationships between the IT function and the rest of the organization and a well-architected infrastructure. This investment failure increases the likelihood that the percentage of projects that fail to deliver value will be higher than it should be.

ANALYSES OF THE IT VALUE CHALLENGE

The IT investment and value challenge plagues all industries. It is not a problem peculiar to health care. The challenge has been with us for forty years, ever since organizations began to spend money on big mainframes. This challenge is complex and persistent, and we should not believe we can fully solve it. We should believe we can be better at dealing with it. This section highlights the conclusions of several studies and articles that have examined this challenge.

Factors That Hinder Value Return

The Committee to Study the Impact of Information Technology on the Performance of Service Activities (1994) found these major contributors to failures to achieve a solid return on IT investments:

- The organization's overall strategy is wrong, or its assessment of its competitive environment is inadequate.
- The strategy is fine, but the necessary IT applications and infrastructure are not defined appropriately. The information system, if it is solving a problem, is solving the wrong problem.
- The organization fails to identify and draw together well all the investments and initiatives necessary to carry out its plans. The IT investment then falters because other changes, such as reorganization or reengineering, fail to occur.
- The organization fails to execute the IT plan well. Poor planning or less than stellar management can diminish the return from any investment.

Value may also be diluted by factors outside the organization's control. Weill and Broadbent (1998) noted that the more strategic the IT investment, the more its value can be diluted. An IT investment directed to increasing market share may have its value diluted by non-IT decisions and events—for example, pricing decisions, competitors' actions, and customers' reactions. IT investments that are less strategic but have business value—for example, improving nursing productivity—may be diluted by outside factors—for example, shortages of nursing staff. And the value of an IT investment directed toward improving infrastructure characteristics may be diluted by outside factors—for example, unanticipated technology immaturity or business difficulties confronting a vendor.

The Investment-Performance Relationship

A study by Strassmann (1990) examined the relationship between IT expenditures and organizational effectiveness. Data from an *Information Week* survey of the top 100 users of information technology were used to correlate IT expenditures per employee with profits per employee. Strassmann concluded that there is no obvious direct relationship between expenditure and organizational performance. This finding has been observed in several other studies (for example, Keen, 1997). It leads to several conclusions:

- Spending more on IT is no guarantee that the organization will be better off. There has never been a direct correlation between spending and outcomes. Paying more for care does not give one correspondingly better care. Clearly, one can spend so little that nothing effective can be done. And one can spend so much that waste is guaranteed. But moving IT expenditures from 2 percent of the operating budget to 3 percent of the operating budget does not inherently lead to a 50 percent increase in desirable outcomes.

- Information technology is a tool, and its utility as a tool is largely determined by the tool user and his or her task. Spending a large amount of money on a chain saw for someone who doesn't know how to use one is a waste. Spending more money on tools for the casual saw user who trims an apple tree every now and then is also a waste. However, skilled loggers might say that if a chain saw blade were longer and the saw's engine more powerful, they would be able to cut 10 percent more trees in a given period of time. The investment needed to enhance the loggers' saws might lead to superior performance. Organizational effectiveness in applying IT has an enormous effect on the likelihood of a useful outcome from increased IT investment.

- Factors other than the appropriateness of the tool to the task also influence the relationship between IT investment and organizational performance. These factors include the nature of the work (for example, IT is likely to have a greater impact on bank performance than on consulting firm performance), the basis of competition in an industry (for example, cost per unit of manufactured output versus prowess in marketing), and an organization's relative competitive position in the market.

The Value of the Overall Investment

Many analyses and academic studies have been directed to answering this broad question, How can an organization assess the value of its overall investments in IT? Assessing the value of the aggregate IT investment is different from assessing the value of a single initiative or other specific investment. And it is also different from assessing the caliber of the IT department. Developing a definitive, accurate, and well-accepted way to answer this question has so far eluded all industries and may continue to be elusive. Nonetheless there are some basic questions that can be asked in pursuit of answering the larger question. Interpreting the answers to these basic questions is a subjective exercise, making it difficult to derive numerical scores. Bresnahan (1998) suggests five questions:

1. How does IT influence the customer experience?

2. Do patients and physicians, for example, find that organizational processes are more efficient, less error prone, and more convenient?

3. Does IT enable or retard growth? Can the IT organization support effectively the demands of a merger? Can IT support the creation of clinical product lines—for example, cardiology—across the IDS?

4. Does IT favorably affect productivity?

5. Does IT advance organizational innovation and learning?

IT as a Commodity

Carr (2003) has equated IT with commodities—soybeans, for example. Carr's argument is that core information technologies, such as fast, inexpensive processors and storage, are readily available to all organizations and hence cannot provide a competitive advantage. Organizations can no more achieve value from IT than an automobile manufacturer can achieve value by buying better steel than a competitor does or a grocer can achieve value by stocking better sugar than a competitor does. In this view, IT, steel, and sugar are all commodities.

Responding to Carr's argument, Brown and Hagel (2003) make three observations about IT value:

1. "Extracting value from IT requires innovation in business practices." If an organization merely computerizes existing processes without rectifying (or at times eliminating) process problems, it may have merely made process problems occur faster. In addition those processes are now more expensive because there is a computer system to support. Providing appointment scheduling systems may not make waiting times any shorter or enhance patients' ability to get an appointment when they need one.

All IT initiatives should be accompanied by efforts to materially improve the processes that the system is designed to support. IT often enables the organization to think differently about a process or expand its options for improving a process. If the process thinking is narrow or unimaginative, the value that could have been achieved will have been lost, with the organization settling for an expensive way to achieve minimal gain.

For example, if Amazon.com had thought that the Internet enabled it to simply replace the catalogue and telephone as a way of ordering something, it would have missed ideas such as presenting products to the customer based on data about prior orders or enabling customers to leave their own ratings of books and music.

2. "IT's economic impact comes from incremental innovations rather than from 'big bang' initiatives." Organizations will often introduce very large computer systems and process change "all at once." Two examples of such big bangs are the replacement of all systems related to the revenue cycle and the introduction of a new patient care system over the course of a few weeks.

Big bang implementations are very tricky and highly risky. They may be haunted by series of technical problems. Moreover, these systems introduce an enormous number of process changes affecting many people. It is exceptionally difficult to understand the ramifications of such change during the analysis and design stages that precede implementation. A full understanding is impossible. As a result, the implementing organization risks material damage. This damage destroys value. It may set the organization back, and even if the organization grinds its way through the disruption, the resulting trauma may make the organization unwilling to engage in future ambitious IT initiatives.

In contrast, IT implementations (and related process changes) that are more incremental and iterative reduce the risk of organizational damage and permit the organization to learn. The organization has time to understand the value impact of phase n and then can alter its course before it embarks upon phase $n + 1$. Moreover, incremental change leads the organization's members to understand that change, and realizing value, are a never ending aspect of organizational life rather than something to be endured every couple of years.

3. "The strategic impact of IT investments comes from the cumulative effect of sustained initiatives to innovate business practices in the near term." If economic value is derived from a series of thoughtful, incremental steps, then the aggregate effect of those steps should be a competitive advantage. Most of the time, organizations that wind up dominating an industry do so through incremental movement over the course of several years (Collins, 2001). This observation is consistent with our view in Chapter Twelve. Persistent innovation by a talented team, over the course of years, will result in significant strategic gains. The organization has learned how to improve itself, year in and year out. Strategic value is a marathon. It is a long race that is run and won one mile at a time.

SUMMARY

IT value is complex, multifaceted, and diverse across and within proposed initiatives. The techniques used to analyze value must vary with the nature of the value.

The project proposal is the core means for assessing the potential value of a potential IT initiative. IT proposals have a commonly accepted structure. And approaches exist for comparing proposals with different types of value propositions. Project proposals often present problems in the way they estimate value—for example, they may unrealistically combine fractions of effort saved, fail to appreciate the complex behavior of system users, or underestimate the full costs of the project.

Many factors can dilute the value realized from an IT investment. Poor linkage between the IT agenda and the organizational strategy, the failure to set goals, and the failure to manage the realization of value all contribute to dilution.

There are steps that can be taken to improve the achievement of IT value. Leadership can ensure that project proponents have done their homework, that accountability for results has been established, that formal proposals are used, and that postimplementation audits are conducted. Even though there are many approaches and factors that can enhance the realization of IT-enabled value, the challenges of achieving this value will remain a management issue for the foreseeable future.

Health care organization leaders often feel ill equipped to address the IT investment and value challenge. However, no new management techniques are required to evaluate IT plans, proposals, and progress. Leadership teams are often asked to make decisions that involve strategic hunches (such as a belief that developing a continuum of care would be of value) about areas where they may have limited domain knowledge (new surgical modalities) and where the value is fuzzy (improved morale). Organizational leaders should treat IT investments just as they would treat other types of investments; if they don't understand, believe, or trust the proposal, or its proponent, they shouldn't approve it.

KEY TERMS

Failure to deliver returns
IT project proposals

IT value
Value realization

LEARNING ACTIVITIES

1. Interview the CIO of a local health care provider or payer. Discuss how his or her organization assesses the value of IT investments and ensures that the value is delivered.

2. Select two articles from a health care IT trade journal that describe the value an organization received from its IT investments. Critique and compare the articles.

3. Select two examples of intangible value. Propose one or more approaches that an organization might use to measure each of those values.

4. Prepare a defense of the value of a significant investment in an electronic medical record system.

CHAPTER

16

HEALTH IT LEADERSHIP

A COMPENDIUM OF CASE STUDIES

Faculty and others who teach health administration students are often in search of case studies that can be used to help students apply theory and concepts to real-life IT management situations, encourage problem solving and critical thinking, and foster discussion and collaboration among students. This chapter provides a compendium of case studies from a variety of health care organizations and settings. It is intended to serve as a supplement to the preceding chapters and as a resource to faculty and students. Many of these case studies were originally written by working health care executives enrolled as students in the doctoral program in health administration offered at the Medical University of South Carolina. We wish to acknowledge and thank these students for allowing us to share their stories and experiences with you:

Penney Burlingame	Randall Jones
Barbara Chelton	Catrin Jones-Nazar
Stuart Fine	Ronald Kintz
David Freed	James Kirby
David Gehant	George Mikatarian
Patricia Givens	Lorie Shoemaker
Victoria Harkins	Gary Wilde

Each case begins with background information that includes a description of the setting, the current information system (IS) challenge facing the organization, and the factors that are felt to have contributed to the current situation. (All real names and identifying information have been changed from the original cases to protect the identity of the individuals and organizations involved.) Following each case is a set of recommended discussion questions. To the extent possible, the cases are organized by major theme, such as strategic IS planning, system acquisition, and system implementation. (See Table 16.1.)

TABLE 16.1. **List of Cases and Major Themes**

Title of Case	Major Theme(s)
Case 1: Board Support for a Capital Project	Strategic planning and IT alignment; IT governance
Case 2: The Decision to Develop an IT Strategic Plan	Strategic planning and IT alignment
Case 3: Selection of a Patient Safety Strategy	Strategic planning and IT alignment
Case 4: Strategic IS Planning for the Hospital ED	Strategic planning and IT alignment
Case 5: Planning an EMR Implementation	IT strategy; system implementation
Case 6: Considerations for Voice over IP Telephony	Assessing the value of a health information technology (HIT) investment: use of emerging technologies
Case 7: Implementing a Capacity Management Information System	System acquisition
Case 8: Implementing a Telemedicine Solution	System acquisition; use of emerging technologies
Case 9: Replacing a Practice Management System	IT governance; system implementation
Case 10: Conversion to an EMR Messaging System	System implementation; project management
Case 11: Concerns and Workarounds with a Clinical Documentation System	System implementation; project management
Case 12: Strategies for Implementing CPOE	System implementation; project management
Case 13: Implementing a Syndromic Surveillance System	IT strategy; system implementation
Case 14: The Admitting System Crashes	Disaster recovery
Case 15: Breaching the Security of an Internet Patient Portal	IT security
Case 16: Assessing the Value and Impact of CPOE	Assessing the value of an HIT investment

We hope you find the cases thought-provoking and useful in applying the concepts covered in this book to what is happening in health care organizations throughout our nation.

CASE 1: BOARD SUPPORT FOR A CAPITAL PROJECT

Major themes: strategic planning and IT alignment; IT governance

Background Information

Lakeland Medical Center is a 210-bed public hospital located in the Southeast. It is governed by a politically appointed nine-member board and serves a market of approximately 100,000 people. The hospital has been financially successful, but in recent years several capital investments have not brought high returns. As a result, project investment decisions became more conservative and oriented toward financial returns. Competitive forces have continued to grow in the market, and significant internal expense items (such as the organization's pension program, paid leave bank, and health insurance program) have put strains on Lakeland's financial resources.

Revenue continues to grow at an average rate of about 10 percent each year, but controlling expenses remains a challenge. Bad debt has grown from $5 million last year to a budgeted amount of $14 million this year. The hospital continues to accomplish high patient and employee satisfaction scores, high quality scores, and an A+ credit rating. Debt is approximately $55 million, and cash reserves are approximately $95 million. Total operating revenues are approximately $130 million. The hospital employs 940 staff members. The average length of stay is 4.3 days. Annual capital expenditure is $4 million.

Information Systems Challenge

In 2005, the installation of computed radiography (CR) components to build a picture archiving and communication system (PACS) began, at an estimated total cost of $1 million. In 2006, $400,000 was spent for additional CR components. But in 2007, the board of directors (with three new members) did not approve the request of $1.9 million for completion of the PACS, saying that it represented far too large a percentage of the organization's annual capital budget. A year later Lakeland is still in need of completing the PACS program, with a board that is unlikely to approve the expenditure.

A number of factors are contributing to the board's decision not to authorize the additional $1.9 million for completion of the PACS, including

- Leadership's inability to guarantee to the board's satisfaction a financial return on the proposed investment.
- The board's perception that the radiologists are not committed to the hospital and to the community because none of the radiologists live in the community.

- The board's perception that the cardiologists are not committed to the hospital or to the community. The five cardiologists on staff are considered to be uncooperative among themselves and not supportive of the hospital's goals.
- Poor leadership within the IT department for providing the proper guidance on acquisition and implementation.
- The board's philosophy that Lakeland Medical Center should be more *high-touch* and less *high-tech*, and thus there is a philosophical difference over the need for a PACS.
- Jealousy among the medical staff that the diagnostic imaging department continues to obtain capital approvals for large items representing a major percentage of the annual capital budget. Thus, many influential members of the medical staff, such as surgeons, are not supportive of the expenditure.
- A few vocal employees speaking directly to board members expressing their concern that the PACS implementation will result in job loss for them.
- Leadership's inability to make a connection between this capital project and the strategic goals of the organization.

The chief of staff, Dr. Mary White, firmly believes that a PACS will increase patient and physician satisfaction because waiting times for results will decrease, enhance patient education, improve staff and physician productivity, improve clinical outcomes, improve patient safety, eliminate lost films, reduce medical liability, assist in reducing patient length of stay, and increase revenue potential. She believes it is management's challenge to understand the key issues of the board and to present the necessary supportive information for ultimate approval of the PACS program.

Discussion Questions

1. Conduct a role play. Divide into four teams—the Lakeland Medical Center administrative team, the board, the medical staff, and the hospital and community at large. Assume the role of your constituent group and answer these questions: What are your views on this proposal? What are your major concerns? What questions do you have? And for whom? Do you think this is a case of someone failing to do his or her homework in putting together a sound business plan for the PACS project, or do you think there are bigger issues at play here? Explain your answers as necessary.

2. Assume that the CEO believes that the PACS project is well aligned with Lakeland's strategic goals but that this case hasn't been made clear to the board. How might Lakeland build this case? Who should lead that effort? What work needs to be done that has not occurred yet?

3. Are the board's concerns about medical staff commitment relevant in this case? Why or why not?

4. Develop a strategy for addressing the board's concerns and winning their buy-in and approval for the PACS project. Include in your description the who, what, where, when, and how.

CASE 2: THE DECISION TO DEVELOP AN IT STRATEGIC PLAN

Major themes: strategic planning and IT alignment

Background Information

Meadow Hills Hospital is a 211-bed acute care hospital with 400 members on its medical staff. Meadow serves a population of 300,000. There are three other similarly sized hospitals in the region. As an organization, Meadow Hills is very well run. It has a good reputation in the community and is considered to be technically advanced based on its investments in imaging technology. The organization is also in a strong financial position, with $238 million in reserves.

Meadow Hills has never had an information technology strategic plan.

Information Systems Challenge

The IT function reports to the Meadow Hills chief financial officer (CFO). The CEO and other members of the senior leadership team have largely left IT decisions up to the CFO. As a result the organization's financial systems are very well developed. Computerized provider order entry (CPOE), an electronic medical record (EMR) system, and a PACS have not been implemented. IT support for departments such as nursing, pharmacy, laboratory, imaging, and risk management is limited.

The Meadow Hills IT team is well regarded and the limited IT support for clinical processes has not drawn complaints from the nursing or medical staff. The organization does not currently have a chief information officer (CIO).

The CEO has never felt the need to pay attention to IT. However, he is worried that reimbursement based on care quality will arrive at Meadow Hills soon. He also believes that the Meadow Hills Clinical Laboratory and Imaging Center would be more competitive if it had stronger IT support; rival labs and imaging centers are able to offer electronic access to test results. And he suspects that the lack of IT support may eventually lead to nurses and physicians choosing to practice elsewhere.

Discussion Questions

1. What steps should the CEO take to develop an IT strategy for the organization?
2. Are there unique risks to the ability of Meadow Hills Hospital to develop and implement an IT strategy?
3. Meadow Hills appears to have been successful despite years without an IT strategy. Why is this?

CASE 3: SELECTION OF A PATIENT SAFETY STRATEGY

Major themes: strategic planning and IT alignment

Background Information

Langley Mason Health (LMH) is located in North Reno County, the largest public health care district in the state of Nevada, serving an 850-square-mile area encompassing seven distinctly different communities. The health district was founded in 1937 by a registered nurse and dietician who opened a small medical facility on a former poultry farm. Today the health system comprises Langley Medical Center, a 317-bed tertiary medical center and level II trauma center; Mason Hospital, a 107-bed community hospital; and Mason Continuing Care Center and Villa Langley, two part-skilled nursing facilities (SNFs); a home care division; an ambulatory surgery center; and an outpatient behavioral medicine center.

In anticipation of expected population growth in North Reno County and to meet the state mandated seismic requirements for 2013, LMH developed an aggressive facilities master plan (FMP) that includes plans to build a state-of-the-art 453-bed replacement hospital for its Langley Medical Center campus, double the size of its Mason Hospital, and build satellite clinics in four of its outlying communities. The cost associated with actualizing this FMP is estimated to be $1 billion. In 2004, LMH undertook and successfully passed the largest health care bond measure in the state's history and in so doing secured $496 million in general obligation bonds to help fund its massive facilities expansion project. The remaining funds must come from revenue bonds, growth strategies, philanthropic efforts, and strong operational performance over the next ten years. Additionally, $5 million of routine capital funds will be diverted every fiscal year for the next five years to help offset the huge capital outlay that will be necessary to equip the new facilities. That leaves LMH with only $10 million per year to spend on routine maintenance, equipment and technology for all its facilities. LMH is committed to patient safety and is building what the leadership team hopes will be one of the safest hospital-of-the-future facilities. The challenge is to provide for patient safety and safe medication practices given the minimal capital dollars available to spend today.

LMH developed an IT strategic plan in late 2007, with the following ten goals identified:

- Empower health consumers and physicians.
- Transform data into information.
- Support the expansion of clinical services.
- Expand e-business opportunities.
- Realize the benefits of innovation.
- Maximize the value of IT.
- Improve project outcomes.
- Prepare for the unexpected.

- Deploy a robust and agile technical architecture.
- Digitally enable new facilities, including the new hospital.

Information Systems Challenge

LMH has implemented phase one—an enterprise-wide EMR system developed by Cerner Corporation in 2005 at a cost of $20 million. Phase two of project is to implement computerized provider order entry (CPOE) with decision-support capabilities. This phase was to have been completed in 2007, but has been delayed due to the many challenges associated with phase one, which still must be stabilized and optimized. LMH does have a fully automated pharmacy information system, albeit older technology, and Pyxis medication-dispensing systems on all units in the acute care hospitals. Computerized discharge prescriptions and instructions are available only for patients seen and discharged from the LMH emergency departments.

Currently, the pharmacy and nursing staff at LMH have been working closely on the selection of a smart IV pump to replace all of the health system's aging pumps and have put forth a proposal to spend $4.9 million dollars in the fiscal year beginning July 2009. Smart pumps have been shown to significantly reduce medication administration errors, thus reducing patient harm. This expenditure would consume roughly half of all of the available capital dollars for that fiscal year.

The chief information officer, Marilyn Moore, PhD, understands the pharmacists' and nurses' desire to purchase smart IV pumps but believes the implementation of this technology should not be considered in isolation. She sees the smart pumps as one facet of an overall medication management capital purchase and patient safety strategic plan. Dr. Moore suggests that the pharmacy and nursing leadership team lead a medication management strategic planning process and evaluate a suite of available technologies that taken together could optimize medication safety (for example, CPOE, electronic medication administration records [e-mar], robots, automated pharmacy systems, bar coding, computerized discharge prescriptions and instructions, and smart IV pumps), the costs associated with implementing these technologies, and the organization's readiness to embrace these technologies. Paul Robinson, PharmD, the director of pharmacy, appreciates Dr. Moore's suggestion but feels that smart IV pumps are critical to patient safety and that LMH doesn't have time to go through a long, drawn-out planning process that could take years to implement and the process of gaining board support. Others argue that all new proposals should be placed on hold until CPOE is up and running. They argue there are too many other pressing issues at hand to invest in yet another new technology.

Discussion Questions

1. Describe the current situation as you see it. What are the major issues in this case?
2. Marilyn Moore, CIO, and Paul Robinson, director of pharmacy, have different views of how LMH should proceed. What are the pros and cons of their respective

approaches? Which approach, if either, seems like an appropriate course of action to you? Explain your rationale.

3.   Assume you are to mediate a discussion on this issue and that participants are to come to consensus on how best to proceed. What would you do?

CASE 4: STRATEGIC IS PLANNING FOR THE HOSPITAL ED

Major themes: strategic planning and IT alignment

Background Information

Founded in 1900, Newcastle Hospital today is a 375-bed, not-for-profit community hospital that serves over 200,000 residents of Newcastle County, New York. The hospital is approximately thirty miles from midtown Manhattan. It provides a full range of both primary and secondary medical and surgical services and is an affiliate of one of the large New York City hospital systems for both tertiary referrals and select residency programs. Newcastle Hospital has an independent governing body with 25 trustees; 604 active physicians; and 1,121 full-time equivalent (FTE) staff. Revenues of approximately $130 million per year come from 15,600 inpatient admissions; 71,000 outpatient visits; and 65,000 home care visits. Newcastle Hospital operates in a difficult environment characterized by relatively poor reimbursement and severe competition. There is one other acute care hospital in the county and a total of thirty-five others within a twenty-mile radius.

The sentinel event in the hospital's recent history occurred four years ago—a six-month nursing strike that alienated the workforce, decimated public confidence, and directly cost at least $19.5 million, effectively eradicating the hospital's capital reserves. Most of the senior management was replaced after the strike. When hired, the new CEO and CFO uncovered extensive inaccuracies that resulted in a reduction of reported net assets by almost $30 million and the near-bankruptcy of the hospital. The new management restated financial statements; began resolving extensive litigation; and set out to reestablish immediate operations, future finances, and long-term strategy. The new CEO states that "years of board and management neglect, plus the ravages of the strike complicated recovery, because standards, systems, and middle managers were universally absent or ineffective."

Among its many challenges, the challenges within the hospital's emergency department (ED) are particularly important to the overall recovery effort. The ED is described by the hospital CEO as the organization's "financial, clinical and public relations backbone." The ED sees 34,000 patients per year and admits 24 percent of them, constituting 51 percent of all inpatient admissions. In addition, the ED is a clinically distinguished Level II trauma center, with a long legacy of outcomes that compare favorably against regional, state, and national benchmarks. Finally, most community members have experience with the ED and consider it a proxy for the hospital as a whole, whether or not they have experienced an inpatient stay.

Currently, Newcastle ED patient satisfaction compared to patient satisfaction among peer organizations ranks at the fourteenth percentile in the Press Ganey New York State survey and the 5th percentile in national surveys. Since 1997, three organized initiatives to improve these results (especially regarding walkouts and waiting times) have failed, even though two involved prestigious consultants. After the management change, the new CEO diagnosed two core barriers to overcoming the ED problems: first, inflexibility and unwillingness to change among the ED physician management group that had been in place since 1987 and, second, an almost complete absence of the data required to define, measure, and improve the ED's service performance. The first barrier was addressed via an RFP process that resulted in engaging a new physician management group two years ago.

Information Systems Challenge

The present IS challenge follows directly from Newcastle Hospital's overarching strategic objectives: "satisfying patients and staff," "supporting ourselves," and "getting better every day" (that is, improving performance). The ED as presently structured has ill-defined manual processes and no information system. The challenge is selecting an ED information system with an emphasis on informing, not just automating, key ED processes, in order to support the overall strategic initiatives of the organization.

Several organizational and IT system factors that affect this IT challenge have been identified by the hospital CEO:

Organizational Factors

- Undefined strategy. Newcastle Hospital operated without a formal strategic action plan and corresponding tactics until two years ago. As a result, systematic prioritization and measurement of institutional imperatives such as improving the ED did not occur.

- Data integrity. Data throughout the hospital were undefined and unreliable. For example, two irreconcilable daily census reports made timely bed placement from the ED impossible.

- Culture. "Looking good," that is, escaping accountability, was valued more highly than "doing good," that is, substantively improving performance. Serious problems in the ED were often masked or dismissed as anecdotes, even in the face of regulatory citations and six- to eight-hour waiting times. The previous ED contract had contained no quality standards, and the ED physicians claimed to be busy "saving lives" whenever their poor service performance was questioned.

IT System Factors

- IT strategy. Paralleling the hospital, the IS department had no defined strategies, objectives, or processes. Alignment with hospital strategy and IT performance measurement were not considered. Although some progress has been made, this remains an area needing attention.

- IT governance. There is no IT steering committee at either the board or management levels. IT policies, service-level agreements, decision criteria, and user roles and responsibilities do not exist.

■ Functionality. The IT applications portfolio is missing critical elements (for example, order entry, case management, nursing documentation, radiology) that would greatly benefit the ED, even without a dedicated ED system. The hospital's core information system is three versions out of date and certain functions have been bypassed by users altogether.

■ IT infrastructure and architecture. The data center and most IT staff are located twelve miles away from the hospital, isolating IT both physically and culturally from users and patients. Software and networks have been arbitrarily and extensively customized over the years, without documentation, and inadequate hardware capacity has often been given as an excuse for not pursuing an ED system.

■ IT organization and resources. IT spending has been, on average, less than 1 percent of the hospital's budget and IT staff have lacked essential training in critical applications and tools. Newcastle Hospital has been dependent on multiple IT vendors for a variety of implementation and operations support activities.

Discussion Questions

1. Outline the steps you would take to initiate a strategic planning process for improving the ED information system. How will you ensure that this plan is in alignment with the hospital's and department's overall strategic plans?

2. Multiple factors have contributed to the current state of the ED at Newcastle Hospital and are listed in the case. Which of these do you think will be the most difficult to overcome? Why?

3. The new CEO has good insight into the ED issues. Assuming that his assessment of the situation is accurate, discuss how his continued support could affect the outcome of any ED IS strategic plan.

4. Assume the CEO has appointed you to spearhead the ED IS strategic planning effort. What are the first steps you will take? Outline a general plan of action for the next three months. Indicate, by title, whom you would involve in the process. Explain your choices.

CASE 5: PLANNING AN EMR IMPLEMENTATION

Major themes: IT strategy; system implementation

Background Information

The Leonard Williams Medical Center (LWMC) is a 240-bed, community acute care hospital operating in a small urban area in upstate New York. The medical center offers tertiary services and has a captive professional corporation, Williams Medical Services (WMS). WMS is a multispecialty group employing approximately fifty primary care and specialty physicians.

WMS has its own board, made up of representatives of the employed physicians. The WMS board nominations for members and officers are subject to the approval of the medical center board. The capital and operating budgets of WMS are reviewed and approved during the LWMC budget process. The WMS board is responsible for governing the day-to-day operations of the group.

LWMC serves a population of approximately 215,000. There are five other hospitals in the region. One of these, aligned with a large clinic, is viewed as the primary competitor.

In its most recent fiscal year, LWMC had an operating margin of 0.4 percent. LWMC has $40 million in investments and has a long-term debt to equity ratio of 25 percent.

Information Systems Challenge

LWMC has been very effective in its IT efforts. It was the first hospital in its region to have a clinical information system. Bedside computing has been available on the inpatient units since the 1990s. The CIO and IT department are highly regarded. LMWC has received several industry recognitions for its efforts.

The LMWC information systems steering committee recently approved the acquisition and implementation of a CPOE system. This decision followed a thorough analysis of organizational strategies, the efforts of other hospitals, and the vendor offerings. LMWC is poised to begin this major initiative.

During a recent steering committee meeting, it was learned that the WMS physicians were anxious to acquire an electronic medical record (EMR) system.

Two years ago a rival physician group had purchased an EMR system. WMS, concerned about a competitive threat, obtained approval of $300,000 to acquire its own EMR. The rival group has since encountered serious difficulties with implementation and has deinstalled the system. This troubled path caused WMS to slow down its efforts.

Now WMS has decided to return to its plans to implement an EMR. The physicians have begun to look at vendor offerings but have not involved the LWMC CIO and IT staff. The physicians have ignored the CIO's technical and integration advice and requirements during their EMR search.

The CEO is concerned about the EMR process and its disconnect from the medical center's IT plans.

Discussion Questions

1. What is your assessment of this situation? What are the physician group's possible reasons for deciding to proceed on an independent path?

2. If you were the CEO, what steps would you take to bring the hospital and physician group IT plans back into alignment? Should the EMR effort proceed or wait until the CPOE initiative is complete? Should you require that both systems come from the same vendor?

3. The LWMC board is concerned that the physicians are being naive about the challenges of EMR implementation, have established no measurable goals for the system, and have only weak incentives to make the implementation successful. How would you address these concerns?

CASE 6: CONSIDERATIONS FOR VOICE OVER IP TELEPHONY

Major themes: assessing the value of an HIT investment; use of emerging technologies

Background Information

Forest Regional Health Care comprises a 420-bed tertiary hospital, outpatient imaging center, outpatient rehabilitation facility, and seven physician practices with a total of 215 physicians. Forest is the largest employer in its region and has a long history of aggressive investment in new technology. Over the recent years Forest has implemented a digital PACS, a fully integrated operating room system, and an electronic medical record system.

Information Systems Challenge

The telephone system that supports Forest is twenty years old and no longer supported by the vendor. Forest obtains support from a third-party vendor that refurbishes used components from discarded telephone systems.

Forest is examining a replacement telephone system based on Voice over Internet Protocol (VoIP) technologies. VoIP replaces the analog voice signal with a digital voice signal. Potential benefits of this approach are

- The ability to use one network infrastructure for both telephony and data (rather than a separate network for each)
- The ability to implement new applications that require a digital voice signal: for example, interactive call centers and message routing based on the ID of the caller.

The Forest vice president of support services manages the telephone system. He has begun to think through his replacement strategy and plans. He could replace the existing old and unsupported telephone system with old but supported technology, or he could move the organization to the newer VoIP technology.

Discussion Questions

1. Should the vice president's approach put greater stress on the need to replace an obsolete system (risk mitigation) or on the desirability of improving the organization's ability to implement new applications (enable new opportunities)?

2. How should he engage the organization in learning about the potential of VoIP and developing plans for potential uses of the technology?

3. If a result of this learning is a belief that the VoIP technology is not fully mature, how should Forest assess whether it should proceed or not?

CASE 7: IMPLEMENTING A CAPACITY MANAGEMENT INFORMATION SYSTEM

Major theme: system acquisition

Background Information

Doctors' Hospital is 162-bed, acute care facility located in a small city in the southeastern United States. The organization had a major financial upheaval six years ago that resulted in the establishment of a new governing structure. The new governing body consists of an eleven-member authority board. The senior management of Doctors' Hospital includes the chief executive officer (CEO), three senior vice presidents, and one vice president. During the restructuring the chief information officer (CIO) was changed from a full-time staff position to a part-time contract position. The CIO spends two days every two weeks at Doctors' Hospital.

Doctors' Hospital is currently in phase one of a three-phase construction project. In phase two the hospital will build a new emergency department (ED) and surgical pavilion, which are scheduled to be completed in eleven months.

Information Systems Challenge

The current ED and outpatient surgery department have experienced tremendous growth in the past several years. ED visits have increased by 50 percent, and similar increases have been seen in outpatient surgery. Management has identified that inefficient patient flow processes, particularly patient transfers and discharges, have resulted in backlogs in both the ED and outpatient areas. The new construction will only exacerbate the current problem.

Nearly one year ago Doctors' Hospital made a commitment to purchase a capacity management software suite to reduce the inefficiencies that have been identified in patient flow processes. The original timeline was to have the new system pilot-tested prior to the opening of the new ED and surgical pavilion. However, with the competing priorities its members face as they deal with major construction, the original project steering committee has stalled. At its last meeting, nearly six months ago, the steering committee identified the vendor and product suite. Budgets and timelines for implementation were proposed but not finalized. No other steps have been taken.

Discussion Questions

1. Do you think the absence of a full-time CIO has had an impact on this acquisition project? Why or why not?

2. What steps should the CIO take to ensure that the capacity management system will be purchased and implemented? What do you see as the critical first step in this process? Why?

3. Discuss who you think should serve on the project steering committee. Who should serve as chair? Why?

4. At this point, what do you think is a realistic time frame for implementation of the capacity management system? What steps can be taken to ensure the new timeline is met despite competing priorities?

CASE 8: IMPLEMENTING A TELEMEDICINE SOLUTION

Major themes: system acquisition; use of emerging technologies

Background Information

Grand Hospital is located in a somewhat rural area of a midwestern state. It is a 209-bed, community, not-for-profit entity offering a broad range of inpatient and outpatient services. Employing approximately 1,600 individuals (1,250 full-time equivalent personnel), and having a medical staff of more than 225 practitioners, Grand has an annual operating budget that exceeds $130 million, possesses net assets of more than $150 million, and is one of only a small number of organizations in this market with an A credit rating from Moody's, Standard & Poor's, and Fitch Ratings. Operating in a remarkably competitive market (there are roughly 100 hospitals within seventy-five minutes driving time of Grand), the organization is one of the few in the region—proprietary or not-for-profit—that have consistently realized positive operating margins. Grand attends on an annual basis to the health care needs of more than 11,000 inpatients and 160,000 outpatients, addressing more than 36 percent of its primary service area's consumption of hospital services. In expansion mode and currently in the midst of $57 million in construction and renovation projects, the hospital is struggling to recruit physicians, both to meet the health care needs of the expanding population of the service area and to succeed retiring physicians.

Grand has been an early adopter of health care information systems and currently employs a proprietary health care information system that provides (among other components)

- Patient registration and revenue management
- Electronic medical records with computerized physician order entry
- Imaging via a PACS
- Laboratory management
- Pharmacy management

Information Systems Challenge

Since 1995, Grand Hospital has transitioned from being an institution that consistently received many more inquiries than could be accommodated concerning physician practice opportunities, to a hospital at which the average age of the medical staff has increased by eight years. There is a widespread perception among physicians that because of such factors as high malpractice insurance costs, an absence of substantive tort reform, and the comparatively unfavorable rates of reimbursement being paid physician specialists by the region's major health insurer, this region constitutes a "physician unfriendly" venue in which to establish a practice. Consequently, a need exists for Grand to investigate and evaluate creative approaches to enhancing its physician coverage for certain specialty services. These potential approaches include the effective implementation of information technology solutions.

The findings and conclusions of a medical staff development plan, which has been endorsed and accepted by Grand's medical executive committee and board of trustees, have indicated that because of needs and circumstances specific to the institution, the first areas of medical practice on which Grand should focus in approaching this challenge are radiology, behavioral health crisis intervention services, and intensivist physician services. In the area of radiology, Grand needs qualified and appropriately credentialed radiologists available to interpret studies 24 hours per day, 7 days per week. Similarly, it needs qualified and appropriately credentialed psychiatrists available on a 24/7 basis to assess whether behavioral health patients who present in the hospital's emergency room are a danger to themselves or to others, as defined by state statute, and whether these patients should be released or committed against their will for further assessment on an inpatient basis. Finally, inasmuch as Grand is a community hospital that relies on its voluntary medical staff to attend to the needs of patients admitted by staff members such as some ED personnel, it also needs to have intensivist physicians available around the clock to assist in assessing and treating patients during times when members of the voluntary attending staff are not present within or immediately available to the intensive care unit.

The leadership at Grand Hospital is investigating the potential application of telemedicine technologies to address the organization's need for enhanced physician coverage in radiology, behavioral health, and critical care medicine.

Discussion Questions

1.   What are the ways in which Grand's early adoption of other health care information system technologies might affect its adoption of telemedicine solutions?

2.   What do you see as the most likely barriers to the success of telemedicine in the areas of radiology, behavioral health, and intensive care? Which of these areas do you think would be the easiest to transition into telemedicine? Which would be the hardest? Why?

3.   If you were charged by Grand to bring telemedicine to the facility within eighteen months, what are the first steps you would take? Whom would you involve in the planning process? Defend your response.

CASE 9: REPLACING A PRACTICE MANAGEMENT SYSTEM

Major themes: IT governance; system implementation

Background Information

University Physician Group (UPG) is a multispecialty group practice plan associated with the College of Osteopathic Medicine (COM). UPG employs 90 physicians and 340 clinical and business support personnel.

UPG has recently been profitable (with revenue from operations this fiscal year of $32 million and a retained profit of $500,000 from operations). However, prior year losses make UPG a breakeven organization.

Management and the physicians are focusing on strengthening the fiscal position of the organization. This focus has led to plans to restructure physician compensation, establish a self-insurance trust for professional liability, and improve the financial budgeting and reporting processes.

UPG has entered into a preliminary agreement to merge with Northern Affiliated Medical Group (NAMG). NAMG is a 150-physician multispecialty group located in the same city as UPG. NAMG holds a contract with the local county hospital to provide indigent care and serve as the faculty for the graduate medical education programs in family medicine.

Both organizations believe that the merged organization would be able to reduce expenses through the elimination of redundant functions and, because of greater geographical coverage and size, would improve their ability to obtain more favorable payer contracts.

Information Systems Challenge

For many years UPG has obtained practice management systems from Gleason Solutions (GS). The applications are hosted in a GC data center, reducing the UPG's need for IT staff.

Prior to the merger, UPG was in the process of examining replacements for GS. UPG had become displeased because of the GS applications' failure to incorporate new technologies and application features, limited ability to generate reports, and inflexible integration approaches to other applications.

Despite its displeasure, UPG now appears to be on the path to renewing the GS contract. GS executives have effectively lobbied several important physicians and administrators, and UPG's limited cash position makes the GS low-cost financial proposal attractive.

NAMG uses the GS applications and has also been examining replacing the system. NAMG has a strong IT department and will be providing IT support to the newly merged organization. After examining the market, NAMG has identified four potential vendors, including GS.

Discussion Questions

1. Would you suspend both organizations' pursuit of a new system until an IT strategic plan for the merged organization has been developed? Why?

2. What steps would you take to integrate the system selection processes of the two organizations?

3. Implementing a practice management system is always challenging. What additional implementation risks are introduced by the merger?

4. Both organizations expect the result of the merger to be lower costs, improved patient service, and increased market power. What steps would you take to make sure that the new practice management system furthers these objectives?

CASE 10: CONVERSION TO AN EMR MESSAGING SYSTEM

Major themes: system implementation; project management

Background Information

Goodwill Health Care Clinic is the clinical arm of Jefferson Health Sciences Center in a large southern city. The clinic was founded in the early 1950s as a place for faculty physicians to engage in clinical practice. Over the years the clinic has grown to 900 faculty physicians and 2,000 employees, with over one million patient visits per year. Clinic services are spread across eleven primary care and specialty care units. Each unit operates somewhat independently but shares a common medical record numbering system that allows consolidation of all documentation across units. Paper charts were used until two years ago when the clinic adopted an electronic medical record (EMR) system.

Goodwill Health Care Clinic uses a centralized call center to receive all patient calls. Patients call a central switchboard to schedule appointments, request medication refills, or speak to anyone in any of the eleven units. Call center staff are responsible for tracking all calls to ensure that each is dealt with appropriately. Currently the call center uses a customized Lotus Notes system that can be accessed by anyone in the system who needs to process messages. Messages can be tracked and then *closed* when the appropriate action has been taken. Notes created from closed messages are printed and filed in the appropriate patients' paper records. These notes cannot be accessed via the EMR.

Clinic staff are very comfortable with the current Lotus Notes system and it is used routinely by all units.

Information Systems Challenge

Goodwill Health Care Clinic requires all medication lists and refill information to be kept up to date in the EMR. Therefore, the existence of the current Lotus Notes system means that the same information must be documented in two locations—first in the call center note and then in the EMR. This leads to duplication of effort and documentation errors. The potential for serious error is present. Physicians and other health care providers look in the EMR for the most up-to-date medication information.

Although the adoption of the EMR has been fairly successful, not all units use all of the available components of the EMR. A companion paper record is needed for miscellaneous notes, messages, and so forth. All units are recording office visits into the EMR, but not all have activated the lab results or the prescription writing features. Several units have been experiencing physician resistance to adding more EMR functions.

The EMR system has a messaging component that works like a closed e-mail system. Messages can be sent, received, and stored by EMR authenticated users. Pertinent patient care messages are automatically stored in the correct patient record. In addition, the EMR messaging system works seamlessly with the prescription writing module, which includes patient safety checks such as allergy checks and drug interactions.

The challenge for Goodwill Health Care Clinic is to implement the messaging feature and prescription writing component (where it is not currently being used) of their current EMR in the call center and the clinical units, replacing the existing Lotus Notes system and improving the quality of the documentation, not only of medication refills but of all patient-related calls.

Discussion Questions

1. Outline the steps that you would take to ensure a successful conversion from the existing call center system to the new EMR compatible system. Defend your response.

2. Who should be involved in the conversion planning and implementation? Discuss the roles of the people on your list and your reasons for selecting them.

3. What are some strategies that you would employ to minimize physicians' and other users' resistance to the conversion?

4. Do you think that making sure all units are running the same EMR functions is a necessary precursor to the conversion to the messaging and prescription writing components? What information would be helpful in making this determination?

CASE 11: CONCERNS AND WORKAROUNDS WITH A CLINICAL DOCUMENTATION SYSTEM

Major themes: system implementation; project management

Background Information

Garrison Children's Hospital is a 225-bed hospital. Its 77-bed neonatal intensive care unit (NICU) provides care to the most fragile patients, premature and critically ill neonates. The 28-bed pediatric intensive care unit (PICU) cares for critically ill children from birth to eighteen years of age. Patients in this unit include those with life-threatening conditions that are acquired (trauma, child abuse, burns, surgical complications, and so forth) or congenital (congenital heart defects, craniofacial malformations, genetic disorders, inborn errors of metabolism, and so forth).

Garrison is part of Premier Health Care, an academic medical center complex located in the Southeast. Premier Health Care also includes an adult hospital, a psychiatric hospital, and a full spectrum of adult and pediatric outpatient clinics. Within the past six months or so, Premier has implemented an electronic clinical documentation system in its adult hospital. More recently the same clinical documentation system has been implemented at Garrison in both pediatric medical and surgery units and intensive care units. Electronic scheduling is to be implemented next.

The adult hospital drives the decisions for the pediatric hospital, a circumstance that led to the adult hospital's CPOE vendor being chosen as the documentation vendor for both hospitals. A CPOE system was implemented at Garrison Children's Hospital several years prior to implementation of the electronic clinical documentation system, which began in 2007.

Information Systems Challenge

A pressing challenge facing Garrison Children's Hospital is that nurses are very concerned and dissatisfied with the new clinical documentation system. They have voiced concerns formally to several nurse managers, and one nurse went directly to the chief nursing officer (CNO) stating that the "flow sheets" on the new system are grossly inadequate and she fears using them could lead to patient safety issues. Lunchroom conversations among nurses tend to center on their having no clear understanding of why the organization is automating clinical documentation or what it hopes to achieve. Nurses in the NICU and PICU seem to be most vocal about their concerns. They claim there is inconsistency in what is being documented and lack of standardization of content. The computer workstations are located outside the patients' rooms, so nurses generally document their notes on paper and then enter the data at the end of the shift or when they have time.

The system support team, consisting of nurses as well as technology specialists, began the workflow analysis, system installation, staff training, and go-live first with a small number of units in both the adult hospital and the children's hospital, beginning in January 2007. The NICU and PICU did not implement the system until May and June 2007. System support personnel moved rapidly through each unit, working to train and to manage questions. The timeline for each unit implementation was based on the number of beds in the unit and the number of staff to be trained. No consideration was given to staff members' prior experience with computers and keyboarding skills or to complexity of documentation and existing work processes.

Although there are similarities between the adult and pediatric settings, there are also many differences in terms of unit design, computer resources (hardware), level of computer literacy, information documented, and work processes, not to mention patient populations. Little time was spent evaluating or planning for these differences and completing a thorough workflow analysis. After the initial units went live less and less time was spent on training and addressing unit-specific needs, due to the demands placed upon training staff to stay on the timeline in preparation for the next system implementation involving electronic scheduling.

The clinical documentation system was implemented to the great consternation and dissatisfaction of the end users (physicians, nurses, social workers, and so forth) at Garrison, yet the Premier clinicians are happy with it. Many Garrison physicians and nurses initially refused to use the system, stating it was "unsafe," "added to workload," and was not intuitive. A decision to stop using the system and return to the paper documentation process was not then and is not now an option. Physician "champions" were encouraged to work with those who were recalcitrant and nursing staff were encouraged to "stick it out," in hopes that system use would "get easier."

As a result, with their concerns and complaints essentially forced underground, Garrison clinical staff developed *workarounds*, morale was negatively affected, and the expectation that everyone would eventually "get it" and adapt has not become a reality. Instead, staff are writing on a self-created paper system and then translating those notes to the computer system; physicians are unable to retrieve important, timely patient information; and the time team members spend trying to retrieve pertinent patient information has increased. There have been clear instances where patient safety has been affected due to the problems with the appropriate use of this system.

Discussion Questions

1. What is the major problem in this case? What factors seem to have contributed to the current situation?

2. The nurses at Garrison argue that pediatric hospitals and intensive care units, in particular, are different from adult hospitals and that these differences should be clearly addressed in the implementation of a new clinical documentation system. Do you agree with this argument? Why or why not? Give examples from the literature to support your views.

3. How might the workflow issues and concerns mentioned in this case been detected earlier?

4. Assume you part of the leadership team at Garrison. How would you assess the current situation? What would you do first? Next? Explain what steps you would take and why you feel your approach is necessary.

5. What lessons can be learned from this case and applied to other settings?

CASE 12: STRATEGIES FOR IMPLEMENTING CPOE

Major themes: system implementation; project management

Background

Health Matters is a newly formed nonprofit health system comprising two community hospitals (Cooper Memorial Hospital and Ashley Valley Hospital), nine ambulatory care clinics, and three imaging centers. Since its inception two years ago, the information services department has merged and consolidated all computer systems under one umbrella. Each of the facilities within the health system is connected electronically with the others through a fiber optic network. The organizational structure of the two hospitals is such that each has its own executive leadership team and board.

Seven years ago, the leadership team at Cooper Memorial Hospital made the strategic decision to choose Meditech as the vendor of choice for its clinical and financial applications. The philosophy of the leadership team was to solicit a single vendor solution so that the hospital could minimize the number of disparate systems and interfaces. Since then, Meditech has been deployed throughout the health system and applications have been kept current with the latest releases. Most nursing and clinical ancillary documentation is electronic, as is the medication administration record. Health Matters does have several ancillary systems that interface with Meditech; these include a picture archiving and communication system (PACS), a fully automated laboratory system, an emergency department tracking board, and an electronic bed board system. The leadership team at Ashley Valley Hospital chose to select non-Meditech products, because at the time Meditech did not offer these applications or its products were considered inadequate by clinicians. However, the current sentiment among the leadership team is to continue to go with one predominant vendor, in this case, Meditech, for any upgrades, new functionality, or new products.

The information system (IS) group at Health Matters consists of a director of information systems (who reports to the chief financial officer) and fifteen staff members. The IS staff are highly skilled in networking and computer operations but have only moderate skill as program analysts and project managers. The CEO, Steve Forthright, plans to hire a chief information officer (CIO) to provide senior-level leadership in developing and implementing a strategic IS plan that is congruent with strategic goals of Health Matters.

Currently, the senior leadership team at Health Matters has identified the following as the organization's top three IS challenges. The current director of information systems has been somewhat involved in discussions related to the establishment of these priorities.

- To implement successfully computerized provider order entry (CPOE)
- To increase the variety and availability of computing devices (workstations or hand-held devices) at each nursing station
- To implement successfully medication administration using bar-coding technology

Information Systems Challenge

The most pressing IS challenge is to move forward with the implementation of CPOE. The decision has already been made to implement the Meditech CPOE application. Several internal and external driving forces are at play. Internally, the physician leaders believe that CPOE will further reduce medication errors and promote patient safety. The board has established patient safety as a strategic goal for the organization. Externally, groups such as Leapfrog and the Pacific Business Group on Health have strongly encouraged CPOE implementation. The CEO Steve Forthright has concerns, however, because Health Matters does not yet have a CIO on board and he feels the CIO should play a pivotal role. Much of Steve's concern stems from his experience with CPOE implementation at another institution, with a different vendor and product. Steve had organized a project implementation committee, established an appropriate governance structure, and the senior leadership team thought it had "covered the bases." However, according to Steve, "The surgeons embraced the new CPOE system, largely because they felt the postoperative order sets were easy to use, but the internists and hospitalists rebelled. The CPOE project stalled and the system was never fully implemented." Steve is not the only person reeling from a failed implementation. The clinical information committee at Health Matters is chaired by Mary White who was involved in a failed CPOE rollout at another hospital in 2003. She was a strong supporter of the system at the time, but now speaks of the risks and challenges associated with getting physician buy-in and support throughout the health system.

Members of the medical staff at Cooper Memorial Hospital have access to laboratory and radiology results electronically. They have access through workstations in the hospital; most physicians also access clinical results remotely through personal digital assistants (PDAs). An estimated 35 percent of the physicians take full advantage of the system's capabilities. Almost all active physicians use the PACS to view images, and most use a computer to look up lab values. Fewer than half of the physicians use electronic signatures to sign transcribed reports.

Discussion Questions

1. Assume you are part of a team charged with leading the implementation of CPOE within Health Matters. How would you approach the task? What would you do first? Next? Who should be involved in the team? Lead the team?

2. The CIO hasn't been hired yet. Do you see that as a problem? Why or why not? What role, if any, might the CIO have in the CPOE implementation project?

3. To what extent does that fact that Health Matters is a relatively new health system simplify or complicate the CPOE implementation project? How do other health systems typically implement CPOE or other clinical information system projects of this magnitude?

4. How might you solicit the wisdom and expertise of others who may have undergone CPOE projects like this one? Or who have used Meditech's CPOE application? How might Steve Forthright and Mary White's prior experiences with partially and fully failed implementations affect their views in this case?

5. Develop a high-level implementation plan of key tasks and activities that will need to be done. How will you estimate the time frame? The resources needed? What role does the vendor have in establishing this plan?

CASE STUDY 13: IMPLEMENTING A SYNDROMIC SURVEILLANCE SYSTEM

Major themes: IT strategy; system implementation

Background Information

Syndromic surveillance systems collect and analyze prediagnostic and nonclinical disease indicators, drawing on preexisting electronic data that can be found in systems such as electronic health records, school absenteeism records, and pharmacy systems.

These surveillance systems are intended to identify specific symptoms within a population that may indicate a public health event or emergency. For example, the data being collected by a surveillance system might reveal a sharp increase in diarrhea in a community and that could signal an outbreak of an infectious disease.

The infectious disease epidemiology section of a state's public health agency has been given the task of implementing the Early Aberration Reporting System of the Centers for Disease Control and Prevention. The agency views this system as significantly improving its ability to monitor and respond to potential problematic bioterrorism, food poisoning, and infectious disease outbreaks.

The implementation of the system is also seen as a vehicle for improving collaboration between the agency, health care providers, information technology vendors, researchers, and the business community.

Information Systems Challenge

The agency and its infectious disease epidemiology section face several major challenges.

First, the necessary data must be collected largely from hospitals and in particular emergency rooms. Developing and supporting necessary interfaces to the applications in a large number of hospitals is very challenging. These hospitals have different application vendors, diverse data standards, and uneven willingness to divert IT staff and budget to the implementation of these interfaces.

To help address this challenge, the section will acquire a commercial package or build the needed software to ease the integration challenge. In addition, the section will provide each hospital with information it can use to assess its own mix of patients and their presenting problems.

The agency is also contemplating the development of regulations that would require the hospitals to report the necessary data.

Second, the system must be designed so that patient privacy is protected and the system is secure.

Third, the implementation and support of the system will be funded initially through federal grants. The agency will need to develop strategies for ensuring the financial sustainability of the application and related analysis capabilities should federal funding end.

Fourth, the agency needs to ensure that the section has the staff and tools necessary to appropriately analyze the data. Distinguishing true problems from the "noise" of a normal increase in colds during the winter, for example, can be very difficult. The agency could damage the public's confidence in the system if it overreacts or underreacts to the data it collects.

Discussion Questions

1. If you were the head of the agency's epidemiology section how would you address the four challenges described here?

2. Which of the challenges is the most important to address? Why?

3. If you were a hospital CEO being asked to redirect IT resources for this project, what would you want in return from the agency to ensure that this system provided value to your organization and clinicians?

4. A strong privacy advocacy group has expressed alarm about the potential problems that the system could create. How would you respond to those concerns?

CASE STUDY 14: THE ADMITTING SYSTEM CRASHES

Major theme: disaster recovery

Background Information

Jones Regional Medical Center is a large academic health center. With 900 beds, Jones had 47,000 admissions in 2007. Jones frequently has occupancy in excess of 100 percent; requiring diversion of ambulances. In addition, Jones had 1,300,000 ambulatory and emergency room visits in 2007.

Jones is internationally renowned for its research and teaching programs.

The IT staff at Jones are highly regarded. They support over 300 applications and 12,000 workstations.

The admitting system at Jones is provided by the vendor Technology Med (TechMed). The TechMed system supports master patient index; registration; inpatient charge and payment entry; medical records abstracting and coding; hospital billing and patient accounting; reporting; and admission, discharge and transfer capabilities.

The TechMed system was implemented in 1995 and uses now obsolete technology, including a rudimentary database management system. The organization is concerned about the fragility of the application and has begun plans to replace the TechMed system two years from now.

Information Systems Challenge

On December 20, the link between the main data center (where the TechMed servers were housed) and the disaster recovery center was taken down to conduct performance testing.

On December 21, power was lost to the disaster recovery center but emergency power was instantly put in place. However, as a precaution, a backup of the TechMed database was performed.

During the afternoon of December 21, the TechMed system became sluggish and then unresponsive. Database corruption was discovered. The backup performed earlier in the day was also corrupt. The link to the disaster recovery data center had not been restored following the performance testing.

Because there was no viable backup copy of the database, the Jones IT and hospital staff began the arduous process of a full database recovery from journaled transactions. This process was completed the evening of December 22.

The loss of the TechMed system for over thirty-six hours and the failure during that time of registration transactions to update patient care and ancillary department systems resulted in a wide variety of operational problems. The patient census had to be maintained manually. Reports of results were delayed. Paper orders were needed for patient who were admitted on December 21 and 22. Charge collection lagged.

Once the TechMed system was restored, additional hospital staff were brought in to enter, into multiple systems, the data that had been manually captured during the outage. By December 25, normal hospital operations were restored. No patient care incidents are believed to have resulted.

Discussion Questions

1. If you were the CIO of Jones Regional Medical Center during this system failure, what steps would you take during the outage? What steps would you take after the outage to reduce the likelihood of a reoccurrence of this problem?

2. The root cause analysis of the outage showed that process, technology, and staffing factors all contributed to the problem. What are some of the likely factors? Which of these factors do you believe are likely to have been the most important?

3. If you were a member of the audit committee of the Jones board of trustees, what questions would you ask the CIO?

4. What issues and problems should a disaster recovery plan prepare for? How does an organization determine how much to spend to reduce the occurrence and severity of such episodes?

CASE STUDY 15: BREACHING THE SECURITY OF AN INTERNET PATIENT PORTAL

Major theme: IT security

Information for this case was taken from J. C. Collmann and T. Cooper, "Breaching the Security of the Kaiser Permanente Internet Patient Portal: The Organizational Foundations of Information Security," *Journal of the American Medical Informatics Association*, 2007, *14*(2), 239–243.

Background Information

Kaiser Permanente is an integrated health delivery system that serves over eight million members in nine states and the District of Columbia. In the late 1990s Kaiser Permanente introduced an Internet Patient Portal, Kaiser Permanente Online (also known as KP Online.) Members can use KP Online to request appointments, request prescription refills, obtain health care service information, seek clinical advice, and participate in patient forums.

Information Systems Challenge

In August 2000, there was a serious breach in the security of the KP Online pharmacy refill application. Programmers wrote a flawed script that actually concatenated over

800 individual e-mail messages containing individually identifiable patient information, instead of separating them as intended. As a result, nineteen members received e-mail messages with private information about multiple other members. Kaiser became aware of the problem when two members notified the organization that they had received the concatenated e-mail messages. Kaiser leadership considered this incident a significant breach of confidentiality and security. The organization immediately took steps to investigate and to offer apologies to those affected.

On the same day the first member notified Kaiser about receiving the problem e-mail, a crisis team was formed. The crisis team began a root cause analysis and a *mitigation assessment* process. Three days later Kaiser began notifying its members and issued a press release.

The investigation of the cause of the breach uncovered issues at the technical, individual, group, and organizational levels. At the technical level, Kaiser was using new Web-based tools, applications, and processes. The pharmacy module had been evaluated in a test environment that was not equivalent to the production environment. At the individual level, two programmers, one from the e-mail group and one from the development group, working together for the first time in a new environment and working under intense pressure to quickly fix a serious problem, failed to adequately test code they produced as a patch for the pharmacy application. Three groups within Kaiser had responsibilities for KP Online, operations, e-mail and development. Traditionally these groups worked independently and had distinct missions and organizational cultures. The breach revealed the differences in the way groups approached priorities. For example, the development group often let meeting deadlines dictate priorities. At the organizational level, Kaiser IT had a very complex organizational structure leading to what Collmann and Cooper 2007 call "compartmentalized sensemaking." Each IT group "developed highly localized definitions of a situation, which created the possibility for failure when integrated in a common infrastructure."

Discussion Questions

1. How serious was this e-mail security breach? Why did the Kaiser Permanente leadership react so quickly to mitigate the possible damage done by the breach?

2. Assume that you were appointed as the administrative member of the crisis team created the day the breach was uncovered. After the initial apologies, what recommendations would you make for investigating the root cause(s) of the breach? Outline your suggested investigative steps.

3. How likely do you think future security breaches would be if Kaiser Permanente did not take steps to resolve underlying group and organizational issues? Why?

4. What role should the administrative leadership of Kaiser Permanente take in ensuring that KP Online is secure? Apart from security and HIPAA training for all personnel, what steps can be taken at the organizational level to improve the security of KP Online?

CASE STUDY 16: ASSESSING THE VALUE AND IMPACT OF CPOE

Major theme: assessing the value of an HIT investment

Background Information

The University Health Care System is an academic medical center with over 1,200 licensed beds and over 9,000 employees. The system comprises the University Hospital, Winston Geriatric Hospital, Jefferson Rehabilitation Hospital, and two outpatient centers in the metropolitan area. The system has a history of being a patriarchal, physician-driven organization. When University Health Care first started taking patients, it was viewed as a Mecca to which community physicians throughout the South referred difficult-to-treat patients. That referral mentality persisted for decades, so physicians within the system had had a difficult time making the transition to an organization that had to compete for patients with other health care entities in the region.

In recent years, University Health Care System has evolved and given physicians proportionately more clout in decision making, in part because the health care leadership team has not stepped forward. Creating a balance between clinician providers and administrative leadership is a real issue. In the midst of the difficulty, both groups have agreed to embark on the electronic medical record (EMR) journey. Currently about 55 percent of the system's patient record is electronic; the remainder is on paper. The physicians as a whole, however, have embraced technology and view the EMR as the "right road" to take in achieving the organization's goal of providing high quality, safe, cost-effective patient care.

Information Systems Challenge

Currently, the University Health Care System is in the midst of rolling out the CPOE portion of the EMR project. The multidisciplinary decision-making project was established before beginning the initiative, and leaders and clinicians tried to educate themselves on what the CPOE project would entail. They were familiar with cases such as one at Cedars-Sinai where CPOE was halted after a physician uproar over the time it took to use and patient safety concerns. To help ensure this did not happen at the University Health Care System, the leadership team decided to take a slower, phased-in approach. Team members visited similar organizations that had implemented CPOE, attended vendor user-group conferences, consulted with colleagues from across the nation, and articulated the following project goals:

- Optimize patient safety
- Improve quality outcomes and reduce variation in practice through the use of evidence-based practice guidelines
- Reduce risk for errors
- Accommodate regulatory standards expectations

- Enhance patient satisfaction
- Standardize processes
- Improve efficiency

The board has made it very clear that it wants regular updates on the progress of the project and expects to see what the return on the investment has been.

Discussion Questions

1. How might you evaluate the CPOE implementation process at University Health Care System? Give examples of different methods or strategies you might employ.

2. How would you respond to the board's desire for a "return on investment" from this initiative? Is it a reasonable request? Why or why not?

3. Assume you are to lead the evaluation component of this project. You have reviewed the goals for the project. What *process* would you use to develop a plan for assessing the value of CPOE? Who would be involved? What roles would they play? How would you decide on what metrics to use? What baseline data would you want to collect or review?

APPENDIX

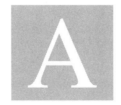

OVERVIEW OF THE HEALTH CARE IT INDUSTRY

There is a health care information technology (IT) industry. This industry is composed of companies that provide hardware, software, and a wide range of services, including consulting and outsourcing, to health care organizations. The industry also includes associations that support the professional advancement of the health care IT professional, organizations that put on industry conferences and publications that cover current topics and issues in the industry.

It is not possible to develop an IT strategy and implement that strategy without engaging this industry.

This appendix provides an overview of this industry. It will discuss

- The size, structure, and composition of the health care IT industry, and characteristics of health care that affect the application of IT products and services
- Sources of information about that industry
- Health care IT associations

THE HEALTH CARE IT INDUSTRY

Health care is the largest sector of the U.S. economy ($2.1 trillion in 2006). It is not surprising that a large, diverse, and robust industry has developed to provide IT products and services to that sector. The health care IT industry is generally viewed as having three major markets; health care providers, health care insurance companies, and health care suppliers: for example, pharmaceutical companies, medical supply distribution companies, and health care device manufacturers. Some industry analyses cover the global health care IT market, and others focus on the market in the United States. We will focus on the health care provider market in the United States.

Size of the Industry

In 2007, health care providers spent $26 billion on IT hardware, software, and services (Gartner, 2008). This spending is expected to increase at a 5 percent compounded annual growth rate for the next several years. Health care was the fastest growing IT market worldwide in 2007. In general, growth in IT spending among health care providers is attributed to providers' pursuing IT "answers" to a range of challenges and issues facing them:

- Concerns over patient safety can lead to investments in CPOE and medication administration record systems.

- Cost pressures can lead to the use of IT to improve organizational efficiency.

- Problems with shortages of health care professionals and cost pressures can result in efforts to use IT to improve operational efficiency and reduce staff workloads.

- Compliance with new health care regulations, such as rules designed to improve the security of information systems or reduce fraudulent billing, often requires an IT response.

- Desires to improve patient service can lead to new systems designed to improve the process of obtaining an appointment or to reduce test result turnaround time.

Such answers are identified during the IT strategy and alignment process that was discussed in Chapter Twelve.

The typical health care provider's IT spending is proportioned across the categories listed in Table A.1.

IT Spending Relative to Other Industries

Health care organizations will spend, on average, about 2.7 percent of their revenues on IT. This spending includes the cost of internal IT staff and the cost of purchasing products and services from the market. Other industries spend more: for example, banks will spend 5.1 percent of their revenues on IT (Gartner, 2008).

TABLE A.1. **Typical Provider Distribution of IT Spending**

Expenditure Category	Percentage of IT Spending
Hardware	10
Internal services	22
Software	7
Telecommunications[a]	28
IT services[b]	33

[a]Networks, Internet connections, and telephone costs.
[b]Implementation, consulting, and product maintenance services.
Source: Gartner, 2007.

Why does health care have this apparently lower level of IT spending than other information-intensive industries? To some degree the percentages reflect the cost structure of health care. Being a health care provider is a very labor- and capital-intensive business. Provider organizations must have a large number of relatively expensive staff such as physicians, nurses, and other health care professionals. Few other industries have this density of expensive workers. Health care providers, particularly hospitals, must invest large sums of money in buildings, supplies, and equipment. Manufacturers are also capital intensive; they must invest in plants and manufacturing equipment. However, most service organizations—for example, law firms, consulting organizations, and financial institutions—do not have the same levels of demand for buildings and equipment.

Hence the relatively low percentages result from the need to make significant investments and bear significant ongoing costs in other aspects of the organization. The salaries of health care professionals and the costs of buildings, supplies, and equipment overshadow health care IT costs.

Other factors also play a role in producing relatively low levels of health care investment in IT:

- For many years health care organizations viewed IT as important for supporting day-to-day operations but not important strategically. An organization might believe that it was strategically more important to establish a new imaging center than it was to invest in an electronic medical record system. To a degree this orientation is changing as health care organizations realize that they cannot accomplish care improvement (and many other) goals without substantial IT investments. However, it can also be argued that IT is indeed less important in health care than in other industries. If a bank's computer systems stop working, the bank immediately stops working. No checks can be cashed. Taking deposits becomes difficult. In contrast, if a hospital's systems stop working, surgery can go on, medications can be given, and phlebotomists can draw blood.

- Health care organizations have fewer ways than other types of organizations do to obtain capital. Publicly traded organizations can issue stock. Health care organizations often have small operating margins that make it difficult for them to obtain debt from the bond market. This often-limited ability to obtain capital hinders these organizations' ability to make large IT investments.

- Many health care organizations are very small, having revenues of less than $100 million. Small organizations face a very difficult time hiring and retaining talented IT staff. This problem can make an organization hesitant to pursue IT investments because it is not sure that it can support the systems.

- IT investments often have their most significant impact when the operations that they are to support are complex and have large volumes of activity. For a small health care organization, the volume and complexity of activity may be sufficiently limited that an IT investment would not result in enough gain to justify that investment.

Structure of the Health Care Market

Table A.2 displays the taxonomy of the health care industry as defined by the North American Industry Classification System (NAICS). The NAICS outlines three major industry segments: payers, providers, and government health care. Each of the sectors in this classification (with each sector having a different NAICS code) represents a different submarket in health care. Some IT companies focus on the federal health care system, others on nursing homes, and yet others on physician offices. Some focus even more narrowly. Within the hospital sector (NAICS code 6222), for example, some IT companies focus on large academic medical centers and others focus on small community hospitals.

The health care IT market is not homogeneous. Different companies serve different segments. Some companies serve multiple segments by carrying diverse product lines or offering systems that will work in multiple sectors: for example, a clinical

TABLE A.2. Health Care Vertical Market: NAICS Taxonomy

Health care providers	Ambulatory services	Physician offices Dentist offices Other health Outpatient centers Laboratories Home health
	Hospitals	General medical and surgical Psychiatric and substance abuse Specialty hospitals
	Nursing and residential care	Nursing care Mental care Elderly care
Insurance	Health	Accident and health insurance Hospital and medical Service plans
Government health		Federal hospitals Local hospitals Government psychiatric and long-term care

Source: Gartner 2008.

laboratory system is of interest to civilian and federal hospitals, large physician groups, and freestanding clinical laboratories.

A rough taxonomy of companies that serve health care can be constructed:

- Some companies strive to have a product and service line that covers the full spectrum of health care settings. Hence these companies will offer hospital information systems, physician office systems, nursing home applications, and applications for ancillary departments, such as radiology.

- Several companies focus on a specific setting: for example, hospitals or the physician's office, but not both.

- Some companies offer products that support an application needed by multiple sectors: for example, pharmacy systems or systems that support claims electronic data interchange between providers and payers.

- Some companies offer infrastructure: for example, workstations, networks, and servers that are used by all sectors. These companies usually do not offer applications.

- Several companies offer services used by multiple sectors: for example, IT strategic planning, application implementation, and consulting services.

- Some companies focus their service offerings on a specific type of organization—for example, improving the operations of physician practices—or a specific type of service—for example, improving collections of overdue payments for a provider billing office.

There are literally thousands of companies that support the IT needs of the health care industry. In any given year, hundreds of companies may go out of business and hundreds of new companies may emerge. You can gain an appreciation of the diversity of health care IT companies by attending a large health care IT conference, such as the annual conference of the Healthcare Information and Management Systems Society (HIMSS), and visiting the exhibit hall.

Later in this appendix, we will present sources of IT information. These sources often discuss the products and services of health care IT companies.

Major Suppliers of Health Care IT Products and Services

Table A.3 provides a summary of the top vendors in the industry. These data, collected by the publication *Healthcare Informatics* (2008), rank companies according to their health information technology (HIT) revenue. Use such lists with caution of course. In any given year, some companies will be acquired, and others will experience dramatic upturns and downturns in financial performance. Companies will disappear from the list, and companies will arrive on the list over the course of time. The products and services listed in Table A.3 are illustrative but do not make up a comprehensive list. Moreover, the fact that a company is large does not mean that it has the best solution for a particular need of a particular organization.

TABLE A.3. **Major Health Care IT Vendors: Ranked by Revenue**

Company	HIT Revenue	Types of Products and Services
McKesson	$1.9B	Applications, consulting services
Cerner	$1.5B	Applications
Siemens	$1.5B	Applications, imaging
CSC	$1.3B	System integration, outsourcing
Perot Systems	$1.3B	Consulting, process improvement
Ingenix	$1.3B	Care analyses
GE	$1.0B	Applications, imaging
Emdeon	$800M	Revenue cycle and clinical applications
Agfa	$650M	Imaging
Misys	$570M	Applications

Source: Company and revenue data from *Healthcare Informatics*, 2008.

Nonetheless, the data in Table A.3 are interesting for several reasons:

- Health care leadership should know the names and have a reasonable understanding of the major IT vendors that serve their type of organization; sooner or later the organization will be doing business with some of these vendors.

- The size of some of these companies is apparent, with several companies taking in over $1 billion in revenue.

- The diversity of products and services is also apparent. Some companies focus on applications, whereas others focus on consulting, outsourcing, data analysis, or transcription services.

When an organization needs to turn to the market for applications, infrastructure, or services, its leadership would be well served by reviewing several of the sources of information described in this appendix, talking to colleagues who may have recently pursued similar IT products and services, and engaging the services of consultants who keep close tabs on the health care IT industry.

SOURCES OF INDUSTRY INFORMATION

It is essential for the health care professional to identify sources that he or she can trust for current information on health care IT. This textbook cannot examine all the terrain covered by this industry. Moreover, the face of the industry can change quickly. New companies arrive as others disappear. New technologies emerge, and people's understanding of current technologies improves. Federal legislation that affects what health care IT is expected to do can surface rapidly.

These sources of information should be diverse: colleagues, consultants, vendors, conferences, and trade press. It takes time and some effort to identify your best sources. You will find some consultants helpful and others not so helpful. You will note that some publications are insightful and others are not.

The following sections provide a brief overview of publications you may find useful.

Periodicals

Among the high-quality health care information technology periodicals (journals and magazines) are

- *ADVANCE for Health Information Executives*
- *Health Data Management*
- *Health Management Technology*
- *Healthcare Informatics*
- *Healthcare IT News*

All the associations discussed later in this appendix also publish journals, magazines, or newsletters.

These publications can be supplemented with periodicals that cover the overall IT industry. They include

- *CIO*
- *Computerworld*
- *Information Week*
- *CIO Insight*

Several periodicals focus on vertical segments of technology; *Database Management, Network World*, and *eWeek* are examples.

Several periodicals address cross-industry management issues, including IT. These publications include

- *BusinessWeek*
- *The Economist*
- *The Harvard Business Review*
- *MIS Quarterly*
- *MIT Sloan Management Review*

In addition, there are magazines and journals that cover health care broadly. They often publish articles and stories on IT issues:

- *Health Affairs*
- *Hospitals & Health Networks*
- *Modern Healthcare*

You can obtain subscription information for these publications by visiting their Web sites. A visit to a university library, medical library, or large public library and an afternoon spent perusing these publications would be worthwhile.

Books

In any given year, several books that cover various aspects of health care IT are published. Publishers that routinely produce such books and publish conference proceedings include

- Elsevier
- Healthcare Information and Management Systems Society
- Jossey-Bass
- Springer-Verlag
- John Wiley & Sons

Industry Research Firms

Finally, there are industry research firms that routinely cover IT generally and health care specifically. Such firms include Forrester, Gartner, and HIMSS Analytics. These firms, and others, do a nice job of analyzing industry trends, critiquing the products and services of major vendors, and assessing emerging technologies and technology issues. They provide written analyses, conferences, and access to their analysts.

HEALTH CARE IT ASSOCIATIONS

All health care professionals should join associations that are dedicated to advancing and educating their profession. Health care chief financial officers (CFOs) often join the Healthcare Financial Management Association, and health care executives routinely join the American College of Healthcare Executives.

These associations serve several useful purposes for the person who joins. They provide

- Publications on topics of interest to the profession
- Conferences, symposiums, and other educational programs
- Information on career opportunities and career development opportunities
- Data that can be used to compare performance across organizations
- Opportunities to meet colleagues who share similar jobs and hence have similar challenges and interests
- Staff who work with legislators and regulators on issues that affect the profession

These association products and services can be invaluable sources of information and experience for any organization or individual.

The health care IT industry has several associations that serve the needs of the health care IT professional. People who are not health care IT professionals will find that their own profession's association also routinely provides periodical articles and conference sessions that cover IT issues. For example, the Healthcare Financial Management Association may present conference sessions on IT advances in analyzing the costs of care or in streamlining patient accounting and billing processes.

The health care IT industry associations are discussed in the following sections. Additional information on these associations can be obtained through each association's Web site.

American Health Information Management Association (AHIMA)

AHIMA is an association of health information management professionals. AHIMA serves largely what has historically been known as the medical records professional. AHIMA's members confront a diverse range of issues associated with both the paper and the electronic medical record, including privacy, data standards and coding, management of the record, appropriate uses of medical record information, and state and federal regulations that govern the medical record.

AHIMA sponsors an annual conference, produces publications, makes a series of knowledge resources available (news, practice guidelines, and competency tests), posts job opportunities, supports distance learning opportunities, and engages in federal and state policy lobbying. AHIMA also offers local and state chapters, which have their own conferences and resources.

The medical records profession has a process for certifying the skill levels of its professionals. AHIMA manages that certification process.

American Medical Informatics Association (AMIA)

AMIA is an association of individuals and organizations "dedicated to developing and using information technologies to improve health care." AMIA focuses on clinical information systems, and a large portion of its membership has an interest and training in the academic discipline of medical informatics. AMIA brings together an interesting mixture of practitioners and academics.

AMIA offers an annual symposium, a spring congress, a journal, a series of working groups and special interest groups, and a resource center with job opportunities, publications, and news. AMIA carries out initiatives designed to influence federal policy on health care IT issues.

College of Healthcare Information Management Executives (CHIME)

CHIME is an association dedicated to advancing the health care chief information officer (CIO) profession and improving the strategic use of IT in health care (CIOs were discussed in Chapter Thirteen). CHIME provides two annual forums, a newsletter, employment information, a data warehouse of information contributed by its members and vendors, distance learning sessions, and classroom-style training. CHIME is partially supported by the CHIME Foundation, established as a nonprofit organization by a group of vendors and consultants committed to advancing the CIO profession.

Healthcare Information and Management Systems Society (HIMSS)

HIMSS is an association dedicated to "providing leadership for the optimal use of health care information technology and management systems for the betterment of human health." HIMSS members are diverse, covering all segments and professions in the health care IT industry.

HIMSS sponsors an annual conference and series of symposiums and smaller conferences. It publishes books, a journal, and newsletters. HIMSS member services include employment information, industry and vendor information, certification programs, distance learning, and white papers. The association has special interest groups and local chapters, and it is actively working with the federal government to develop policy.

Other Industry Groups and Associations

Within the health care IT industry, organizations also exist that serve the needs of health care organizations (in contrast to the individual professional). This section will not attempt to list and describe them. However, examples include the University HealthSystem Consortium, which serves academic health centers; Voluntary Hospitals of America, which provides services to hospitals; and the Scottsdale Institute, whose members are large integrated delivery systems. These and other similar organizations have a partial or dedicated focus on health care IT.

All the associations and groups mentioned in this discussion provide publications and conferences. In addition, companies whose business is putting on conferences sometimes offer health care IT events. Quality publications in addition to those listed previously are available. The reader who is interested in developing a deeper appreciation of the wealth of conference and publication opportunities can type "healthcare IT publications" and "healthcare IT conferences" into a Web search engine to locate many online sources of information.

SUMMARY

The health care IT industry is large and growing. The many pressures on health care organizations to perform and comply are leading them to invest in IT. The industry is served by a multitude of companies that provide products and services. These companies are diverse, both in revenue and in their choice of focus within the submarkets that compose the health care industry.

Professionals in the health care IT industry have formed associations that serve their information and development needs. These associations and industry publications are terrific sources of information on industry issues, emerging technologies, and the strengths and weaknesses of companies serving the industry. The industry faces a core challenge in its application of IT to improve health care; the complexities of care processes, medical data, and health care are often proving to have no boundaries.

LEARNING ACTIVITIES

1. Identify two companies that serve the health care IT market. Write a summary that lists each company's products, services, market focus, and size. Compare the two companies.

2. Pick one of the health care IT associations listed in this appendix. Develop a summary that describes the association's membership, activities, products, and services.

3. Select two periodicals that serve the health care IT industry and review an issue of each one. Comment on the types of topics and issues that these publications address.

APPENDIX

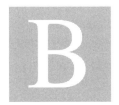

SAMPLE PROJECT CHARTER

Information Systems

Mobile Mammography Van

Project Charter

Version 1.0

Created: 08/01/2008

Printed:

Prepared by: Sam Smith

Presented to: Karen Zimmerman

Project Charter Table of Contents

VISION OF THE SOLUTION

    Vision Statement

    Major Features

    Assumptions and Dependencies

    Related Projects

SCOPE AND LIMITATIONS

    Scope of Initial Release

    Scope of Subsequent Releases

    Out of Scope

PROJECT SUCCESS FACTORS

BUDGET HIGHLIGHTS

TIMELINE

PROJECT ORGANIZATION

PROJECT MANAGEMENT STRATEGIES

    Project Meetings

    Issue Management

    Scope Change Management

    Training Strategy

    Documentation Development Strategy

    Project Work Paper Organization and Coordination

REVISION HISTORY

TABLE B.1.

Name	Date	Reason for Changes	Ver./Rev.

FOREWORD

The purpose of a Project Charter is to document what the Project Team is committed to deliver. It specifies the project timeline, resources, and implementation standards. The Project Charter is the cornerstone of the project, and is used for managing the expectations of all project stakeholders.

A Project Charter represents a formal commitment among Business Sponsors, Steering Committees, the Project Manager, and the Project Team. Therefore it is the professional responsibility of all project members to treat this agreement seriously and make every effort to meet the commitment it represents.

BUSINESS REQUIREMENTS

Background

Sponsored by the Dana Farber Cancer Institute (DFCI) in partnership with the Boston Public Health Commission, neighborhood health centers, and community groups, Boston's Mammography Van provides mammography screening and breast health education throughout the City of Boston to all women, regardless of ability to pay, with a priority on serving uninsured and underserved women right in their neighborhoods. The Mammography Van program began in April of 2008, using GE software for registration, scheduling, and billing. All clinical documentation of the mammography screening has been performed manually since April 2008. Statistical reports generated to maintain state and federal guidelines are all done manually.

Project Overview

The project has two major objectives:

- Implementation of Mammography Patient Manager software to allow for on-line documentation of the clinical encounter with the patient.
- Implementation of a wireless solution on the van at the time of the new software implementation. This will allow real-time updating of the patient appointment information as well as registering walk-on patients on the spot. Online documentation will allow ease of reporting to the state and federal agencies.

The products evaluated for implementation are specific to the needs of a mobile program and will meet most, if not all, of the needs of the program.

Project Objectives

Boston's Mobile Mammography Van program will benefit monetarily with a software system because of the reporting capabilities available with online documentation. Grant money, as well as state and federal money, is available to the program if evidence is produced to support the needs of the grant and/or the state and federal guidelines of mammography programs. The program will be more easily able to report on the information required by grants and governments to receive funding. There is also the current possibility that we are losing funding as a result of our current manual reporting practice.

The current program's resources spend valuable time manually calculating statistics. A software system will automate these processes, thus freeing the resources to perform more valuable functions. The van's mammography technician spends a lot of time manually updating and calculating which clients require additional follow-up. A software system will allow real-time reporting of which clients require which type of follow-up. This will decrease the amount of time the technician will spend manually determining which patient requires which follow-up letter. The program will be secure in its adherence to state and federal reporting guidelines for the van program as well as for the technicians working in the program.

Value Provided to Customers

- Improved productivity and reduced rework
- Streamlined business processes
- Automation of previously manual tasks
- Ability to perform entirely new tasks or functions
- Conformance to current standards or regulations
- Improved access to patient clinical and demographic information via remote access
- Reduced frustration level compared to current process

Business Risks

The major risk associated with the implementation is the selection of an incompatible vendor. There is always the concern that with a program that is new to the institution, the understanding needed to fully anticipate the needs of the program is incomplete. In addition, there is the risk that the software solution will increase workload as it offers more functions than are currently available to the user in a manual system.

Risk mitigation action items include this charter, which should clearly state the "in scope" objectives of the implementation. This should address both risks identified here.

VISION OF THE SOLUTION

Vision Statement

The Mobile Mammography Van program will be a more efficient and safe environment. The current lack of a software system introduces risks due to potential regulatory issues, patient safety issues due to potential missed follow-up, as well as program risks due to potential loss of funding. The proposed implementation of a software system alleviates these risks as well as introduces the prospect of future expansion of the program that is not easily achieved in the current environment.

The program should be able to handle more patients with the new software. The registration and scheduling process will stay the same, but the introduction of remote access will increase efficiency. Changes to appointments or patient demographic data can now occur on the van. An interface with the GE scheduling and registration software to the mobile mammography software will ensure no duplicate entry of patient data. The ability to document patient history online on the van will decrease the amount of paperwork filled out at the end of the day by the technician. There will also be the opportunity to track patients better by entering data during the day rather than at the end of the day.

The current transcription process is not expected to change. Films will still be read in the current manner, but reports will be saved to a common database. This will allow the technician or program staff to access the reports on line. Entry of the BIRAD result (mammography result) will occur much more quickly and efficiently. Patient follow-up based on the BIRAD will be done more quickly as well. Letters can be automatically generated based on the results and printed in batches. All patient follow-up, including phone calls, letters, and certified letters can be captured in the system with a complete audit trail. This ensures the program's compliance with regulations concerning patient follow-up.

The film-tracking functions will also allow more accurate tracking of the patient's films. Accurate film tracking will increase the turnaround time for film comparisons and patient follow-up.

The ability to customize the software will increase the grant funding possibilities for the program. The program can introduce new variables or queries to the clients in order to produce statistical reports based on the gathered information. Increases in funding can lead to increases in the program's expansion. The increased expansion will increase the availability of free mammography to underprivileged women.

Major Features

- Interface can be implemented from GE system to OmniCare system (OmniCare supports clinical documentation) for registration information.
- Mammography history questionnaires can be preprinted and brought on the van for the patient to fill out.
- OmniCare will allow entry of BIRAD results.
- Transcribed reports can be uploaded or cut and pasted into OmniCare from the common database.
- Patient letters are generated from and maintained in OmniCare.
- Follow-up including pathology results will be maintained in OmniCare.
- Communication management functions will be maintained with full audit trail.
- Film tracking will be done in OmniCare.
- Statistical reporting will be facilitated.

Assumptions and Dependencies

The assumptions and dependencies for this project are few, but all are crucial to the success of the implementation. The software and hardware to be purchased for this implementation are key aspects of the project. The project is dependent on the remote access satellite hardware working as expected. The software vendor chosen during the vendor selection project is assumed to be the best fit for this program. The GE interface is a crucial assumption in this project. This working interface is key to the efficiencies this program is looking to achieve with the implementation. Resources are an assumption inherent in the budget. Appropriate resources to effectively implement the solution are important to the success of the implementation.

Related Projects

There are no related projects for this project. All needed work is included in this implementation project.

SCOPE AND LIMITATIONS

Scope of Initial Release

- GE interface for patient demographic and registration information
- Film tracking (possible bar coding for film tracking)
- Mammography history questionnaires
- BIRAD result entry
- Patient follow-up management
- Communications management
- Statistical reporting
- Custom fields management
- Remote access satellite installation

Interface Scope

- GE registration data

Organizational Scope

- The OmniCare implementation will focus on the implementation of the software with the DFCI (Dana Farber Cancer Institute) program of the Boston Mobile Mammography Van. No other partner institutions are involved for the rollout. The film reads done at Faulkner Hospital are not included in this scope.

Conversion Scope

- No data conversion is planned for this project.

Scope of Subsequent Releases

- Future releases may try to include the Faulkner Hospital radiologists. Currently as Faulkner reads the film, the radiologist dictates and the text is transcribed. It would be more efficient in the future if the readings were automatically part of OmniCare.

Out of Scope

- Billing functions are not within the scope of this implementation. Billing is currently done via the GE system and will continue this way.
- A results interface is not within the scope of this implementation. The results of the mammograms will be available only on paper in the medical record or within the OmniCare solution. There will be no integration with the Results application.
- Scheduling and registration functions are not in scope for this implementation. These functions are currently done via the GE system. An interface from GE to provide this information in the OmniCare solution is planned.
- Entry of radiologists' data is not in scope for this implementation. It is listed as a possible scope of subsequent releases.

PROJECT SUCCESS FACTORS

- Increased turnaround time for patient follow-up
- Decreased turnaround time with films by film tracking
- Decreased time creating and managing reports
- Increased numbers of mammographies taken
- Decreased time spent by staff on administrative tasks

BUDGET HIGHLIGHTS

Capital budget	**$52,550**
Hardware	$10,000
Software	$30,000
Remote access	$6,200
1st yr. remote svc.	$1,350
Contingency	$5,000

Project Staff Resources

IS analyst = .50 FTE for 6 months

Network services = .25 for 3–6 months

Karen = 8 hr./wk. for 4 months

Program asst. (Sarah) = 12 hr./wk. for 4 months

New person to be hired

Temp to do data entry conversion

TIMELINE

Project will commence on November 1, 2008, and be completed July 1, 2009.
Approximate date of completion of major phases:

Analysis	January 1, 2009
Satellite installation	February 1, 2009
Registration interface	March 1, 2009
Film tracking	March 1, 2009
History questionnaires	May 1, 2009
Result entry	June 1, 2009
Communications mgmt	June 1, 2009
Patient follow-up	June 1, 2009
Reporting	June 15, 2009

PROJECT ORGANIZATION

Business Sponsor(s) Anne Jones, VP of External Affairs

Business Owner(s) Karen Ruderman, Program Director

Steering Committee Karen Zimmerman, Program Director
Anne Johnson, Director of Planning
Jerry Melini, Technical Director of Radiology

Project Manager Charles Leoman

Project Team IS analysts TBD
Network Services IS staff TBD
Karen Zimmerman, Program Director
Sarah Smithson, Program Assistant
Data Entry temporary staff

PROJECT MANAGEMENT STRATEGIES

Project Meetings

In order to maintain effective communication with Project Team members and the
Mobile Mammography Van community, a series of standing meetings will be conducted.
Meeting minutes will be documented and stored on the shared core team directory. The
following meetings and facilitated sessions will be held:

Issue Management

Issue identification, management, and resolution are important project management activities. The Project Manager is responsible for the issue management process and works with the Project Team and Steering Committee (if needed) to agree on the resolution of issues.

Effective issue management enables

- A visible decision-making process
- A means for resolving questions concerning the project
- A project issue audit trail

The standard IS project issue management process and forms will be used and attached to this charter as needed.

TABLE B.2.

Decision-Making Level	Steering Committee	Project Team

Role	■ Resolves show-stopper issues and changes in scope.
	
	■ Acts as a sounding board for decisions and actions that affect user acceptance of the project. This includes anything that affects project milestones and outcomes.
	
	■ Reviews decisions, recommendations, and requests that are high in integration and complexity and that are not resolved at the Project Team level.
	
	■ Scope management and planning.
	
	■ Chaired by Business Sponsor.
		■ Governs the actual work and the progress of the project.
		
		■ Reviews project work and status:
		
		  Resource issues
		
		  Vendor issues
		
		  Project risks
		
		■ Serves as working or focus group to report daily progress.
		
		■ Responsible for implementation decisions that have integration impact and that are of medium or high complexity.
		
		■ Cochaired by IS Project Manager and Business Owner.

Participants	Key stakeholders on business and IS sides.	All resources assigned to the project.
Meeting frequency	Meets regularly to ensure steady project progress.	Meets, as needed, weekly to monthly, for project status and updates.

Scope Change Management

Scope change management is essential to ensure that the project is managed to the original scope, as defined in this charter. The purpose of a scope management process is to constructively manage the pressure to expand scope.

Scope expansion is acceptable as long as

- Users agree that the new requirements are justified.

- Impact to the project is analyzed and understood.

- Resulting changes to project (cost, timing, resources, quality) are approved and properly implemented.

Any member of the Project Team or other member of the Mobile Mammography Van community may propose a change to the scope of the project. The requester will initiate the process by completing a Change Request Definition Form. When necessary, the Project Manager will review and seek advice from the Steering Committee on scope changes that affect the project schedule or budget, or both.

The standard IS project scope management process and forms will be used and attached as appendixes to this charter, as needed.

Training Strategy

Training Scope   The program personnel consist of a program administrator, one mammography technician, one assistant to the administrator, and one patient educator and administration person. All of the employees will receive training for their specific role related to the process. The program administrator will learn all of the roles in order to fill in when needed. Additional training will be given to the other employees for backup purposes.

Training Approach   The vendor will provide the training during the initial implementation. The employees of the program will then train new employees.

Training Material Development   The vendor will provide training materials.

Documentation Development Strategy

The team will develop the following documentation:

- Technical operations procedure manual
- Policies and procedures related to the use and management of the system
- Application manuals, if needed
- OmniCare technical and application maintenance and support manuals, if needed

Project Work Paper Organization and Coordination

In order to keep the project documentation, meeting minutes, and deliverables organized and accessible to the core team, a project folder on the shared network will be established and maintained.

REFERENCES

Accreditation Association for Ambulatory Health Care. (2003). *About AAAHC*. Retrieved June 1, 2004, from http://www.aaahc.org/about/about2.shtml.

Accredited Standards Committee X12. (2008). *X12N/TG2—Health care purpose and scope*. Retrieved August 1, 2008, from http://www.x12.org/x12org/subcommittees.

Adler-Milstein, J., McAfee, A., Bates, D., Jha, A. (2007). The state of Regional Health Information Organizations: Current activities and financing. *Health Affairs, Web Exclusives*, *27*(1), w60.

Agarwal, R., & Sambamurthy, V. (2002). *Organizing the IT function for business innovation leadership*. Chicago: Society for Information Management.

Agency for Healthcare Research and Quality. (2001). *Reducing and preventing adverse drug events to decrease hospital costs*. Retrieved May 26, 2004, from http://www.ahrq.gov/qual/aderia/aderia.htm.

Ahmad, A., Teater, P., Bentley, T., Kuehn, L., Kumar, R., Thomas, A., et al. (2002). Key attributes of a successful physician order entry system implementation in a multi-hospital environment. *Journal of the American Medical Informatics Association*, *9*, 16–24.

Alter, A. (2007, December). Top trends for 2008. *CIO Insight*, *88*, 37–40.

Altis, Inc. (2004). *Engines defined*. Retrieved November 2004 from http://www.altisinc.com/IE/defined.html.

Amatayakul, M., et al. (2001). *Definition of the health record for legal purposes* (AHIMA Practice Brief). Retrieved December 2004 from http://library.ahima.org/xpedio/groups/publics/documents/ahima/pub_bok1_009223.html.

American Health Information Management Association. (2002a). *Destruction of patient health information (updated)* (AHIMA Practice Brief). Retrieved November 2004 from http://library.ahima.org/xpedio/groups/public/documents/ahima/pub_bok1_016468.html.

American Health Information Management Association. (2002b). *Retention of health information* (AHIMA Practice Brief). Retrieved June 1, 2004, from http://library.ahima.org/xpedio/groups/publics/documents/ahima/pub_bok1_012545.html.

American Health Information Management Association. (2003a). *Final rule for HIPAA security standards*. Chicago: Author.

American Health Information Management Association. (2003b). *Implementing electronic signatures* (AHIMA Practice Brief). Retrieved June 1, 2004, from http://library.ahima.org/intradoc-cgi/idc_cgi_isapi.dll?IdcService = GET_HIGHLIGHT_INF.

American Health Information Management Association. (2008). *What does your personal health record contain?* Retrieved February 2008 from http://www.myphr.com/what/contents.asp.

American Health Information Management Association, Data Quality Management Task Force. (1998). *Data quality management model* (AHIMA Practice Brief). Retrieved January 8, 2004, from http://library.ahima.org/xpedio/groups/public/documents/ahima/pub_bok1_000066.html.

American Hospital Association. (2007). *Continued progress: Hospital use of information technology*. Chicago. Author.

American Medical Association. (2003). Guidelines for physician-patient electronic communications. Retrieved August 9, 2008, from http://www.ama-assn.org/ama/pub/category/2386.html.

American National Standard Institute. (2007). *HL7 EHR system functional model release*. Retrieved August 1, 2008, from http://www.hl7.org/ehr/downloads/index_2007.asp.

American Telemedicine Association. (2003). *Report on reimbursement*. Washington, DC: Author.

American Telemedicine Association. (2007). *Defining telemedicine*. Retrieved October 21, 2008, from http://www.atmeda.org/news/definition.html.

Applegate, L., Austin, R., & McFarlan, W. (2003). *Corporate information strategy and management* (6th ed.). Boston: McGraw-Hill.

Arlotto, P., & Oakes, J. (2003). *Return on investment: Maximizing the value of healthcare information technology*. Chicago: Healthcare Information and Management Systems Society.

Arts, D., DeKeizer, N., & Scheffer, G. (2002). Defining and improving data quality in medical registries: A literature review, case study, and generic framework. *Journal of the American Medical Informatics Association*, *9*(6), 600–611.

Ash, J. S., Anderson, N. R., & Tarczy-Hornoch, P. (2008). People and organization issues in research systems implementation. *Journal of the American Medical Informatics Association*, *15*, 283–289.

Ash, J. S., Sittig, D. F., Poon, E. G., Guappone, K., Campbell, E., & Dykstra, R. (2007). The extent and importance of unintended consequences related to computerized provider order entry. *Journal of the American Medical Informatics Association*, *14*(4), 415–423.

Ash, J. S., Stavri, P., Dykstra, R., & Fournier, L. (2003). Implementing computerized physician order entry: The importance of special people. *International Journal of Medical Informatics*, *69*(2–3), 235–250.

Associated Press. (1995a, February 28). *7 Get fake HIV-positive calls*. Retrieved December 2004 from http://www.aegis.com/news/ap/1995/AP950248.html

ASTM International. (2008). *ASTM E2369-05 standard specification for Continuity of Care Record (CCR)*. Retrieved August 1, 2008, from http://www.astm.org/Standards/E2369.htm.

Baker, L., Wagner, T. H., Singer, S., & Bundorf, M. K. (2003). Use of the Internet and e-mail for health care information: Results from a national survey. *JAMA*, *289*, 2400–2406.

Balas, D., Weingarten, S., Garb, C., Blumenthal, D., Boren, S., & Brown, G. (2000). Improving preventive care by prompting physicians. *Archives of Internal Medicine*, *160*(3), 301–308.

Ball, M. J., Smith, C., & Bakalar, R. S. (2007). Personal health records: Empowering consumers. *Journal of Healthcare Information Management*, *21*(1), 76–85.

Barlow, J., Singh, D., Bayer, S., & Curry, R. (2007). A systematic review of the benefits of home telecare for frail elderly people and those with long-term conditions. *Journal of Telemedicine & Telecare*, *13*(4), 172–179.

Barlow, S., Johnson, J., & Steck, J. (2004). The economic effect of implementing an EMR in an outpatient clinical setting. *Journal of Healthcare Information Management*, *18*(1), 46–51.

Baron, R. J., Fabens, E. L., Schiffman, M., & Wolf, E. (2005). Electronic health records: Just around the corner? Or over the cliff? *Annals of Internal Medicine*, *143*(3), 222–226.

Bates, D., & Gawande, A. (2003). Improving safety with information technology. *New England Journal of Medicine*, *348*(25), 2526–2534.

Bates, D., Kuperman, G., Rittenberg, J., Teich, J., Fiskio, J., Ma'luf, N., et al. (1999). A randomized trial of a computer-based intervention to reduce utilization of redundant laboratory tests. *American Journal of Medicine*, *106*(2), 144–150.

Bates, D. W., Kuperman, G. J., Wang, J., Gandhi, T., Kittler, A., Volk, L., et al. (2003). Ten commandments for effective clinical decision support: Making the practice of evidence-based medicine a reality. *Journal of the American Medical Informatics Association*, *10*, 523–530.

Bates, D., Leape, L., Cullen, D., Laird, N., Peterson, L., Teich, J., et al. (1998). Effect of computerized physician order entry and a team intervention on prevention of serious medication errors. *JAMA*, *280*, 1311–1316.

Bazzoli, F. (2004, May). NAHIT IT standards directory aims to provide common ground. *Healthcare IT News*, p. 5.

Bensaou, M., & Earl, M. (1998). The right mind-set for managing information technology. *Harvard Business Review*, *76*(5), 119–128.

Berkman, E. (2002, February 1). How to stay ahead of the curve. *CIO*. Retrieved December 2004 from http://www.cio.com/archive/020102/enterprise.html.

Berman, J., Zaran, F., & Rybak, M. (1992). Pharmacy-based antimicrobial-monitoring service. *American Journal of Hospital Pharmacy*, *49*, 1701–1706.

Bleich, H., Safran, C., & Slack, W. (1989). Departmental and laboratory computing in two hospitals. *M.D. Computing*, *6*(3), 149–155.

Blumenthal, D., & Glaser, J. P. (2007). Information technology comes to medicine. *New England Journal of Medicine*, *356*(24), 2527–2534.

Brailer, D., & Terasawa, E. (2003). *Use and adoption of computer-based patient records*. Oakland, CA: California HealthCare Foundation.

Bresnahan, J. (1998, July 15). What good is technology? *CIO Enterprise*, pp. 25–26, 28, 30.

Briney, A. (2000). *2000 information security industry survey*. Retrieved November 2004 from http://www.infosecuritymag.com.

Brown, C., & Sambamurthy, V. (1999). *Repositioning the IT organization to enable business transformation*. Chicago: Society for Information Management.

Brown, J., & Hagel, J. (2003). Does IT matter? *Harvard Business Review*, *81*, 109–112.

Brown, N. (2003). *Telemedicine Research Center: What is telemedicine?* Retrieved October 14, 2003, from http://trc.telemed.org/telemedicine/primer.asp.

Bu, D., Pan, E., Johnston, D., Walker, J., Alder-Milstein, J., Kendrick, D., et al. (2007). *The value of information technology-enabled disease management*. Wellesley, MA: Center for Information Technology Leadership.

Burke, J., & Pestotnik, S. (1999). Antibiotic use and microbial resistance in intensive care units: Impact of computer-assisted decision support. *Journal of Chemotherapy*, *11*(6), 530–535.

Burnum, J. (1989). The misinformation era: The fall of the medical record. *Annals of Internal Medicine*, *110*, 482–484.

Burt, C., Hing, E., & Woodwell, D. (2005). *Electronic medical record use by office-based physicians: United States, 2005*. Retrieved August 9, 2008, from http://www.cdc.gov/nchs/products/pubs/pubd/hestats /electronic/electronic.htm.

California HealthCare Foundation. (2005). *National consumer health privacy survey 2005*. Retrieved August 1, 2008, from http://www.chcf.org/topics/view.cfm?itemID = 115694.

Carr, N. (2003). IT doesn't matter. *Harvard Business Review*, *81*, 41–49.

Cash, J., McFarlan, W., & McKenney, J. (1992). *Corporate information systems management: The issues facing senior executives*. Burr Ridge, IL: Irwin.

Cecil, J., & Goldstein, M. (1990). Sustaining competitive advantage from IT. *McKinsey Quarterly*, *4*, 74–89.

Centers for Medicare and Medicaid Services. (2002). *Standards for privacy of individually identifiable health information: Final rule*. Retrieved February 2005 from http://www.hhs.gov/ocr/hippa/prirulepd.pdf.

Centers for Medicare and Medicaid Services. (2004). *HIPAA administrative simplification: Security: Final rule*. Retrieved November 2004 from http://www.cms.hhs.gov/hipaa/hipaa2/regulations/security.

Centers for Medicare and Medicaid Services. (2006, November 3). *CMS manual system* (Pub 100-04 Medicare Claims Processing). Retrieved February 2008 from http://www.cms.hhs.gov/Transmittals/Downloads/R1104CP .pdf.

Centers for Medicare and Medicaid Services. (2008). *National Provider Identifier standard (NPI)—Overview*. Retrieved June 2008 from http://www.cms.hhs.gov/NationalProvIdentStand/01_Overview.asp.

Centers for Medicare and Medicaid Services (2006, December 28). *Security Guidance*. Retrieved November 17, 2008 from http://www.cms.hhs.gov/SecurityStandard.

Certification Commission for Healthcare Information Technology. (2008). [Home page.] Retrieved November 6, 2008, from www.cchit.org.

Chamberlain, D. A. (2007). *NCPDP 101*. Retrieved August 1, 2008, from http://www.ncpdp.org/PDF/NCPDP_ 101.pdf.

Chaudhry, B., Wang, J., Wu, S., Maglione, M., Mojica, W., Roth, E., et al. (2006). Systematic review: Impact of health information technology on quality, efficiency, and costs of medical care. *Annals of Internal Medicine*, *144*(10), 742–752.

Chin, T. (2003). Doctors pull plug on paperless systems. Retrieved February 17, 2003, from http://www.ama-assn.org/amednews/2003/02/17/bil20217.htm.

Christensen, C. (1997). *The innovator's dilemma*. Boston: Harvard Business School Press.

Christensen, C. (2001). The past and future of competitive advantage. *MIT Sloan Management Review*, *42*(2), 105–109.

College of Healthcare Information Management Executives. (1998). *The healthcare CIO: A decade of growth*. Ann Arbor, MI: Author.

College of Healthcare Information Management Executives. (2008). *The seven CIO success factors*. Retrieved April, 21, 2008, from http://www.cio-chime.org/events/ciobootcamp/measure.asp.

Collins, J. (2001). *Good to great*. New York: HarperCollins.

Collmann, J. C., & Cooper, T. (2007). Breaching the security of the Kaiser Permanente Internet patient portal: The organizational foundations of information security. *Journal of the American Medical Informatics Association*, *14*(2), 239–243.

Commission on Accreditation of Rehabilitation Facilities. (2004). *What does CARF accredit?* Retrieved June 1, 2004, from http://www.carf.org/consumer.aspx?Content = Content/ConsumerServices/cs05en.html&ID = 5.

Committee on Workforce Needs in Information Technology. (2001). *Building a workforce for the information economy*. Washington, DC: National Academies Press.

Committee to Study the Impact of Information Technology on the Performance of Service Activities. (1994). *Information technology in the service society*. Washington, DC: National Academies Press.

Conn, J. (2007, February 26). Annual survey shows little budget change. *Modern Healthcare*. http:// modernhealthcare.com/apps/pbcs.dll/article?AID = /20070226/REG/70222012/-1/toc26.02.07.

Cook, R. (2007, July 20). How to spot a failing project. *CIO*. Retrieved November 8, 2008, from http://www.cio .com/article/124309/How_to_Spot_a_Failing_Project.

Cummings, J., Bush, P., Smith, D., & Matuszewski, K. (2005). Bar-coding medication overview and consensus recommendations. *American Journal of Health-Systems Pharmacy*, *62*, 2626–2629.

Cusack, C. M., & Poon, E. G. (2007). *Evaluation toolkit: Health information technology*. Boston: AHRQ National Resource Center for Health Information Technology.

Cutler, D. M., Feldman, N. E., & Horwitz, J. R. (2005). U.S. adoption of computerized physician order entry systems. *Health Affairs*, *24*(6), 1654–1663.

Dartmouth Institute for Health Policy & Clinical Practice. (2008). "Benchmarking." In *Dartmouth Atlas of Health Care*. Retrieved August 12, 2008, from http://www.dartmouthatlas.org/index.shtm.

DeLuca, J., & Enmark, R. (2002). *The CEO's guide to health care information systems* (2nd ed.). San Francisco: Jossey-Bass.

Department of Health and Human Services (2006). New regulations to facilitate adoption of health information technology. Retrieved November 22, 2008 from http://www.hhs.gov/news/press/2006pres/20060801.html.

Department of Health and Human Services. (2008a). *E-prescribing overview*. Retrieved August 1, 2008 from http://www.cms.hhs.gov/eprescribing/

Department of Health and Human Services. (2008b). *Health information technology*. Retrieved August 1, 2008 from http://www.hhs.gov/healthit/.

Department of Health and Human Services. (2008c). *Hospital compare*. Retrieved June 2008 from http://www .hospitalcompare.hhs.gov.

Department of Health and Human Services. (2008d). *The ONC-coordinated federal health information technology strategic plan: 2008–2012*. Retrieved August 1, 2008, from http://www.hhs.gov/healthit/resources /HITStrategicPlanSummary.pdf.

Department of Health and Human Services, Office of Inspector General. (2004). *Fraud prevention and detection. Compliance guidance*. Retrieved November 2004 from www.oig.hhs.gov.

Department of Labor, Bureau of Labor Statistics. (2008). Retrieved November 22, 2008 from http://data.bls.gov/oep/servlet/oep.nioem.servlet.ActionServlet.

DesRoches, C.M., Campbell, E.G., Rao, S.R., Donelan, K., Ferris, T.G., Jha, A., Kaushal, R., Levy, D.E., Rosenbaum, S., Shields, A., Blumenthal, D. (2008). Electronic health records in ambulatory care—A national survey of physicians. *New England Journal of Medicine*, *359*(1), 50–60.

Donald, J. (1989). Prescribing costs when computers are used to issue all prescriptions. *British Medical Journal*, *299*, 28–30.

Dougherty, M. (2001). On the line: Professional practice solutions. *Journal of AHIMA*, *72*(10), 72–73.

Downes, L., & Mui, C. (1998). *Unleashing the killer app*. Boston: Harvard Business School Press.

Dragoon, A. (2003, August 15). Deciding factors. *CIO*, pp. 49–59.

Drazen, E., & Straisor, D. (1995). *Information support in an integrated delivery system*. Paper presented at the 1995 annual HIMSS conference, Chicago.

Duxbury, B. (1982). Therapeutic control of anticoagulant treatment. *British Medical Journal*, *284*, 702.

Dvorak, R., Holen, E., Mark, D., & Meehan, W., III. (1997). Six principles of high- performance IT. *McKinsey Quarterly*, *3*, 164–177.

Earl, M. (1993). Experiences in strategic information systems planning. *MIS Quarterly*, *17*(1), 1–24.

Earl, M., & Feeney, D. (1995). Is your CIO adding value? *McKinsey Quarterly*, *2*, 144–161.

Earl, M., & Feeney, D. (2000). How to be a CEO for the information age. *MIT Sloan Management Review*, *41*(2), 11–23.

Edwards, P. J., Huang, D. T., Metcalfe, L. N., & Sainfort, F. (2008). Maximizing your investment in EHR: Utilizing EHRs to inform continuous quality improvement. *Journal of Healthcare Information Management*, *22*(1), 32–37.

eHealth Initiative. (2007). *Fourth annual survey of health information exchange at the state, regional and community levels*. Retrieved November 6, 2008, from http://www.ehealthinitiative.org/HIESurvey/2007Survey.mspx.

Eng, J. (2001). Computer network security for the radiology enterprise. *Radiology*, *220*(2), 304–309.

Etheridge, Y. (2001). PKI: How and why it works. *Health Management Technology*, pp. 20–21.

Evans, J., & Hayashi, A. (1994, September-October). Implementing on-line medical records. *Document Management*, pp. 12–17.

Evans, R., Pestotnik, S., Classen, D., & Burke, J. (1993). Development of an automated antibiotic consultant. *M.D. Computing*, *10*(1), 17–22.

Feld, C., & Stoddard, D. (2004). Getting IT right. *Harvard Business Review*, *82*(2), 72–79.

Fluke Networks. (2003). *Wireless security notes: A brief analysis of risks*. Retrieved December 2004 from http://wp.bitpipe.com/resource/org_1014144860_961/fnet_wireless_security_bpx.pdf.

Fonkych, K., & Taylor, R. (2005). *The state and pattern of health information technology adoption*. Santa Monica, CA: Rand Health.

Fortin, J., & MacDonald, K. (2006). *Physician practices: Are application service providers right for you?* Oakland, CA: California HealthCare Foundation.

Freedman, D. (1991, July). The myth of strategic I.S. *CIO*, pp. 34–41.

Gadd, C., & Penrod, L. (2000). Dichotomy between physicians' and patients' attitudes regarding EMR use during outpatient encounters. *Proceedings/AMIA Annual Symposium*, pp. 275–279.

Gambetta, M., Dunn, P., Nelson, D., Herron, B., & Arena, R. (2007). Impact of the implementation of telemanagement on a disease management program in an elderly heart failure cohort. *Progress in Cardiovascular Nursing*, 22(4), 196–200.

Gans, D., Kralewski, J., Hammons, T., & Dowd, B. (2005). Medical groups' adoption of electronic health records and information systems. *Health Affairs*, 24(5), 1323–1333.

Garrett, L., Jr., Hammond, W., & Stead, W. (1986). The effects of computerized medical records on provider efficiency and quality of care. *Methods of Information in Medicine*, 25(3), 151–157.

Gartner, Inc. (2007). *2006–2007 IT spending and staffing report: North America*. Stamford, CT: Author.

Gartner, Inc. (2008). *Forecast: Healthcare IT spending worldwide, 2006–2011*. Stamford, CT: Author.

Gearon, C.J. (2007). *Perspectives on the future of personal health records*. California HealthCare Foundation.

Glaser, J. (2002). *The strategic application of information technology in health care organizations* (2nd ed.). San Francisco: Jossey-Bass.

Glaser, J. (2003a, March). Analyzing information technology value. *Healthcare Financial Management*, pp. 98–104.

Glaser, J. (2003b, September). When IT excellence goes the distance. *Healthcare Financial Management*, pp. 102–106.

Glaser, J. (2006, January). Assessing the IT function in less than one day. *Healthcare Financial Management*, pp. 104–108.

Glaser, J. (2008a, April). Creating IT agility. *Healthcare Financial Management*, pp. 36–39.

Glaser, J. (2008b, February 6). The four cornerstones of innovation. *Most Wired Online*.

Glaser, J., DeBor, G., & Stuntz, L. (2003). The New England healthcare EDI network. *Journal of Healthcare Information Management*, 17(4), 42–50.

Glaser, J. and Williams, R. (2007). The definitive evolution of the role of the CIO. *Journal of Healthcare Information Management*, 21(1), 9–11.

Goldsmith, J. (2003). *Digital medicine implications for healthcare leaders*. Chicago: Health Administration Press.

Gopalakrishna, R. (2000). *Audit trails*. Retrieved July 21, 2004, from http://www.cerias.purdue.edu/homes/rgk/at.html.

Government Accountability Office. (2007, April). *Hospital data quality: HHS should specify steps and time frame for using information technology to collect and submit data* (GOA-07-320). Retrieved July 2008 from www.gao.gov/cgi-bin/getrpt?GAO-07-320.

Grieger, D. L., Cohen, S. H., & Krusch, D. A. (2007). A pilot study to document the return on investment for implementing an ambulatory electronic health record at an academic medical center. *Journal of the American College of Surgeons*, 205(1), 89–96.

Halamka, J. D., Mandl, K. D., & Tang, P. C. (2008). Early experiences with personal health records. *Journal of the American Medical Informatics Association*, 15(1), 1–7.

Hammond, W., & Cimino, J. (2001). *Standards in medical informatics*. In E. Shortliffe & L. Perreault (Eds.), *Medical informatics computer applications in health care and biomedicine* (pp. 212–256). New York: Springer-Verlag.

Han, Y. Y., Carcillo, J. A., Venkataraman, S. T., Clark, R., Watson, R. S., Nguyen, T. C., et al. (2005). Unexpected increased mortality after implementation of a commercially sold computerized physician order entry system. *Pediatrics*, 116(6), 1506–1512.

Hankin, R. (2002). *Bar coding in healthcare: A critical solution*. Retrieved July 19, 2004, from http://www.bbriefings.com/cdps/cditem.cfm?NID=753&CID=5&CFID=250074&CFTO.

Hatoum, H., Catizone, C., Hutchinson, R., & Purohit, A. (1986). An eleven-year review of the pharmacy literature: Documentation of the value and acceptance of clinical pharmacy. *Drug Intelligence and Clinical Pharmacy*, 20, 33–48.

Health Privacy Project. (2007). *Health privacy stories*. Retrieved August 1, 2008, from http://www.healthprivacy.org/usr_doc/Privacystories.pdf.

Healthcare Informatics. (2007, June). *Healthcare Informatics 100*. Retrieved November 14, 2008, from http://www.healthcare-informatics.com/ME2/dirmod.asp?sid=&nm=&type=Publishing&mod=Publications%3A%3AArticle&mid=8F3A7027421841978F18BE895F87F791&tier=4&id=CE9E6AE27E3941248B56585E26929FF9.

Healthcare Information and Management Systems Society. (2003a). *15th Annual HIMSS Leadership Survey sponsored by Superior Consultant Company*. Retrieved November 2004 from http://www.himss.org/2004survey/ASP/healthcarecio_home.asp.

Healthcare Information and Management Systems Society. (2003b). *Implementation guide for the use of bar code technology in healthcare*. Chicago: Author.

Healthcare Information and Management Systems Society. (2008a). *19th Annual HIMSS Leadership Survey, sponsored by Cisco. Retrieved November 2008 from* http://www.himss.org/2008Survey/healthcareCIO_final.asp.

Healthcare Information and Management Systems Society. (2008b). *Davies award*. Retrieved October 21, 2008, from http://www.himss.org/davies/index.asp.

Healthcare Information Technology Standards Panel. (2008c). [Home page.] Retrieved November 6, 2008, from www.hitsp.org.

Henderson, J., & Venkatraman, N. (1993). Strategic alignment: Leveraging information technology for transforming organizations. *IBM Systems Journal*, *32*(1), 4–16.

Hersh, W. and Wright, A. (2008). *Characterizing the health information technology workforce: Analysis from the HIMSS Analytics Database*. Retrieved October 21, 2008 from http://davinci.ohsu.edu/~hersh/hit-workforce-hersh.pdf.

Hershey, C., McAloon, M., & Bertram, D. (1989). The new medical practice environment: Internists' view of the future. *Archives of Internal Medicine*, *149*, 1745–1749.

Herzlinger, R. (1997). *Market-driven health care*. Reading, MA: Addison-Wesley.

Holdsworth, M. T., Fichtl, R., Raisch, D., Hewryk, A., Behta, M., Mendez-Rico, E., et al. (2007). Impact of computerized prescriber order entry on the incidence of adverse drug events in pediatric inpatients. *Pediatrics*, *120*(5), 1058–1066.

Hudak, S., & Sharkey, S. (2007). *Health information technology: Are long term care providers ready?* Oakland, CA: California HealthCare Foundation.

Institute of Medicine. (1991). *The computer-based patient record: An essential technology for health care*. Washington, DC: National Academies Press.

Institute of Medicine. (2000). *To err is human: Building a safer health system*. Washington, DC: National Academies Press.

Institute of Medicine. (2001). *Crossing the quality chasm: A new health system for the 21st century*. Washington, DC: National Academies Press.

Institute of Medicine, Committee on Data Standards for Patient Safety. (2003a). *Key capabilities of an electronic health record system*. Washington, DC: Institute of Medicine.

Institute of Medicine, Committee on Data Standards for Patient Safety. (2003b). *Reducing medical errors requires national computerized information systems: Data standards are crucial to improving patient safety*. Retrieved November 20, 2003, from http://www4.nationalacademies.org.

Institute of Medicine, Committee on Data Standards for Patient Safety. (2004). *Patient safety: Achieving a new standard for care*. Washington, DC: National Academies Press.

International Organization for Standardization. (2008). ISO/IEC 15408-1, 2nd ed.: Information Technology—Security techniques—Evaluation criteria for IT security, Part 1, Introduction and General Model. Retrieved November 17, 2008 from http://standards.iso.org/ittf/PubliclyAvailableStandards/index.html.

Jensen, J. (2006). The effects of computerized provider order entry on medication turn-around time: A time-to-first dose study at the Providence Portland Medical Center. *Proceedings/AMIA Annual Symposium*, pp. 384–388.

Jha, A. K., Ferris, T. G., Donelan, K., DesRoches, C., Shields, A., Rosenbaum, S., et al. (2006). How common are electronic health records in the United States? A summary of the evidence. *Health Affairs*, *25*, 496–507.

Johns, M. (1997). *Information management for health professionals*. Albany, NY: Delmar.

Johnston, B., Wheeler, L., Deuser, J., & Sousa, K. (2000). Outcomes of the Kaiser Permanente tele-home health research project. *Archives of Family Medicine*, *9*(1), 40–45.

Johnston, D., Pan, E., Walker, J., Bates, D., & Middleton, B. (2003). *The value of computerized provider order entry in ambulatory settings*. Chicago: Healthcare Information and Management Systems Society.

Johnston, D., Pan, E., Walker, J., Bates, D., & Middleton, B. (2004). *Patient safety in the physician's office: Assessing the value of ambulatory CPOE*. Oakland, CA: California HealthCare Foundation.

Joint Commission on Accreditation of Healthcare Organizations. (2004). *JCAHO hospital accreditation manual 2004*. Oakbrook Terrace, IL: Author.

The Joint Commission. (2008a). *Facts about Quality Check® and quality reports*. Retrieved June 2008 from http://www.jointcommission.org/QualityCheck/06_qc_facts.htm.

The Joint Commission. (2008b). *Facts about scoring and accreditation decisions*. Retrieved August 1, 2008, from: http://www.jointcommission.org/AboutUs/Fact_Sheets/scoring_qa.htm.

The Joint Commission. (2008c). *Facts about the Joint Commission*. Retrieved August 1, 2008, from: http://www.jointcommission.org/AboutUs/Fact_Sheets/joint_commission_facts.htm.

The Joint Commission. (2008d). *The Joint Commission hospital accreditation manual 2008*. Oakbrook Terrace, IL: Author.

Karson, A., Kuperman, G., Horsky, J., Fairchild, D., Fiskio, J., & Bates, D. (1999, April). Patient-specific computerized outpatient reminders to improve physician compliance with clinical guidelines. *Journal of General Internal Medicine*, *14*(Suppl. 2), 126.

Karygiannis, T., & Owens, L. (2002). *Wireless network security: 802.11, Bluetooth and handheld devices* (Special Publication 800-48). Gaithersburg, MD: National Institute of Standards and Technology.

Kaushal, R., & Bates, D. (2002). Information technology and medication safety: What is the benefit? *Quality and Safety in Health Care*, *11*, 261–265.

Keen, P. (1997). *The process edge*. Boston: Harvard Business School Press.

Kelly, D. (2007). *Applying quality management in healthcare: A process improvement* (2nd ed.). Chicago: Health Administration Press.

Kennedy, O., Davis, G., & Heda, S. (1992). Clinical information systems: 25-year history and the future. *Journal of the Society for Health Systems*, *3*(4), 49–60.

Kilbridge, P. M., Classen, D., Bates, D. W., & Denham, C. R. (2006). The National Quality Forum safe practice standard for computerized physician order entry: Updating a critical patient safety practice. *Journal of Patient Safety*, *2*(4), 183–190.

Kuperman, G., Teich, J., Gandhi, T., & Bates, D. (2001). Patient safety and computerized medication ordering at Brigham and Women's Hospital. *Joint Commission Journal on Quality Improvement*, *27*(10), 509–521.

Kurtz, M. (2002). HL7 Version 3.0: A preview for CIOs, managers, and programmers. *Journal of Healthcare Information Management*, *16*(4), 22–23.

Lake, K. (1998). Cashing in on your ATM network. *McKinsey Quarterly*, *1*, 173–178.

Landis, S., Hulkower, S., & Pierson, S. (1992). Enhancing adherence with mammography through patient letters and physician prompts: A pilot study. *North Carolina Medical Journal*, *53*(11), 575–578.

Langberg, M. (2004). *Challenges to implementing CPOE: A case study of a work in progress at Cedars-Sinai*. Retrieved April, 2004, from http://www.modernphysician.com/page.cms?pageId = 216.

LaTour, K. (2002). *Healthcare information standards*. In K. LaTour & S. Eichenwald (Eds.), *Health information management concepts, principles, and practice* (pp. 121–136). Chicago: American Health Information Management Association.

Lee, F. W. (2002). *Data and information management*. In K. LaTour & S. Eichenwald (Eds.), *Health information management concepts, principles, and practice* (pp. 83–100). Chicago: American Health Information Management Association.

Legler, J., & Oates, R. (1993). Patients' reactions to physician use of a computerized medical record system during clinical encounters. *Journal of Family Practice*, *37*(3), 241–244.

Levinson, M. (2001, February 1). Jackpot. *CIO*. Retrieved November 2004 from http://www.cio.com /archive/020103/tl_profile.html.

Leviss, J., Kremsdorf, R., & Mohaideen, M. F. (2006). The CMIO: A new leader for health systems. *Journal of the American Medical Informatics Association*, *13*(5), 573–578.

Levit, K., Cowan, C., Lazenby, H., Sensenig, A., McDonnell, P., Stiller, J., et al. (2000). Health spending in 1998: Signals of change. *Health Affairs*, *19*(1), 124–132.

Libicki, M., Schneider, J., Frelinger, D., & Slomovic, A. (2000). *Scaffolding the new Web: Standards and standards policy for the digital economy*. Santa Monica, CA: Rand.

Liederman, E., Lee, J., Baquero, V., & Seites, P. (2005). Patient-physician Web messaging: The impact on message volume and satisfaction. *Journal of General Internal Medicine*, *20*, 52–57.

Lipton, M. (1996). Opinion: Demystifying the development of an organizational vision. *MIT Sloan Management Review*, *37*(4), 83–92.

Litzelman, D., Dittus, R., Miller, M., & Tierney, W. (1993, June). Requiring physicians to respond to computerized reminders improved their compliance with preventive care protocols. *Journal of General Internal Medicine, 8*, 311–317.

Logical Observation Identifiers Names and Codes. (2008a). *LOINC Background*. Retrieved August 1, 2008 from http://loinc.org/background.

Logical Observation Identifiers Names and Codes. (2008b). *Structure of LOINC codes and names*. Retrieved August 1, 2008, from http://loinc.org/downloads/files/LOINCManual.pdf.

MacDonald, K. (2003). *Online patient-provider communication tools: An overview*. Oakland, CA: California HealthCare Foundation.

Marotta, D. (2000). *Healthcare informatics: HL7 in the 21st century*. Retrieved March 4, 2004, from http://www.healthcare-informatics.com/issues/2000/04_00/h17.htm.

Marshall, P., & Chin, H. (1998). *The effects of an electronic medical record on patient care: Clinician attitudes in a large HMO*. Paper presented at the AMIA Annual Symposium, Portland, OR.

Massaro, T. (1993a). Introducing physician order entry at a major academic medical center: I. Impact on organizational culture and behavior. *Academic Medicine, 68*(1), 20–25.

Massaro, T. (1993b). Introducing physician order entry at a major academic medical center: II. Impact on medical education. *Academic Medicine, 68*(1), 25–30.

McAfee, A. (2003). When too much IT knowledge is a dangerous thing. *MIT Sloan Management Review, 44*(2), 83–89.

McDonald, C., Hui, S., Smith, D., Tierney, W., Cohen, S., Weinberger, M., et al. (1984). Reminders to physicians from an introspective computer medical record: A two-year randomized trial. *Annals of Internal Medicine, 100*, 130–138.

McDowell, S., Wahl, R., & Michelson, J. (2003). Herding cats: The challenges of EMR vendor selection. *Journal of Healthcare Information Management, 17*(3), 63–71.

McGowan, J. J., Cusack, C. M., & Poon, E. G. (2008). Formative evaluation: A critical component in EHR implementation. *Journal of the American Medical Informatics Association, 15*, 297–301.

McKenney, J., Copeland, D., & Mason, R. (1995). *Waves of change: Business evolution through information technology*. Boston: Harvard Business School Press.

McPhee, S., Bird, J. A., Jenkins, C. N., & Fordham, D. (1989). Promoting cancer screening: A randomized, controlled trial of three interventions. *Archives of Internal Medicine, 149*, 1866–1872.

McPhee, S., Bird, J. A., Fordham, D., Rodnick, J., & Osborn, E. (1991). Promoting cancer prevention activities by primary care physicians: Results of a randomized, controlled trial. *JAMA, 266* (4), 538–544.

Medical Records Institute. (2004). *Healthcare documentation: A report on information capture and report generation*. Boston: Author.

Mendelson, D. (2003, December 7). *Financial incentive programs for health information technology: Lessons learned*. Paper presented at the eHealth Initiative Summit, Washington, DC.

Metzger, J., & Fortin, J. (2003). *Computerized physician order entry in community hospitals: Lessons from the field*. Oakland, CA: California HealthCare Foundation.

Metzger, J., & Turisco, F. (2001). *Computerized physician order entry: A look at the marketplace and getting started*. Washington, DC, and New York: Leapfrog Group and First Consulting Group.

Miller, R. H., & Sim, I. (2004). Physicians' use of electronic medical records: Barriers and solutions. *Health Affairs, 23*(2), 116–126.

Miller, R. H., Sim, I., & Newman, J. (2003). *Electronic medical records: Lessons from small physician practices*. Oakland, CA: California HealthCare Foundation.

Miller, R. H., West, C., Brown, T., Sim, I., & Ganchoff, C. (2005). The value of electronic health records in solo or small group practices. *Health Affairs, 24*(5), 1127–1137.

Mills, P. D., Neily, J., Mims, E., Burkhardt, M. E., & Bagian, J. (2006). Improving the bar-coded medication administration system at the Department of Veterans Affairs. *American Journal of Health-Systems Pharmacy, 63*, 1442–1447.

Modai, I., Jabarin, M., Kurs, R., Barak, P., Hanan, I., & Kitain, L. (2006). Cost effectiveness, safety, and satisfaction with video telepsychiatry versus face-to-face care in ambulatory settings. *Telemedicine & E-Health, 12*(5), 515–520.

Moyer, C., Stern, D., Dobias, K., Cox, D., & Katz, S. (2002, May). Bridging the electronic divide: Patient and provider perspectives on e-mail communication in primary care. *American Journal of Managed Care*, pp. 427–433.

National Alliance for Health Information Technology. (2008, April 28). *Report to the Office of the National Coordinator for Health Information Technology on defining key health information technology terms*. Department of Health and Human Services. Retrieved August 1, http://www.nahit.org/docs/hittermsfinalreport_051508.pdf.

National Committee for Quality Assurance. (2008a). *Accreditation*. Retrieved August 1, 2008, from http://www.ncqa.org/tabid/66/Default.aspx.

National Committee for Quality Assurance. (2008b). *Accreditation levels*. Retrieved August 1, 2008, from http://www.ncqa.org/tabid/197/Default.aspxNational Committee for Quality Assurance.

(2008d). *HEDIS 2008*. Retrieved June 2008 from http://www.ncqa.org/tabid/536/Default.aspx.

National Committee for Quality Assurance. (2008e). *MCO/PPO accreditation programs*. Retrieved August 1, 2008, from http://www.ncqa.org/tabid/67/Default.aspx.

National Committee on Vital and Health Statistics. (2003, November 5). *Letter to the secretary: Recommendations for PMRI terminology standards*. Retrieved December 2004 from http://www.ncvhs.hhs.gov/031105lt3.pdf.

National Electrical Manufacturers Association. (2003). *Digital imaging and communications in medicine (DICOM): Part 1. Introduction and overview*. Rosslyn, VA: Author.

National Library of Medicine. (2003). *Fact sheet: Unified Medical Language System*. Retrieved March 3, 2004, from http://www.nlm.nih.gov/pubs/factsheets/umls.html.

National Library of Medicine. (2008). *Unified Medical Language System: SNOMED clinical terms (SNOMED CT)*. Retrieved August 1, 2008, from http://www.nlm.nih.gov/research/umls/Snomed/snomed_main.html.

National Uniform Billing Committee. (1999). *The history of the NUBC*. Retrieved July 20, 2004, from http://www.nubc.org/history.html.

National Uniform Claim Committee. (2008). *Who are we?* Retrieved June 2008 from http://www.nucc.org/index.php?option = com_frontpage&Itemid = 1.

Ornstein, S., & Bearden, A. (1994). Patient perspectives on computer-based medical records. *Journal of Family Practice*, *38*(6), 606–610.

Ornstein, S., Garr, D., Jenkins, R., Rust, P., & Arnon, A. (1991). Computer-generated physician and patient reminders: Tools to improve population adherence to selected preventive services. *Journal of Family Practice*, *32*(1), 82–90.

Overhage, J., Tierney, W., Zhou, X., & McDonald, C. (1997). A randomized trial of "corollary orders" to prevent errors of omission. *Journal of the American Medical Informatics Association*, *4*(5), 364–375.

Oz, E. (2004). *Management information systems: Instructor edition* (4th ed.). Boston: Course Technology.

Oz, E. (2006). *Management information systems: Instructor edition* (5th ed.). Boston: Course Technology.

Paoletti, R. D., Suess, T. M., Lesko, M. G., Feroli, A. A., Kennel, J. A., Mahler, J. M., et al. (2007). Using bar-code technology and medication observation methodology for safer medication administration. *American Journal of Health-Systems Pharmacy*, *64*, 536–543.

Pastore, R. (2003, February 1). Cruise control. *CIO*. Retrieved December 2004 from http://www.cio.com/archive/020103/overview.html.

Pearson, W. S., & Bercovitz, A. R. (2006). Use of computerized medical records in home health and hospice agencies. *Vital Health Statistics*, *13*, 161, 1–14.

Poissant, L., Pereira, J., Tamblyn, R., & Kawasumi, Y. (2005). The impact of electronic health records on time efficiency of physicians and nurses: A systematic review. *Journal of the American Medical Informatics Association*, *12*(5), 505–516.

Poon, E. G., Blumenthal, D., Jaggi, T., Honour, M., Balas, D., & Kaushal, R. (2004). Overcoming barriers to adopting and implementing computerized physician order entry systems in U.S. hospitals. *Health Affairs*, *23*(4), 184–190.

Poon, E. G., Cina, J. L., Churchill, W., Patel, N., Featherstone, E., Rothschild, J. M., et al. (2006). Medication dispensing errors and potential adverse drug events before and after implementing bar code technology in the pharmacy. *Annals of Internal Medicine*, *145*, 426–434.

Poon, E. G., Jha, A. K., Christino, M., Honour, M. M., Fernandopulle, R., Middleton, B., et al. (2006). *BMC Medical Informatics and Decision Making*, *6*(1).

Porter, M. (1980). *Competitive strategy*. New York: Free Press.

Porter, M. (2001). Strategy and the Internet. *Harvard Business Review*, *79*(3), 63–78.

Quinsley, C. A. (2004). A HIPAA security overview (AHIMA Practice Brief). *Journal of AHIMA*, *75*(4), 56A–56C.

Raymond, B., & Dold, C. (2002). *Clinical information systems: Achieving the vision*. Oakland, CA: Kaiser Permanente Institute for Health Policy.

Renner, K. (1996). Cost-justifying electronic medical records. *Healthcare Financial Management*, *50*(10), 63–64, 66, 68, 70.

Reynolds, R.B. (2009). *Fundamentals of Law for Health Informatics and Information Management*. In Brodnick, M.S. et al. (Eds.), *The HIPAA Security Rule* (pp. 195–236). Chicago: American Health Information Management Association.

Ridsdale, L., & Hudd, S. (1994). Computers in the consultation: The patient's view. *British Journal of General Practice*, *44*, 367–369.

Rob, P., & Coronel, C. (2004). *Database systems: Design, implementation, and management* (6th ed.). Boston: Course Technology.

Roberts, A., & Sebastian, M. (2006). The future is now: Implementation of a tele-internsivist system. *Journal of Nursing Administration*, *36*(1), 49–54.

Rosen, P., & Kwoh, C. (2007). Patient-physician e-mail: An opportunity to transform pediatric health care delivery. *Pediatrics*, *120*(4), 701–706.

Ross, J., & Beath, C. (2002). Beyond the business case: New approaches to IT investment. *MIT Sloan Management Review*, *43*(2), 51–59.

Ross, J., Beath, C., & Goodhue, D. (1996). Develop long-term competitiveness through IT assets. *MIT Sloan Management Review*, *38*(1), 31–42.

Sakowski, J., Leonard, T., Colburn, S., Michaelsen, B., Schiro, T., Schneider, J., et al. (2005). Using a bar-coded medication administration system to prevent medication errors in a community hospital network. *American Journal of Health-Systems Pharmacy*, *62*, 2619–2625.

Sambamurthy, V., & Zmud, R. (1996). *Information technology and innovation: Strategies for success*. Morristown, NJ: Financial Executives Research Foundation.

Saving lives, reducing costs: CPOE lessons learned in community hospitals. (2006). Westborough, MA: Massachusetts Technology Collaborative in Partnership with New England Healthcare Institute.

Schoen, C., Osborn, R., Doty, M. M., Bishop, M., Peugh, J., & Murukutla, N. (2007). Toward higher-performance health systems: Adults' health care experiences in seven countries, 2007. *Health Affairs*, 717–734.

Schott, S. (2003, April). How poor documentation does damage in the courtroom. *Journal of AHIMA*, *74*(4), 20–24.

Sciamanna, C., Rogers, M., Shenassa, E., & Houston, T. (2007). Patient access to U.S. physicians who conduct Internet or e-mail consults. *Journal of General Internal Medicine*, *22*, 378–381.

Shakir, A. (1999). Tools for defining data. *Journal of AHIMA*, *70*(8), 48–53.

Shamliyan, T., Duval, S., Jing, D., & Kane, R. (2008). Just what the doctor ordered: Review of the evidence of the impact of computerized provider order entry on medication errors. *Health Services Research*, *43*(1), 32–53.

Simon, S. R., Kaushal, R., Cleary, P. D., Jenter, C. A., Volk, L. A., Orav, E. J., et al. (2007). Physicians and electronic health records: a statewide survey. *Archives of Internal Medicine*, *167*(5), 507–512.

Smith, H. (2001). *A context-based access control model for HIPAA privacy and security compliance* (SANS Institute, Information Security Reading Room). Retrieved December 2004 from http://www.sans .org/rr/whitepapers/legal/44.php.

Solomon, G., & Dechter, M. (1995). Are patients pleased with computer use in the examination room? *Journal of Family Practice*, *41*(3), 241–244.

Spurr, C. (2003). *Information systems project management at Partners HealthCare*. Internal document, Partners HealthCare.

Stair, R., & Reynolds, G. (2003). *Principles of information systems* (6th ed.). Boston: Course Technology.

Stone, J. (2007). Communication between physicians and patients in the era of e-medicine. *New England Journal of Medicine*, *356*(24), 2451–2454.

Stouffer, R. (2008). Doctor use of patient e-mail still low despite benefits. *Pittsburgh Tribune-Review*. Retrieved November 6. 2008, from http://www.pittsburghlive.com/x/pittsburghtrib/business/s_580825.html.

Strassman, P. (1990). *The business value of computers*. New Canaan, CT: Information Economics Press.

Superior Consultant Company. (2004). *Best strategies for selecting a clinical information system*. Dearborn, MI: Author.

Tang, P. C., Ash, J. S., Bates, D. W., Overhage, J. M., & Sands, D. Z. (2006). Personal health records: Definitions, benefits, and strategies for overcoming barriers to adoption. *Journal of the American Medical Informatics Association*, *13*(2), 121–126.

Tang, P. C., & Lansky, D. (2005). The missing link: Bridging the patient-provider health information gap. *Health Affairs*, *24*(5), 1290–1295.

Tate, K., Gardner, R., & Weaver, L. (1990). A computerized laboratory alerting system. *M.D. Computing*, *7*(5), 296–301.

Teich, J., Merchia, P., Schmiz, J., Kuperman, G., Spurr, C., & Bates, D. (2000). Effects of computerized physician order entry on prescribing practices. *Archives of Internal Medicine, 160*, 2741–2747.

Tierney, W., McDonald, C., Hui, S., & Martin, D. (1988). Computer predictions of abnormal test results. *JAMA, 259*, 1194–1198.

Tierney, W., Miller, M., & McDonald, C. (1990). The effect on test ordering of informing physicians of the charges for outpatient diagnostic tests. *New England Journal of Medicine, 322*, 1499–1504.

Tierney, W., Miller, M., Overhage, J. M., & McDonald, C. (1993). Physician inpatient order writing on micro-computer workstations: Effects on resource utilization. *JAMA, 269*, 379–383.

Toole, J. (2003). *The need for transformation.* In *Health care technology* (Vol. *1*). San Francisco: Montgomery Research.

Wager, K. A., & Lee, F. W. (2006). *Introduction to healthcare information systems.* In M. Johns (Ed.), *Health information management technology: An applied approach* (2nd ed.). Chicago: American Health Information Management Association.

Wager, K. A., Lee, F., White, A., Ward, D., & Ornstein, S. (2000). Impact of an electronic medical record system on community-based primary care practices. *Journal of the American Board of Family Practice, 13*(5), 338–348.

Wager, K. A., Ward, D. M., Lee, F. W., White, A. W., Davis, K. S., & Clancy, D. (2005). Physicians, patients and EHRs: When it comes to a consultation, is three a crowd? *Journal of the American Health Information Management Association, 76*(4), 38–41.

Wager, K. A., Zoller, J. S., Soper, D. E., Smith, J. B., Waller, J. L., & Clark, F. C. (2008). Assessing physician and nurse satisfaction with an ambulatory care EMR: One facility's approach. *International Journal of Healthcare Information Systems and Informatics, 3*(1), 63–74.

Walsh, T. (2003). Best practices for compliance with the final Security Rule. *Journal of Healthcare Information Management, 17*(3), 14–18.

Walsh, K., Landrigan, C., Adams, W., Vinci, R., Chessare, J., Cooper, M., et al. (2008). Effect of computer order entry on prevention of serious medication errors in hospitalized children. *Pediatrics, 121*(3), e421–427.

Wang, S., Middleton, B., Prosser, L., Bardon, C., Spurr, C., & Carchidi, P. (2003). A cost-benefit analysis of the electronic medical record in primary care. *American Journal of Medicine, 114*, 397–403.

Webopedia. (2004a). *Audit trail.* Retrieved November 2004 from http://www.webopedia.com/TERM/a/audit_trail.html.

Webopedia. (2004). *The seven layers of the OSI model.* Retrieved November 2004 from http://www.webopedia.com/quick_ref/OSI_Layers.asp.

Webopedia. (2004c). *Token-ring network.* Retrieved November 2004 from http://www.webopedia.com/TERM/T/token_ring_network.html.

Weil, S. (2004). *The final HIPAA Security Rule: Conducting effective risk analysis.* Retrieved April 13, 2004, from http://www.hipaadvisory.com/action/Security/riskanalysis.htm.

Weill, P., & Broadbent, M. (1998). *Leveraging the new infrastructure.* Boston: Harvard Business School Press.

Weill, P., & Ross, J. (2004). *IT governance: How top performers manage IT decision rights for superior results.* Boston: Harvard Business School Press.

Whatis?com. (2002). *The Whatis?com encyclopedia of technology terms.* Indianapolis, IN: Que.

White, C. (2001). *Data communications and computer networks: A business user's approach.* Boston: Course Technology.

The White House. (2006, August). *Fact sheet: Health care transparency: Empowering consumers to save on quality care.* Retrieved November 6, 2008, from http://www.whitehouse.gov/news/releases/2006/08/20060822.html.

Whitten, J., & Bentley, L. (2005). *Systems analysis and design methods* (7th ed.). New York: McGraw-Hill/Irwin.

Whitten, J., & Bentley, L. (2007). *Systems analysis and design methods* (8th ed.). New York: McGraw-Hill/Irwin.

Wise, P., & Mon, D. (2004). *EHR functional outline review & validation.* Retrieved October 2004 from http://www.hl7.org/ehr/documents/public/presentations/18.

Yarnall, K., Rimer, B., Hynes, D., Watson, G., Lyna, P., Woods-Powell, C., et al. (1998). Computerized prompts for cancer screening in a community health center. *Journal of the American Board of Family Practice, 11*(2), 96–104.

INDEX

Page references followed by *fig* indicate illustrated figures; followed by *t* indicate tables; followed by *e* indicate exhibits.

THE BEST SELLING TEXT IN THE FIELD UPDATED FOR THE NEW ERA OF HEALTH CARE IT

"This is the most comprehensive and authoritative book available for the field today."
— Mark L. Diana, PhD, assistant professor and MHA program director, School of Public Health and Tropical Medicine, Tulane University

"With health care information technology now in the national policy spotlight, this book should be required reading for every health care administrator and student."
— Mark Leavitt, MD, PhD, chairman, Certification Commission for Healthcare Information Technology

"The book provides an excellent overview of foundational principles and practical strategies—a valuable reference for health administration and health informatics students and professionals."
— Eta S. Berner, EdD, professor, Department of Health Services Administration, University of Alabama, Birmingham

"The authors skillfully provide the tools necessary to facilitate movement from a paper-based to an electronic health record environment while championing the importance of managing in such an environment."
— Melanie S. Brodnik, PhD, director and associate professor, School of Allied Medical Professions, Ohio State University

"Deploying health care information technology today is like navigating whitewater in the midst of a raging storm. Leveraging investments while introducing significant change is no easy task. It requires focused attention, a spirit of collaboration, and a willingness to learn from others. This book is written for the IT leader who is willing to tackle these challenges."
— Stephanie Reel, CIO and vice provost for Information Technologies, Johns Hopkins University

KAREN A. WAGER, DBA, is executive director of student affairs and associate professor, College of Health Professions, Medical University of South Carolina.

FRANCES WICKHAM LEE, DBA, is director of instructional operations for the Clinical Effectiveness and Patient Safety Center and associate professor, College of Health Professions and College of Medicine, Medical University of South Carolina.

JOHN P. GLASER, PHD, is vice president and chief information officer, Partners HealthCare, Boston, Massachusetts.

HEALTH CARE SERVICES AND POLICY

ISBN 978-0-470-38780-1

www.josseybass.com
JOSSEY-BASS™
An Imprint of
WILEY

9 780470 387801
90000

Cover design by: Michael Rutkowski